Postgraduate Ophthalmology Exam Success

This book serves as a core revision resource for candidates preparing for ophthalmology exams, presenting content in a clear and logical format. It covers ophthalmic instruments, surgical steps, while also addressing related viva voce questions, including surgical techniques and potential complications. Ophthalmic specialist trainees, residents, and specialty doctors will find this guide essential for revising oral and clinical-based exams in ophthalmology.

Key Features:

- Comprehensive coverage of ophthalmic instruments, including a groundbreaking section on OPD instruments and an in-depth description of surgical instruments with corresponding viva questions.
- Includes a dedicated section on sterilization techniques, ensuring a thorough understanding of best practices.
- Offers invaluable guidance to trainees and residents on presenting answers clearly, succinctly, and confidently.
- Emphasizes crucial yet often overlooked topics, in a viva voce.

For more information about this series please visit:
www.routledge.com/MasterPass/book-series/CRCMASPASS

Postgraduate Ophthalmology Exam Success

Maneck Nicholson, Anjali Nicholson,
and Syed Faraaz Hussain

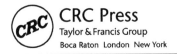

CRC Press
Taylor & Francis Group
Boca Raton London New York

CRC Press is an imprint of the
Taylor & Francis Group, an **informa** business

Designed cover image: Shutterstock

First edition published 2025
by CRC Press
2385 NW Executive Center Drive, Suite 320, Boca Raton FL 33431

and by CRC Press
4 Park Square, Milton Park, Abingdon, Oxon, OX14 4RN

CRC Press is an imprint of Taylor & Francis Group, LLC

© 2025 Maneck Nicholson, Anjali Nicholson, Syed Faraaz Hussain

Library of Congress Cataloging-in-Publication Data
Names: Nicholson, Maneck, author. | Nicholson, Anjali, author. | Hussain, Syed Faraaz, author.
Title: Postgraduate ophthalmology exam success / Maneck Nicholson, Anjali Nicholson, and Syed Faraaz Hussain.
   Other titles: Master pass.
Description: First edition. | Boca Raton, FL : CRC Press, 2024. | Series: MasterPass series | Includes bibliographical references and index. | Summary: "This book provides a core revision resource for candidates preparing for ophthalmology exams in a direct and logical format. Covering not just Ophthalmology instruments, drugs, emergencies, charts, etc. in detail, but also the related questions that such viva exams may ultimately lead to, like the community, legal and ethical aspects. Ophthalmic specialist trainees, residents, and speciality doctors will find this book to be an essential guide to revising for oral and clinical-based exams in Ophthalmology. Key Features: 1. Covers community Ophthalmology with highlights on legal and ethical issues. 2. Provides invaluable guidance to ophthalmic trainees and residents in presenting their answers in a logical, succinct, and elegant manner. 3. Highlights the essential aspects of often neglected topics like emergencies, trials, etc"—Provided by publisher.
Identifiers: LCCN 2024002979 (print) | LCCN 2024002980 (ebook) | ISBN 9781032596624 (hardback) | ISBN 9781032592749 (paperback) | ISBN 9781003455646 (ebook)
Subjects: MESH: Ophthalmology—education | Ophthalmology—ethics | Clinical Decision-Making—ethics | Examination Questions
Classification: LCC RE49 (print) | LCC RE49 (ebook) | NLM WW 18.2 | DDC 617.70076—dc23/eng/20240408
LC record available at https://lccn.loc.gov/2024002979
LC ebook record available at https://lccn.loc.gov/2024002980

ISBN: 978-1-032-59662-4 (hbk)
ISBN: 978-1-032-59274-9 (pbk)
ISBN: 978-1-003-45564-6 (ebk)

DOI: 10.1201/9781003455646

Typeset in Minion Pro
by Apex CoVantage, LLC

Contents

About the authors

Maneck Nicholson, DNB, FRCS (Glasgow), FICO (UK), FAICO (Refractive Surgery), DHA
Dr. Maneck Nicholson is an ophthalmic surgeon currently practicing in Mumbai. She has completed her fellowship in cataract and refractive surgery from the Narayana Nethralaya Eye Institute, following which she completed a fellowship at the Massachusetts Eye and Ear Infirmary, Harvard Medical School, Boston. She worked as a consultant in the Department of Cataract and Refractive Surgery at the LV Prasad Eye Institute and at that time headed the Aurobindo Geriatric Eye Foundation. As the head of education there, she took an avid interest in teaching and has provided cataract training to numerous ophthalmologists at national and international forums. She currently serves as faculty in the Department of Cataract and Refractive Surgery at the Shantilal Shanghvi Eye Institute. She is also passionate about public health and community ophthalmology.

Anjali Nicholson, MS, FVRS, DOMS, CHA, DNB
Dr. Anjali Nicholson, a trained retina surgeon from the Sankara Nethralaya Eye Institute in Chennai, has received numerous awards for her contribution to ophthalmology. As an ex-head of the Department of the Ophthalmology Services at TN Medical College and BYL Nair Hospital, she has been instrumental in training and mentoring numerous ophthalmologists. Her areas of interest include retina, pediatric ophthalmology, squint, and neuro-ophthalmology, apart from her work as a comprehensive and seasoned ophthalmologist. She is also an avid reader, speaker, and orator. She has in-depth experience as examiner and teacher of over 30 years conducting undergraduate and postgraduate MS and DNB exams. Currently she is practicing at Nicholson Eye Clinic in Mumbai.

Syed Faraaz Hussain, MS, FVRS, FPOS (USA), FICO (UK), FAICO, FCPS
Dr. Syed Faraaz Hussain is a trained fellow in strabismus and pediatric ophthalmology (under Dr. Burton Kushner, Wisconsin University, Madison, USA) and in vitreoretinal surgeries (from BYL Nair Hospital, Mumbai), having completed his MS in ophthalmology under Dr. A. D. Nicholson and Dr. A. B. Ingole and MBBS graduation from Seth GS Medical College and KEM Hospital, Mumbai. He has worked in various charitable and educational institutes, including the Municipal Eye Hospital (MEH) under MCGM, and is now working as a consultant eye surgeon at Fazal Clinic and as Associate Professor at MGM Medical College & Hospital, Kamothe, as well as an honorary consultant at NMMC Hospital, Vashi. He is passionate about teaching and takes an active interest in neuro-ophthalmology, along with retina and pediatric ophthalmology.

Foreword

It gives me great pleasure to write a foreword to *Postgraduate Ophthalmology Exam Success*, authored by my colleagues Dr. Maneck Nicholson, Dr. Anjali Nicholson, and Dr. S. Faraaz Hussain.

The wealth of information imparted in an original format, with recently updated and relevant material compiled in a well-illustrated, concise manner, along with the well described, step-by-step guidelines on the decision-making process, will no doubt be of immense value to our ophthalmic fraternity, especially the postgraduates, trainees, residents, exam takers, healthcare providers, and clinicians. A vast array of subjects has been covered—from a compilation of the efforts made by our predecessors and their training and collective recommendations to current medical and technological trends.

In this era of fast changing therapies, a concise, easily readable book that respects tradition but welcomes change is bound to benefit the readers. I wish success to the authors, to the readers, and to those they look after.

In the words of Alexander Pope, "Be not the first by whom the new are tried, nor yet the last to put the old aside."

Dr. Rumi P. Jehangir

Preface

Success in ophthalmology requires not only a profound understanding of theoretical knowledge but also the ability to apply that knowledge effectively in practical examinations. As an ophthalmology teacher for several decades, I have witnessed the struggles of postgraduate students as they navigate the complex world of ophthalmic surgical instruments and clinical examinations. It is with the sincere desire to bridge the gap between theory and practice that I present to you, *Postgraduate Ophthalmology Exam Success*.

In my years of teaching, I have observed a common pattern among students—they often falter when faced with the tricks and challenges posed by examiners. While some students managed to excel, many struggled to showcase their true potential. Furthermore, preparing for viva voce examinations necessitated referring to numerous textbooks that covered different practical aspects, making the process cumbersome and time-consuming.

This book aims to consolidate my vast experience as a teacher and examiner, spanning three decades, into one concise volume. It is designed to equip you, the postgraduate student, with the necessary knowledge and techniques to excel in clinical examinations while providing practical insights relevant to the field of ophthalmology. By offering a comprehensive resource, I hope to guide you in mastering the art of answering and scoring well in practical assessments, all while deepening your understanding of clinical ophthalmology.

I am indebted to the distinguished ophthalmologists who have been instrumental in fueling the flame of education and curiosity within me.

Among them, Dr. S. Badrinath holds a special place as my eternal inspiration and mentor. His wisdom and guidance have played a crucial role in shaping my approach to ophthalmology education.

I am immensely grateful to the entire team at Taylor & Francis Group for their unwavering support, invaluable guidance, and encouragement throughout the process of bringing this book to life. Their dedication to promoting excellence in medical education has been instrumental in making this endeavor possible.

Furthermore, I extend my heartfelt appreciation to my co-authors, Dr. S. Faraaz Hussain and Dr. Maneck Nicholson, whose expertise and collaboration have been invaluable in shaping the contents of this book. Without their contributions, this project would not have come to fruition.

Lastly, I express my gratitude to the countless students at KEM, Nair, and Sion Hospital. Your unwavering enthusiasm and commitment to learning have been the driving force behind this book. Your feedback, insights, and shared experiences have enriched its content and ensured its relevance to the challenges faced by aspiring ophthalmologists.

In writing this book, I hope to empower you, the student, not only to master ophthalmic surgical instruments but also to find joy in the process of learning and exploring the fascinating world of clinical ophthalmology. May this guide be your trusted companion on your journey to becoming a skilled and compassionate ophthalmologist.

Dr. Anjali Nicholson

Special contributions

DARIUS NICHOLSON, MS, DOMS, FRCS (EDINBURGH)

Dr. Darius Nicholson has undergone numerous specialized fellowships in cataract and refractive surgery in Germany and Japan. His areas of specialization include advanced cataract surgery and laser vision correction. He is currently practicing at Nicholson Eye Clinic and Hospital.

SHIVANAND SHETH, MS, FICO, FAICO, FRANZCO

Dr. Shivanand Sheth graduated from Medicine at Mumbai, India, in 2007 and completed his ophthalmology training from BYL Nair Charitable Hospital and Topiwala National Medical College, Mumbai, after which he undertook further advanced training/fellowships in pediatric ophthalmology, strabismus, and neuro-ophthalmology in India, the USA, and Australia. He is a pediatric ophthalmologist at the Royal Children's Hospital. His expertise covers most aspects of pediatric ophthalmology, along with strabismus and neuro-ophthalmology in patients of all ages.

GARGI SHAH, MS, FCPS, FICO (UK)

Dr. Gargi Shah has been trained in pediatric ophthalmology, squint surgery, and neuro-ophthalmology at the Aravind Eye Hospital in Madurai. She is a gold medallist in MS in ophthalmology and DOMS. She is currently practicing in Mumbai.

REVIEWERS AND SPECIAL ACKNOWLEDGMENTS

Cornea and Ocular Surface: Charuta Puranik, DNB, DO
Vitreo-Retina: Bhavik Panchal, DNB
Glaucoma: Kiranmaye Turaga, MS
Lens: Vivek Singh, DNB
Oculoplasty: Komal Bakal, DNB
OPD Instruments and related: Hardik Nanavati, DNB

SPECIAL THANKS TO THE FOLLOWING

Bhavisha Beed, MS
Navin Soni, MS
Manvi Sobti, MS
Anamika Agrawal, MS
Avinash Ingole, MS
Darshana Rathod, MS
Atul Seth, MS
Siddharth Dikshit, DO, DNB
Shamika Wagh, MD
Kruti Mody Shah, MS
Prajakta Dandekar, DNB
Priyanka Walvekar, DNB
Ankit Bhopalka, MS
Deepak Bhatt, MD

And special thanks to all the students from TNMC and Nair Hospital and LTMGH Hospital who, over the years have, helped in making this book.

We extend our sincere gratitude to Appasamy Associates and Volk India for allowing us to use their images.

We are deeply thankful to Dr. Taraprasad Das for his invaluable help and guidance.

1

Introduction

- Each instrument has a diagnostic or surgical role and can be used either as holding (forceps, needle holders) or tissue modifying (cutting) instruments. They are broadly divided into sharps (scissors, blades, knives) and blunts (speculums, hooks).
- The nomenclature of instruments follows guidelines depending on the name of the inventor (Barraquer's speculum), functions it performs (forceps, scissors), its appearance (cat's paw retractors) or a scientific name related to surgery (chalazion clamp).
- Understanding the rationale behind this helps in understanding its action and subsequent use.

1. How must one answer in a practical exam?

- Have basic knowledge pertinent to the instrument and its use.
- Know all related relevant questions with their common answers.
- Don't miss out on life-threatening and sight-threatening problems.
- Have a practical approach in describing the instruments.
- Mention the common conditions first, and mention the rare ones last.
- Classify your answers properly as it shows an organized state of mind.
- Every student appearing for an exam is well read. What is important is how he or she is presenting the subject before the examiner.

2. What are the different instrument materials used?

- Stainless steel: Most commonly used to make instruments.

- Titanium: Lighter, harder, and stronger, but costlier. The rigidity of the instrument can be exploited to make fine teeth or tips.
- Fiber optics: Used for transmitting light from the source to the target organ. LIO for retinal surgeries and nasal endoscopes.
- Diamond: Used to make keratomes and retinal diamond-dusted brushes.
- Tungsten carbide: Contains carbon and tungsten in equal parts.

3. What are the points one must consider when handed an instrument?

- Name of the instrument
- Identifying characteristics
- Uses of that instrument
- Surgeries the instrument is used in
- Indications and contraindications of the surgery
- Salient or important steps of the surgery
- Complications of the surgery

4. What are additional important tips?

- Very often the examiners ask candidates to pick up an instrument of their choice. At this time, it is better to pick up an instrument used for a specific purpose (e.g., enucleation scissors) as against a general instrument (e.g., 1 × 2 fixation forceps). This is because the questions faced by the candidate will be far more specific with the former.
- All complications must always be classified as those occurring during the surgery and as postoperative complications.
- During the surgery
  - Anesthesia related
  - Surgery related

DOI: 10.1201/9781003455646-1

- – Sight threatening
- – Life threatening
- Postoperative
  - – Early
  - – Delayed
- Always remember the specific complications related to a particular surgery (e.g., false passage during lacrimal sac probing).
- If you cannot remember any complications, always remember three things common to all surgeries:
  - Hemorrhage
  - Infection
  - Failure of surgery
- Always prepare answers for the causes of failure of the surgery, and keep in mind the factors may be preoperative, intraoperative, postoperative.

- In the following chapters, certain questions pertaining to each instrument have been mentioned. The list may not be complete; however, being common questions, they should be useful to any candidate.
- Listen to all the questions carefully, avoid answering other related questions if not aware of the one asked.
- Maintain eye contact and speak clearly.
- Give short, precise answers.
- If you do not know an answer, say so and move on to the next question.
- Practice talking about various instruments and common charts prior to the exam with your contemporaries.
- Stay positive even if you have performed poorly at one station.

2

General instruments and sterilization

2.1 TOPICS

- Speculums
- Forceps
- Scissors
- Needle holders
- Cautery
- Calipers
- Desmarres lid retractor
- Bard–Parker blade handle and blade
- Merocel sponge
- Sterilization of instruments
- Operation room construction and sterility
- Needles
- Suture materials

2.2 SPECULUMS

Introduction

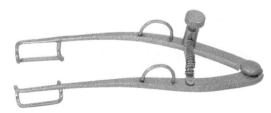

Figure 2.1 Weiss eyelid speculum with open blades

- A speculum has 2 limbs joined at the end.
- It can either have open/closed/wire/solid blades at the open end.
- Uses of speculums:
  - Slit-lamp procedures (FB removal, suture removal)
  - Examining children
  - Intraocular surgeries (cataract, glaucoma)
- Extraocular surgeries (squint, oculoplasty)
- Retinal laser procedures

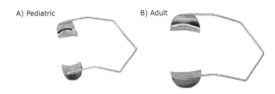

Figure 2.2 Barraquer wire speculum with solid blades: (A) pediatric; (B) adult

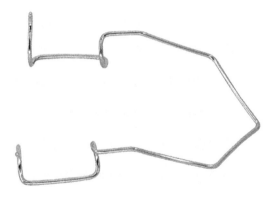

Figure 2.3 Barraquer wire speculum

- A variety of Barraquer eye speculums in both adult and pediatric sizes are available with solid, closed, and open blades that are both temporal and nasal in approach.
- Uses:
  - For better exposure during intraocular surgery
  - Corneal foreign body removal or examination in cases of chemical injury
  - Examination in OPD of uncooperative or young patients

DOI: 10.1201/9781003455646-2

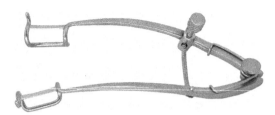

Figure 2.4 Williams eye speculum with open blades

- Holds the speculum open through screw adjustments
- Controlled retraction
- Causes a greater rise of IOP
- Use: For extraocular surgeries
- Keeping lashes away from the field of surgery

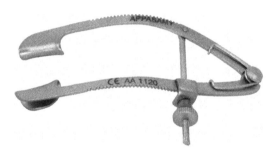

Figure 2.5 Lancaster eye speculum with solid blades

- Uses:
  - Predominantly in squint surgery
  - In the examination of uncooperative children and for the retraction of soft tissues

2.3 FORCEPS

Introduction

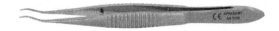

Figure 2.6 Lims forceps

- Tip: Plain, serrated, notched, smooth or toothed, with or without tying platform
- Shaft: Straight, curved, angled, cross-action
- Handle: Round or flat, with or without grip
- Curved forceps with 1 × 2 teeth at the tip for holding tissue

- Fenestrated tying platform for holding and suture tying
- Use: For holding the corneal or scleral edge while suturing

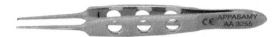

Figure 2.7 Bishop–Harmon tissue forceps

- 2 × 1 tooth aligned at right angles
- Use: For holding tissues in oculoplasty surgery

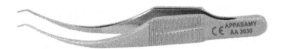

Figure 2.8 Colibri forceps

- Italic word which means "bird"
- Grooved handle with straight tip with 0.8 mm wide jaws and fine tooth 1 × 2
- Use: For holding the cornea and sclera while suturing (keratoplasty)

Figure 2.9 Kelman–McPherson forceps

- Fine, medium-sized, plain, angled forceps
- Angled at 8 mm to 15 mm from the tip
- Has a tying platform
- Uses:
  - In IOL implantation and explantation and in suturing and suture burial
  - In fine suturing in keratoplasty and trabeculectomy
  - To hold flaps/sutures in trabeculectomy

Figure 2.10 Plain forceps

- Blunt tip with vertical and horizontal serrations
- No teeth, flat platform
- Uses:
  - To hold conjunctiva and scleral flap in a non-traumatic manner

- To hold nasal mucosal flaps in DCR surgery
- As suture tying forceps

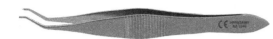

Figure 2.11 Superior rectus holding forceps/ Dastoor forceps

- S-shaped double curve near the tip
- Tip: 7.7 mm from the fulcrum; insertion of superior rectus: 7.7 mm from the limbus
- Uses
  - To fix the globe in downward gaze while holding superior rectus tendon
  - Complications while taking the superior rectus (bridle) suture:
    - Globe perforation
    - Muscle injury
    - Hematoma formation

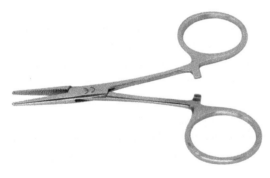

Figure 2.12 Hartman hemostatic artery forceps/ clamp

- Serrated jaws with ratchet lock in a scissor-like fashion
- Uses:
  - To achieve hemostasis in oculoplastic surgery
  - To clamp and crush the extraocular muscle before cutting in resection
  - To crush the lateral canthal tendon during a lateral canthotomy
  - Curved jaws used to crush a bleeding optic nerve stump and help in lifting the globe out of the orbit in enucleation
  - Curved jaws used during Fasanella–Servat surgery: Two forceps used to hold the superior edge of the tarsal plate

2.4 SCISSORS

Introduction

- Tip: Sharp or blunt, straight or curved or angled
- Jaw: Straight, curved, or angled
- Handle: Spring action, bow ribbon, or hinge based
- Delicate tip—do not touch

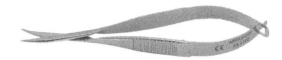

Figure 2.13 Westcott tenotomy scissors

- 21 mm blade, gently curved/straight
- Sharp/blunt pointed tips
- Use: To open the conjunctiva and tenons prior to making scleral flap

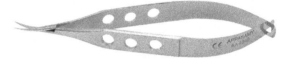

Figure 2.14 Castroviejo corneal scissors

- Blades are kept apart by spring action.
- Lighter than Westcott spring scissors
- Types:
  - Universal: Both blades equal in length
  - Right and left scissors: Lower blade is longer by 0.5 mm
- Uses:
  - For wound enlargement in ECCE surgery
  - Keratoplasty
  - Evisceration

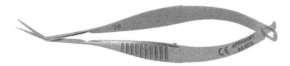

Figure 2.15 Vannas scissors

- Micro blades
- 6 mm long with a sharp tip
- Spring mechanism
- Straight, curved, or angled

- Uses:
  - To make the sclerostomy in trabeculectomy surgery
  - Can be used instead of iridectomy scissors to make the iridectomy
  - To cut fine sutures, capsular bag tag
- Precautions to be taken during suture removal:
  - Take all aseptic precautions.
  - Cut the suture near the scleral end and pull it out by holding the longer corneal end, to prevent the exposed part of suture from entering the anterior chamber.
- Complications of suture removal:
  - Infiltration at suture site
  - Endophthalmitis
  - Shallowing of the anterior chamber

2.5 NEEDLE HOLDERS

Introduction

- Tip: Fine, standard, or heavy
- Jaw: Straight or curved
- Handle: Locking or non-locking—secures the needle during suturing
- Use: Used to hold the needle when suturing, make a 26G cystitome during cataract surgery, and hold sutures while tying knots

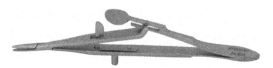

Figure 2.16 Kalt needle holder

- Cross-serrated jaws, with a lock which stabilizes the needle, triangular design with a thumb release.
- Uses:
  - While taking lid sutures and the superior rectus suture
  - To tag the recti muscles
  - To pass scleral sutures during a scleral buckling surgery

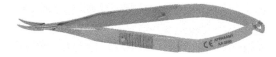

Figure 2.17 Castroviejo's needle holder

- Spring action needle holder
- Working end has straight jaws with serrated handles.
- May or may not have a locking mechanism.
- Uses
  - Suturing corneoscleral incisions and the conjunctiva
  - In the suturing of skin, muscles and to hold fine needles.

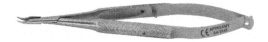

Figure 2.18 Barraquer needle holder

- Spring-action needle holder with narrow curved jaws
- Fine serrations for better grip
- For suturing of cornea, sclera with 10-0 nylon or any fine suture material (to know suture materials, expect possible related questions)

2.6 CAUTERY

- It consists of a radio-frequency cautery unit, electrodes, and connecting wires.
- It can have the following effects on biological tissue:
  - Cutting: Due to intracellular water evaporation and membrane rupture, this occurs when the probe is held slightly away from the tissue.
  - Coagulation: Due to heat denaturation of intra- and extracellular proteins, this occurs when the tissue is held between the two limbs of the probe.
  - Fulguration: This means coagulation of tissues with charring.
- Uses:
  - Used to provide a bloodless ophthalmic field during surgery
  - Electrolysis of trichiatic lashes
  - Cosmetic removal of mole wart
  - During blepharoplasty
  - During surgeries for removal of skin lesions (benign malignant tumors)
  - Coagulate bleeding vessels
- Safety precautions:
  - When using on eyelids, always protect the globe.
  - Increase or decrease in pigmentation of the skin.

- Use carefully in patients with a pacemaker.
- Do not perform very close to oxygen as it can lead to an explosion.

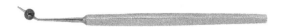

Figure 2.19 Ballpoint cautery

- Types:
  - Stainless steel (5 mm ball) with blunt tip
  - Stainless steel (3 mm ball) with blunt tip
  - Copper (6 mm ball) with blunt long point
- Use: To create a bloodless field prior to making the scleral flap
- Use: Wetfield cautery for hemostasis

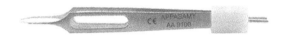

Figure 2.20 Bipolar cautery

- Differences between bipolar and monopolar cautery:
  - Bipolar cautery
    - Both the active and receiving electrodes are placed at the site of cauterization. The probe is shaped to look like forceps with each arm forming the electrodes. The tissue grasped between the electrodes is cauterized.
    - Use: For coagulation of bleeders.
  - Monopolar cautery
    - There is an active electrode from which current is passed and where cauterization occurs, while the patient's body serves as a ground. The grounding pad or returning electrode is usually placed on the person's thigh (body) and carries the current back.
    - Careful application of the patient return electrode is necessary because, if the electrode is not correctly attached, extensive burns can occur which can go undetected.
    - Use: For cutting as well as coagulation.

2.7 CALIPERS

- 20 mm
- Straight shaft

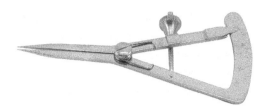

Figure 2.21 Castroviejo caliper (straight)

- For circumferential/horizontal corneal/scleral measurements

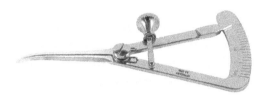

Figure 2.22 Castroviejo caliper (curved)

- 20 mm
- Curved shaft
- For antero-posterior measurements

Uses of calipers

- Diagnostic: Measuring the following:
  - Corneal diameter in children during evaluation under general anesthesia (GA) in buphthalmos, microcornea, macrocornea, sclerocornea
  - Size of lesions (eyelid or skin)
- Intraoperative: Measuring the following:
  - Size of incisions
  - Conjunctival and scleral flap sizes in trabeculectomy
  - Distance from limbus for sclerotomies
  - Muscle length in squint surgery's amount of recession/resection
  - Size of the conjunctival graft or amniotic membrane graft in pterygium surgeries
  - To determine the size and location of the scleral buckle or band
  - To measure the incision length and size of eyelid mass
  - Intraoperative measurements of the size of corneal lesions

Figure 2.23 Desmarres eyelid retractor

- It has a solid smooth C-shaped blades with blunt edges.
- Horizontal width of the blade determines the retractor size.
  - Size 0 = 11 mm wide
  - Size 1 = 13 mm wide
  - Size 2 = 15 mm wide
  - Size 3 = 17 mm wide
- Uses:
  - In the examination of uncooperative children and for the retraction of soft tissues
  - Double eversion of eyelids (chemical burns and fornicial foreign body)
  - To unroll the AMG over the corneal surface
  - In ptosis, orbitotomy, buckling and DCR surgeries to retract tissue
  - To remove ocular prosthesis or blepharospasm examination in an uncooperative patient
- Technique of performing double eversion of the superior eyelid:
  - Patient gently closes the eyelids without force.
  - The evertor is introduced over the upper lid.
  - The lash line is held and everted over the retractor.
  - Now the handle is lowered to expose the superior fornix.
  - Disadvantage: Palpebral conjunctiva gets covered.

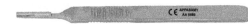

Figure 2.24 Bard–Parker blade handle and no. 15 blade

- Flat serrated handle for grip during surgery.
- Long cylindrical end with a groove to fit a scalpel blade.
- While loading, make sure it is loaded smoothly over the longitudinal grooves.
- While removing the blade, either a scalpel remover or a hemostat forceps can be used.
- You are discouraged to remove the blade by pulling it out.
- Uses:
  - To make scleral and corneal incisions in cataract surgery
  - To make the scleral flap in filtration surgery
  - To make full-thickness wounds during lid sharing procedures such as Cutler–Beard surgery
  - Lamellar corneal and scleral dissection
  - Skin incision in different surgeries, such as DCR and dermoid excision
  - Diagnostic and therapeutic scraping in microbial keratitis
- Alternative: The crescent knife can be used as an alternative to the no. 15 blade.

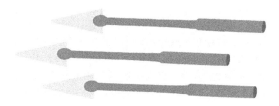

Figure 2.25 Merocel sponge

- Uses:
  - Hemostasis.
  - To maintain dry field during scleral flap formation.
  - To soak aqueous to enhance visibility while making scratch incisions in trabeculotomy.
  - Polyvinyl alcohol swabs are used to apply MMC.
  - To check for filtration through scleral flap after suturing is complete.
  - Can be used to check for vitreous strands during cataract surgery where posterior capsular tear has occurred by dabbing at side port or main port wound margin.

2.8 NEEDLES

Describe the parts of a needle.

- Surgical needles are divided into three parts:
  - Point: From tip to maximum cross-section (can be spatulate, round-bodied/taper point, cutting point, reverse cutting point, and tapered spatulated)
  - Body: Constitutes the needle length and is the area where the needle is grasped, transmitting the penetrating force to the point (shape of the body can be straight, half-curved, curved, or compound-curved)
  - Swage: The part where the suture attaches (In modern-day surgical needles, there is no eye for passing thread.)

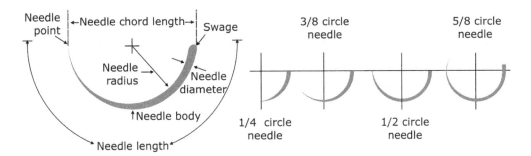

Figure 2.26 Part of a needle

- Needle diameter: Cross-sectional thickness of the needle
- Needle length: Circumferential distance measured along the needle from the point to the swage
- Chord length: Horizontal distance from the point to the swage
- Radius of curvature: Distance from center of the circle constituted by the needle to its edge

- Curvature: Segment of total circle that the needle encompasses, e.g., ½ circle, 1/4 circle, 160°, compound
- Needle length and curvature: Most needles have 3/8th circle; ideal for all applications.

What are the various types of tip designs?

Tip designs in order of frequency of use are as follows (**Table 2.1**):

Table 2.1 Shape of the Needle Tip

Design	Configuration	Characteristic	Uses
Spatulated	4-to-6-sided with cutting edge on sides	Avoids inadvertent penetration of tissue	Most frequently used
	Cuts at tip and sides parallel to tissue plane	Tissue plane marked	Cornea, sclera, squint, RD
		Ideal for cornea and sclera	
		Disadvantage: Passage is larger than suture, so there is increased chance of microleaks.	
Reverse cutting	Triangular with cutting edge at bottom	Suture canal extends deep to path of needle	Descemet's repair
	Cuts at tip and 3 edges	Good for full-thickness suturing	Not good for suturing cornea or sclera as outer cutting-edge damages the deeper tissue

(Continued)

Table 2.1 *(Continued)* Shape of the Needle Tip

Design	Configuration	Characteristic	Uses
		Facilitates tissue penetration	
		May perforate tissue in partial-thickness suturing	
		(e.g., sclera in squint surgery)	
Cutting	Triangular with cutting edge at top	Suture canal extends superficial to path of needle tip	Suturing skin
	Cuts at tip and inner edge so that damage to deeper tissue is avoided	May pull out of tissue as needle is passed	
Round body with taper cut	Round shaft tapered to point	Atraumatic	Use in easily penetrable tissue where trauma should be the least: e.g., Iris
	Cuts at tip only, so easily gets blunted	Less chance of micro-leaks because the needle track is same diameter as the suture	Conjunctiva closure in trabeculectomy, where watertight closure is required

- Spatulated
- Reverse cutting
- Cutting
- Round body with taper point

What are the various body designs of a needle?

- Body: Round, triangular, or ovoid
- Triangular needles: Three cutting edges
- Ovoid needles: Flattened on top or bottom with rounded sides or flattened on all 4 sides
- Body: straight or curved
- Straight needle: Flat or shallow depth skin wounds
- Curved needle: May have 1/2, 1/4, 3/8, or 5/8 circle configuration
- E.g., 5/8 circle needle is commonly used in DCR surgeries

Mention some of the commonly used needles and sutures in eye surgeries.

- Cataract surgery: 3/8 circle, spatulated needle, nylon

- Corneal tears/penetrating keratoplasty: 10-0 nylon spatulated/cutting
- Squint surgeries: 1/4 circle conventional cutting/spatulated, micropoint coated 6-0 Vicryl suture
- DCR: 5/8 circle, taper-cut, 5-0 chromic catgut
- Scleral fixation: 10-0 Prolene, 16 mm straight needle, double armed
- Scleral buckling/encirclage: 4-0 Ethibond, 1/4 circle needle spatulated
- Iris repair: First needle—10-0 Prolene, single-armed straight needle; second needle—curved micropoint/round-bodied 3/8 circle needle
- Lid surgeries: 6-0 silk, reverse cutting point
- Periocular skin: 6-0 nylon for most facial trauma, non-absorbable gives less scarring (6-0 Vicryl preferred in young children to avoid second GA for suture removal)

2.9 SUTURE MATERIALS

Describe an ideal suture material.

- Strong.
- Easy to handle.
- With minimum tissue reaction.
- Tensile strength and duration of the suture depends on material and diameter.

How is the thickness of a suture represented?

- As per metric classification: Thickness of suture material is 1/10 mm.
- Therefore, suture of 0.1 metric number = diameter of 1/1000 mm.

- The notation of 6-0 or 10-0 (0.070–0.0799 mm or 0.020 to 0.029 mm is the diameter range, respectively) is like the sizing of the needles and syringes; i.e., greater the number, smaller the needle.

What are the various non-absorbable suture materials?

- Non-absorbable suture materials are mentioned in **Table 2.2**.
- Even though they are non-absorbable, slow degradation over 1–2 years is known.

What are the various absorbable suture materials?

- Absorbable suture materials are mentioned in **Table 2.3**.

Table 2.2 Non-Absorbable Suture Materials

Suture Material	Duration	Tissue Reaction	Other Characteristics	Uses
Nylon (polyamide)	Loses 10–15% tensile strength per year	Minimal	Monofilament Inert Tensile strength high Elastic	Cornea (10, 9, 8) Sclera: Trabeculectomy Subcuticular Gets vascularized in tissue, therefore not used in IOL fixation
			Suture ends stiff	Resistant to bacterial colonization
			Easy to remove	Not for SFIOL or iris suturing
Silk Virgin natural silk: Fibrin coated with sericin, twisted Advantage over braided: Finer suture material made from virgin silk Braided: De-gummed silk, sericin removed, braided to make it multi-filament	3–6 months	Moderate	Easy to handle Well tolerated by patient	Skin Traction sutures
			Inelastic	Twisted virgin silk can cause sclerokeratitis, therefore not used
			Frays (since braided)	
			Tissue drag present (since braided) Braided (therefore nidus of infection)	

Table 2.2 *(Continued)* Non-Absorbable Suture Materials

Suture Material	Duration	Tissue Reaction	Other Characteristics	Uses
			Braided silk has exceptionally good handling property considered as gold standard	
Polypropylene (Prolene)	Permanent	Minimal	Mono-filament Tensile strength high Maximally elastic Suture ends very stiff Hydrophobic Non-absorbable Good knot security	Non-absorbable, therefore good for IOL fixation (10-0), iris suturing, etc.
Polyester (Mersilene, Dacron, Ethibond, Tecron)	Permanent	Minimal	Monofilament, Braided Tensile strength very high Strongest monofilament Elasticity is less than monofilament Poor Handling	Retinal surgeries Also for SFIOL and iris sutures Certain strabismus surgeries like Periosteal fixation.

Table 2.3 Absorbable Suture Materials

Suture Material	Duration	Tissue Reaction	Other Characteristics	Uses
Polyglactin 910 (Vicryl)	2–3 weeks	Mild (as glycolic and lactic are natural products)	Braided	8–0
Copolymer of glycolic acid and lactic acid (9:1)			Monofilament	Scleral tunnel
Coated Vicryl is 910 coated polyglactin 370 and calcium stearate			Tensile strength high	Pediatric Squint
Advantages of coating: Surface smoother, less tissue drag			Undergoes hydrolytic degradation	

Table 2.3 *(Continued)* Absorbable Suture Materials

Suture Material	Duration	Tissue Reaction	Other Characteristics	Uses
			9-0 and 10-0: Uncoated	10-0
			8-0: Coated	Cataract surgery
			Coated Vicryl is better than Dexon, since it's stronger	Tunnel
			Vicryl Rapide: Rapidly absorbed variant (1–2 weeks), for children's skin	
				6–0 Squint recession 5–0 Resection DCR flaps Orbicularis Levator
Polyglycolic acid (Dexon)	2–3 weeks	Mild	Braided	
Dexon S: Braided without coating, homopolymer of glycolic	Complete absorption by 8–14 weeks		Tensile strength high	
Dexon Plus: Polyglycolic suture treated with surface lubricant poloxamer 185			Undergoes hydrolytic degeneration	
			Good knot security	
Plain gut	1 week	Marked	Allergy	Origin of name: From "kit gut"
From mucosa or submucosa layer of sheep/beef intestine			Undergoes hydrolytic degradation	Kit = Arabian fiddle

(Continued)

Table 2.3 (*Continued*) Absorbable Suture Materials

Suture Material	Duration	Tissue Reaction	Other Characteristics	Uses
			Oldest suture made	Not used due to risk of variant of Creutzfeldt–Jakob disease
Chromic catgut Plain tanned in chromic salt	2–3 weeks	Moderate	Undergoes enzymatic degradation	
Polydioxanone (PDS) (PDS II) Synthetic monofilament			Absorbed by hydrolysis Stronger than Vicryl and Dexon	

2.10 STERILIZATION OF INSTRUMENTS

What is decontamination?

- The term used to describe a combination of processes, including cleaning, disinfection, and/or sterilization incorporated into a process to make reusable items safe for further use.
- Effective decontamination is essential for equipment utilized in surgeries where direct contact with tissues is expected in order to minimize risk of infection and/or other harmful response.

What is sterilization?

- It is an absolute term, meaning complete destruction of all living organisms, including spores.
- It is the removal of all microorganisms (bacteria, viruses, fungi, spores) from an object or culture medium; however, no method of sterilization is 100% effective.
- Examples sterilization methods are steam under pressure, dry heat, ETO gas, hydrogen peroxide gas, plasma, and liquid chemicals.

What is disinfection?

- Disinfection is a process that eliminates many or all pathogenic microorganisms, except bacterial spores, on inanimate objects to a level which is not-harmful to health.

- In healthcare settings, objects usually are disinfected by liquid chemicals (chlorhexidine, betadine, etc.) or wet pasteurization (moist heat).
- Chemical disinfectants may not be effective or be less effective:
  - If used on dirty instruments/equipment (due to inability to make contact with microorganisms or the surface to be decontaminated)
  - If the solution is not freshly made
  - If the solution is made at an incorrect temperature
- All disinfectants must be manufactured, stored, reconstituted, and used in accordance with health and safety regulation.

What is cleaning?

- Cleaning is the removal of dust, dirt, excretions, secretions, organic matter, and all contamination, including harmful and undesirable substances, as well as a large proportion of microorganisms that may be present; this is usually accomplished manually or mechanically by using water with detergents or enzymatic products.
- Cleaning is essential before high-level disinfection and sterilization because inorganic and organic materials remain on the surfaces of

instruments and interfere with the effectiveness of these processes.

- Cleaning must always be thoroughly performed before disinfection or sterilization is
attempted, to remove organic matter that may
compromise the further processes. Automated
methods are preferred unless inappropriate for
the particular device or unavailable.

**Kindly outline in brief how to choose a particu-
lar method for decontamination.**

- This depends on a multitude of factors:
  - Availability and practicality of method
  - Type and level of risk of harm to
    patients
  - Type and level of risk of harm to staff using
    method
  - Manufacturer's instructions for
    decontamination
  - Heat, pressure, moisture, and chemi-
    cal tolerance of the object undergoing
    decontamination
  - Reliability and validity of method
  - Cost-effectiveness
- Ideally, risk assessment and decontamina-
  tion process are outlined during the purchase
  process for the equipment and incorporated in
  the department CSSD (central sterile services
  department).
- Some general guidelines can be as follows:
  (**Table 2.4**).

- Various procedures should be in place in order
  to ensure appropriate decontamination per
  national and local guidelines, the following
  should be ensured (by the Royal College of
  Ophthalmologists [UK]):
  - The decontamination of reusable medical
    devices are done at appropriate facilities.
  - Streamlined procedures are followed for
    the acquisition and maintenance of decon-
    tamination equipment and for managing
    equipment in general.
  - Staff are trained in decontamination pro-
    cesses and hold appropriate competencies
    for their role, with regular update as needed.
  - A monitoring system, usually by indepen-
    dent administration, is in place to ensure
    that decontamination processes are fit for
    purpose and meet the required standard.
  - Appropriate infection control processes and
    staffing are in place, in case of outbreak.
  - There must be appropriate theater facilities,
    in particular the ability to separate clean
    from dirty instruments, as well as separate
    areas for contaminated cases.

**What are the various aspects of instrument
processing?**

- The entire process usually begins from the
  time of acquisition and should be consistent
  across usage till the time of disposal, depending upon the type of device or instrument.

Table 2.4 Determining Risk and Methods for Decontamination

Risk	Usage	Method
High	In close contact with broken skin or broken mucous membrane Introduce into sterile body areas	Cleaning followed by sterilization or Single-use device, where available and practical
Medium	In contact with mucous membranes, contaminated with highly virulent or readily transmissible organisms, before use on immunocompromised patients	Cleaning followed by sterilization or disinfection NB: Where sterilization will damage equipment, cleaning followed by high-level disinfection is an alternative.
Low	In contact with healthy skin not in contact with patient	Cleaning

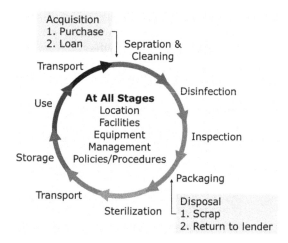

Figure 2.27 Various aspects of instrument processing

- Single-use devices not to be reused because:
    - Inadequate cleaning and decontamination of instrument may occur with reuse due to instrument construction (e.g., small bore), or surface damage due to wear and tear, preventing removal of all debris or organisms.
    - Component materials may become damaged or brittle leading due to reuse to the risk of loose fragments entering the eye during surgery.
    - Some materials can adsorb or absorb certain chemicals, potentially causing harm if repeated tissue contact.
    - Legally, if a single-use item is reused against advice, this may negate the manufacturer's warranty and cause liability to the unit or hospital and the employee under criminal and civil law if damage or injury is caused.
- Single-use instruments are isolated after use and disposed in accordance with manufacturer's guidance and national/local healthcare guidelines, usually as clinical waste.
- Any item that stores patient identifiable information should have this securely erased when the device is prepared for disposal
- Before opening of sterile packages, ensure that:
    - The packaging is intact.
    - The sterilization indicator confirms sterilization, with date mentioned.
    - The expiry date has not passed in case of manufacturer packaging.
- Theater or clinic staff must notify the decontamination unit staff about any concerns regarding problems with instrument or device availability, or the instruments themselves

What are the steps involved in cleaning surgical ophthalmic equipment before sterilization?

- Separation: The instruments are separated from the tubing and the sharp instruments are separated from the blunt instruments.
- Cleaning process: Tissue debris and body fluid deposits must be cleaned from the instruments. Primary mechanical wash is indicated before the following: using ultrasonic cleaner or four bowls technique (mechanical technique).
    - Ultrasonic cleaner (Ultrasonicator Ex):
- This uses distilled water to which an enzyme solution is added to facilitate the cleaning process.
- Sound waves pass at a frequency of 1,00,000 Hz, the waves generate submicroscopic bubbles that implode, causing minute vacuums, and the latter lifts soil off the surface of instruments.
- Ideal cycle time is around 30 minutes, which should be done for sharps every day and for blunt instruments at least once a week.
- All joints of each instrument should be opened to ensure adequate exposure to the ultrasound.
    - Four bowl cleaning (mechanical technique):
- Demineralized water is taken in four bowls.
- The instruments are placed in the first bowl containing a surfactant cleaning solution.
- After cleaning in the first bowl, the instruments are transferred to the next bowl and cleaned one more time.
- The instruments go through all four bowls. A clean soft toothbrush is used to clean the blunt instruments thoroughly.
- Special attention is needed to clean at the hinges and the tips of fine and delicate instruments.
    - The cannulated instruments should be flushed with sterile demineralized water or Ringer lactate solution or BSS solution thrice followed by air. After cleaning, the instruments are dried with hot air, tipped with individual plastic sleeves, and packed in individual perforated boxes/trays. The toothbrush is changed weekly and should be disinfected daily by immersing in a chemical solution like 2% glutaraldehyde.
- Disinfection: As outlined, moist heat is preferred. Sometimes this step is incorporated in the aforementioned process.
- Inspection: This is preferably performed by staff members in the decontamination facility other than those responsible for cleaning them. For fine ophthalmic instruments, it is better

to use magnification, using a loupe system or microscope. The final visual inspection should be made by the operating surgeon before using any instrument.

- Packaging: The guidelines for the particular equipment, size, planned use, and chosen sterilization method must be followed. Some instruments will form part of a multiple package and be packed in suitable trays, in which case if the common seal is opened, the entire set should be considered opened. Others will be individually packed in sealed peel-apart pouches.
- Instruments usually are kept in perforated trays, after covering sharp ends with rubber caps. This set is then double wrapped with thick cloth, such that no part of the tray or inner wrapping is exposed after covering. Each set should have an indicator tape that is in good condition to show sterilization completeness. This is usually documented with date on which sterilization is done.

What are the various cleaning agents used?

- Organic solutions: Slightly acidic pH
- Non-organic solutions: Slightly alkaline pH
- Generally used: Neutral pH

What are the various packaging techniques?

- Sterilization wraps:
  - Woven fabrics
  - Non-woven fabrics
- Peel pouches
- Rigid containers with thick cloth covering
- Plastic disposable pouches for gas sterilization (has unique indicator system)
- After decontaminated instruments are cleaned, assembled, packaged, and labelled, they are ready to be sterilized.

What are the various killing mechanisms in sterilization?

- Denaturation of proteins
- Alkylation
- Oxidation

Mention the various types of sterilization methods.

- Moist heat
- Steam under pressure (autoclaving)

- Toxic gas (ethylene oxide)
- Toxic liquid (hydrogen peroxide)
- Dry heat (hot-air oven)
- Heat impaired by radiation (gamma rays)

What are the commonly used sterilization processes?

- Autoclaving using long cycle or steam sterilization
  - This is the preferred method for ophthalmic equipment.

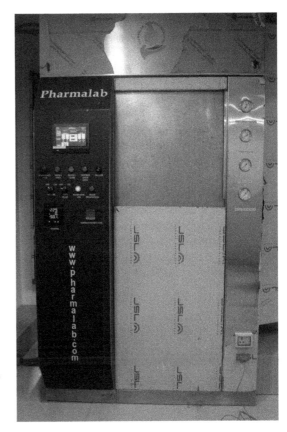

Figure 2.28 Steam sterilization

- Minimum exposure duration for sterilization of wrapped healthcare supplies are 30 minutes at 121°C (250°F) in a gravity displacement sterilizer or 4 minutes at 132°C (270°F) in a pre-vacuum sterilizer.
- In a regular autoclave, linen-wrapped articles are sterilized at 121°C + 20 psi pressure (**Table 2.5**).

Table 2.5 Some Parameters for Autoclaving

Items	Pressure (Pound per Square inch [psi])	Temperature	Holding Time
Blunt instruments, dressing, glass, silicon materials, linen, vessels	20 psi	121°C	20 min
Rubber items	20 psi	121°C	20 min
Liquids	20 psi	110°C	20 min

- After autoclaving, the instruments and other sterilized items should be used within 48 hours, unless they are kept wrapped inside airtight sealed bags. With surgical drums, once opened, the contents must be used immediately.
- If using airtight double packaging after sterilization, instruments can be used within 28 days, but rigorous checks should be ensured.
- Class B autoclaves are recommended for long tubing resterilization.
- Indicator tape should be used in every cycle—as a routine, three tapes should be placed within each of the drums, one each at the bottom, the middle, and the top.
- On the day of surgery, the assisting sterile nurse should check it and hand them over to the running nurse to place them on a register, which should be checked and signed by the surgeon before starting the surgery.
- Gas sterilization or ETO (ethylene oxide sterilization)

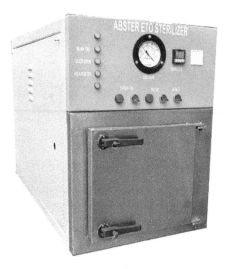

Figure 2.29 Gas sterilization or ETO (ethylene oxide sterilization)

- Gas concentration (450–1,200 mg/L) at temperature (37–63°C) with relative humidity (40–80%) and exposure time (1–6 hours). For ophthalmic equipment, this is preferred for instruments that cannot withstand heat needed for autoclaving, such as cryoprobe, vitrectomy cutter, cautery wire, certain rubber instruments, optical lenses, etc.
- Formalin gas was used earlier, but is now not preferred due to its carcinogenic risk.
- Dry heat sterilization:
- 170°C (340°F) for 60 minutes or 150°C (300°F) for 150 minutes.
- It is done for articles that can be damaged by steam, such as sharp instruments and glass syringes, but not preferred now except in laboratories.
- Chemical sterilization/formalin chamber/cidex are not recommended anymore.

What are the various sterilization techniques for different types of ophthalmic equipment?

What are the commonly used sterilizers?

- Steam sterilization:
  - Specific gravity type
  - Dynamic air removal type (HPHV)
- Ethylene oxide sterilizer:
  - Working at positive pressure with cylinders having EO (12%) combination with CO_2 (88%)
  - Working at negative pressure with 100% pure ethylene oxide in a single-load cartridge

What are the benefits of steam sterilization?

- Better air removal
- Better steam penetration
- Sterilization temperature achieved faster
- Complicated devices can be sterilized
- Better drying

- Total sterilization time can be reduced
- High-speed autoclave
- Linen: 132°C for 10 minutes
- Instruments: 132°C for 15 minutes

What are the steps in ETO sterilization?

- Remove all lubricants from instruments.
- They should be cleaned and should be absolutely dry.
- Pack them in special polythene bags with indicator tape inside the bag.
- As they are carcinogenic and also mutagenic, the equipment should be kept in an isolated room with an exhaust. The exhaust tube from the equipment should be taken and left above the roof of the building.
- Due to their toxic nature, an aeration period of minimum 72 hours for the sterilized items is a mandatory requirement before they are used.
- Sterilized materials should be packaged, labelled, and stored in a manner to ensure sterility, and each item should be marked with the sterilization date. A microbiological control is mandatory.

- Usually, appropriately packaged ETO sterilized equipment is safe to use for 1 year.
- But the date of ETO and packaging should be documented on cover and its correctness ensured rigorously.

What are the advantages and disadvantages of ethylene oxide gas sterilization?

- Advantages:
  - Better air removal
  - Better EO penetration
  - Assured penetration in narrow and long items
  - Faster concentration achievement
  - In case of leakage, toxic gas will not leak out from machine
  - Safer for operator
- Disadvantages:
  - Expensive
  - Double-sealed packing required
  - Aeration time of 7 days (at least 72 hours) required before the treatment can be used
  - Check whether indicator color changes from yellow to black

Table 2.6 Sterilization Techniques

Method	Timing	Advantages	Disadvantages	Use
Autoclaving	45 minutes	Highly effective, inexpensive sporicidal Non-toxic Rapid heating and penetration of instruments	Items must be heat- and moisture-resistant Will not be useful in powders, oils, and ointments	Metals Drapes Gowns Dressing Glass
Dry heat sterilization	30 minutes to 3 hours, depending on holding temperature	Powders Anhydrous oils Glass	Penetrates slowly and unevenly Longer time	Glass Metals Oils Ointments Powders
Ethylene oxide	5 psi—10 hours 10 psi—6 hours	Heat-sensitive instruments, like sharp blades	Dangerous Explosive Carcinogenic Long time Expensive	Heat-labile tubings Laser probes Cryoprobes Vitrectomy cutters

(Continued)

Table 2.6 (*Continued*) Sterilization Techniques

Method	Timing	Advantages	Disadvantages	Use
Glutaraldehyde 2%	Veg pathogens— 15 minutes	Heat-labile equipment	May cause respiratory irritation, asthma, eye and nose irritation, and allergic dermatitis	Airways
	Resistant spores— 3 hours			Endotracheal tubes
				Plastic Glass

What are the variations of sterilization methods that you know of? (Table 2.6)

- Short cycle autoclaving:
  - In between surgeries, the instruments are ideally sterilized using a flash or high-speed autoclave. If not available, a single drum autoclave can be used.
  - The adequate number of surgical instrument sets should be made available, and the practice of boiling should be discontinued.
  - The instruments are cleaned using clean mineral or boiled filtered water and a clean brush. The cannulated instruments should be flushed with sterile BSS/RL solution followed by air before sterilization.
  - The instruments are then placed back in the instrument tray. The trays are placed inside a surgical drum, which can hold up to 6 sets.
  - The drum is placed in the autoclave, and it will take 10 to 12 minutes for the autoclaving to be over.
  - The parameters are 134°C + 30 psi, with 7 to 10 minutes of exposure, which ensures adequate sterilization (the whole process for cleaning and sterilizing 6 sets will take about 20 minutes).
  - In a high-volume setup, at least two nursing personnel should be allocated for this activity.
- Gravity sterilization: Basic sterilization cycle in which steam displaces air in the chamber by gravity (i.e., without mechanical assistance) through a drain port.
- Flash sterilization: A type of gravity downward displacement autoclave, which fills with steam and displaces air downward and forces it out of drainage valve. The cannulas should be cleaned

separately with Ringer lactate solution. The cleaning water should be changed after 4 or 5 sets.
- Pre-vacuum sterilization: Air is mechanically removed from the chamber using a series of vacuum and pressure pulses. This enables the steam to penetrate porous areas of the load that couldn't otherwise be reached with simple gravity displacement.
- Plasma sterilization: Hydrogen peroxide
  - Plasma is defined as highly ionized gas composed of ions, electrons, and neutral particles. Plasma, with respect to sterilization, is generated by introducing a precursor gas or vapor (e.g., hydrogen peroxide or peracetic acid) into a chamber under low-vacuum conditions and then exciting the gas or vapor with microwave or radio-frequency energy.
  - The cycle time is approximately 75 minutes.
  - They have special packaging needs as cellulose containing wrappers are incompatible with hydrogen peroxide processes because they absorb the peroxide and do not allow effective penetration. Commercially available non-woven polypropylene wraps and poly olefin pouches are material of choice.

Mention some pitfalls in sterilization?

- Improper dismantling
- Improper cleaning
- Improper assembling
- Improper packing
- Improper loading
- Malfunctioning sterilizer
- Failures of utilities (like water, steam, compressed air, electricity)
- Post-sterilization drying
- Post-sterilization contamination

- Post-sterilization storage
- Post-sterilization handling

How does one monitor whether sterilization is proper or not?

- Mechanical: Time, temperature, and pressure recording devices and gauges that either graph the relevant parameters on recording charts or provide a printout of values from a digital recorder
- Chemical (three indicators on each tray—1 outside the wrap, 2 inside the wrap, 3 inside the tray)
  - Process indicators: React upon exposure to a specific condition such as heat or change in pH
  - Multivariable indicators: Integrate the effect of temperature and exposure to the actual sterilant over time
  - Integrating indicators: Closely mimic the response of biological indicators to controlled test conditions
  - Chemical indicators do not verify sterility and do not replace the need for weekly spore testing
  - Class 6 indicator/integrator for each load/batch
- Biological (testing indicated every 1–3 months)
  - They are heat-resistant bacterial endospores.
  - *Bacillus stearothermophilus* spores for steam sterilization and *Bacillus subtilis* for dry heat and ETO cycles are used the ampule is put in the load along with other items once a month.
  - It is assumed that if these bacterial endospores have been killed by sterilization, then other microbes have been killed as well.
- All monitoring of sterilization should be diligently maintained in a logbook.
- Surprise checks should be done to ensure adherence.

2.11 OPERATING ROOM CONSTRUCTION AND STERILITY

The establishment of an ophthalmic room (OR) needs specialized planning and coordination, involving a team of civil, mechanical, electrical, and biomedical engineers catering to patient safety and the needs of the surgical/medical team.

What are hospital acquired infections (HAI)?

- Hospital-acquired infection may originate from endogenous or exogenous sources and occur during the hospitalization of the patients.
- For an infection to be defined as hospital-acquired, there must be no evidence that the infection was present or incubating at the time of hospital admission.
- Most frequently acquired hospital-acquired infections are surgical site infections, hospital-acquired pneumonia (urinary tract infection), and blood stream infections.
- Hospital-acquired infections are a major source of concern, and the various protocols formulated have the aim of its prevention.

What are standard precautions?

- Standard precautions combine the major features of universal precautions (UP) and body substance isolation (BSI) and are based on the principle that all blood, body fluids, secretions, excretions (except sweat), non-intact skin, and mucous membranes may contain transmissible infectious agents.
- Standard precautions include a group of infection prevention practices that apply to all patients, regardless of suspected or confirmed infection status, in any setting in which healthcare is delivered.
- These include:
  - Hand hygiene; use of gloves, gown, masks
  - Eye protection or face shield, depending on the anticipated exposure
  - Safe injection practices
- These universal precautions are a set of precautions designed to prevent the transmission of human immunodeficiency virus (HIV), hepatitis B virus (HBV), and other blood-borne pathogens when providing first aid or healthcare (as defined by the CDC).

What is meant by universal precautions?

- Universal precautions, as defined by the CDC, are a set of precautions designed to prevent transmission of human immunodeficiency virus (HIV), hepatitis B virus (HBV), and other blood-borne pathogens when providing first aid or healthcare.
- Under universal precautions, blood and certain body fluids of all patients are considered potentially infectious for HIV, HBV, and other blood-borne pathogens

What are the basic engineering controls to consider while planning prevention of HAI in a hospital setup?

- HAI maybe caused by airborne pathogens and appropriate ventilation is necessary. Circulation of fresh filtered air dilutes and removes airborne (bacterial) contamination, in addition to removing odor.
- All hospital areas and the high-risk areas should be well ventilated as far as possible. Ventilation systems should be designed and maintained in such a manner as to minimize microbial contamination.
- The air conditioner filters should be cleaned periodically, and fans that can spread airborne pathogens should be avoided in high-risk areas.
- Good housekeeping should ensure that unnecessary items like empty boxes and shelves do not clutter and impede ventilation in high-risk areas.
- Positive air pressure is recommended for high-risk areas that must be kept clean.
- Negative air pressure vented to the air is recommended for contaminated areas and is required for the isolation of patients with infections spread by the airborne route.
- Filtration systems (air handling units) designed to provide clean air should have HEPA filters in high-risk areas, including ophthalmic OT setup.
- Unidirectional laminar airflow systems should be available in appropriate areas in the hospital construction.

What are the NABH guidelines for setting up an OT?

- NABH guidelines, though not mandatory yet, have come into effect across the country in view of the over-arching benefit for patient safety standardization as well as possible correlation with IRDA related insurance norms. As a PG, one should be aware of its basics.
- For this purpose, operation theaters have been divided into groups:
  - Super-specialty OT: Super-specialty OT means operation theaters for neurosciences, orthopedics (joint replacement), cardiothoracic surgery, and transplant surgery (kidney, liver etc.).
  - General OT: This includes operation theaters for ophthalmology, district hospital

OT, FRU OT, and all other basic surgical disciplines.
  - Day-care center: Day surgery is the admission of selected patients to hospital for a planned surgical procedure, returning home on the same day, would fall under the category of general OT.
- The following basic assumptions have been kept in view from an ophthalmic viewpoint:
  - Occupancy: Standard occupancy of 5–8 persons at any given point of time inside the OT is considered.
  - Equipment load: Standard equipment load of 5–7 kW considered per OT.
  - Ambient temperature and humidity at each location to be considered while designing the system.
- OT construction:
  - Paint: Antibacterial, antifungal
  - OT door: Automatic/hermetically sealed/touch-free (preferable)
  - General lights: Clean room lights
  - Provision of safety against static charge
  - Separate power circuit for equipment like a phacoemulsification machine, monitors, and microscopes
  - Flooring: Seamless, including skirting, should not be of porous stone as it absorbs moisture and could be a source of bio-burden

What are the general OT guidelines for ophthalmic setup under NABH?

- Air change per hour:
  - Minimum total air changes should be 20, based on international guidelines, although the same will vary with biological load and the location.
  - The fresh air component of the air change is required to be a minimum of 4 air changes (i.e., 16%) out of total minimum 20 air changes.
- Air velocity: This should be same, per the previous guide.
- Positive pressure: There is a requirement to maintain positive pressure differential between OT and adjoining areas to prevent outside air entry into OT. The minimum positive pressure recommended is 15 pascal (0.05 inches of water).
- Air handling/filtration: should be same as previous. When not possible, the OT should be well ventilated with 2 filtrations (pre-filters

and microvee filters should be in position at the AHU).

- Temperature and humidity: The temperature should be maintained at 21°C ± 3°C inside the OT all the time with corresponding relative humidity between 40% and 60%. Appropriate devices to monitor and display these conditions inside the OT may be installed.

What are the design considerations for planning a new operation theater?

- Eye surgeries should ideally be performed in a dedicated eye OT.
- Size should be about 160 square feet per 4 persons (400 square feet as desired by NABH is usually not practically possible).
- The layout of an OR should ensure effective and continued sterilization.
- The OT should be situated in an area away from public movement and ideally should have the following features.
  - The sterile and unsterile areas are segregated, preferably by an air lock or buffer zone.
  - The sterile and unsterilized zones inside the OT are separated by colored lines— scrubbed staff remains in the sterile zone, and the circulating staff and patients remain within the unsterilized zone.
  - Preferably, the entrances for patients and staff should be separate.
  - There should be separate areas for storing sterile and unsterilized items.

- The operating room should preferably have seamless walls and a non-porous floor. (Use of marble is contraindicated.)
- There should not be any surface where dust might accumulate.
- Doors of the OR are always kept closed, and movement must be restricted.
- Restrict the number of personnel to the minimum during surgery.
- The AHU of each OT should be dedicated and should not be linked to air conditioning of any other area.
- During the non-functional hours, AHU blower should be operational round-the-clock (this may be without temperature control). Variable frequency devices (VFD) may be used to conserve energy.
- Window and split AC should not be used in any type of OT because they are pure recirculating units and have pockets for microbial growth, which cannot be sealed.
- The flooring, walls, and ceiling should be non-porous, smooth, seamless without corners (coving) and should be easily cleanable in a repeated manner. The material should be chosen accordingly. Hermetic sealing of the doors is recommended.
- Validation of system to be done per ISO 14664 standards and should include (**Table 2.7**):
  - Temperature and humidity check
  - Air particulate count
  - Air change rate calculation

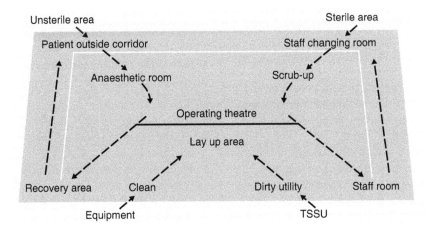

Figure 2.30 OR layout

Table 2.7 Revised Guidelines in Operation Theaters by the National Accreditation Board of Hospital and Healthcare

Parameter	Desired Range
Temperature (°C)	21 ± 3
Relative humidity (%)	40–60
Air movement	From clean to less clean areas
Pressure	Positive air (15 pascals) pressure by manometric control
Air change	Minimum 20 total air changes per hour
Filtration	Air-handling units, high-efficiency particulate air
Air velocity	90–120 feet per minute at the grille/diffuser level

- Air velocity at outlet of terminal filtration units/filters
- Pressure differential levels of the OT with respect to ambient/adjoining areas
- Validation of HEPA filters by appropriate tests like DOP; repeat after 6 months in case HEPA is found healthy.
- Maintenance of the system: Periodic preventive maintenance must be carried out in terms of cleaning of prefilters at the interval of 15 days, per manufacturer recommendations.
- To incorporate the aforementioned features, the OT should be designed in a way that it incorporates four major zones
  - The outer zone acts as a reception area and is accessible to all.
  - The mid-zone/clean zone comprises the changing room and patient preparation room. This is a transfer zone and is accessible only to OT staff.
  - The aseptic zone is a sterile area and includes the space for scrub and gowning, the actual operating area, and the area where instruments are cleaned and sterilized.
  - The disposal zone stores used linen before sending to the laundry. The used disposables are segregated and then disposed off.

What are the recommendations for fumigation?

- Starting OT for the first time, after gap of more than 1 week or after any civil work: At least 3 OT washings followed by fumigations and get 3 consecutive negative cultures of OT from the mandatory swab sites.
- Fumigation is not required if there is positive ventilation in the OT.
  - Running OT: Single fumigation/disinfective mopping/fogging weekly is enough.
  - Use of a fogger machine is preferable.
  - Formalin can be used for fumigation in a low-resource setting, but newer protocols are the following:
- Bacillocid Special (DesNet)
  - Active ingredients are Glutaral 100 mg/g, benzyl-C12-18-alkyldimethylammonium chloride 60 mg/g, and didecyldimethylammonium chloride 60 mg/g.
  - Provides complete asepsis within 30–60 minutes.
  - Cleaning with detergent or carbolic acid is not required if Bacillocid is used
- Bacillocid fumigation
  - Can be done using 2% Bacillocid (100 ml in 5 L of water)
  - Room must be kept closed for 6 hours before entry.
- Bacillol
  - Contains ethanol, 2-propanol, and 1-propanol; used as spray for instant surface disinfection but does not act on spores
  - Ultraviolet radiation (preferable, not mandatory)
  - Daily for 12–16 hours, switched off 2 hours before entering OT

What are the recommendations for cleaning maintenance with regard to an ophthalmic OT? (Table 2.8)

- Clean AC filters every week.
- AC servicing and cleaning every month, with documentation.
- Floor, microscope, surfaces, sinks, and drains to be cleaned daily.
- Walls, if tiled, should be washed up to minimum 4 feet height.
- Floor may be washed/wet-mopped at end of OT list.

Table 2.8 Regimen for Cleaning, Disinfection, and Sterilization

Procedure and Agents	Routine	Efficacy
Disinfection of OT floor, walls, tables, and trolleys with 1% sodium hypochlorite or antiseptic	Every day	Generally effective against a wide range of gram-positive and gram-negative bacteria but not as useful against endospores and viruses
Washing of OT walls, floor, tables, trolleys, etc., with detergent	Once a week	Useful to eliminate accumulated contamination. Enhances the effect of daily cleaning and disinfection
Fumigation of the operating room with formaldehyde or another agent	Weekly or after surgery on the infected cases	Efficacy is not proven in temperature <20°C and relative humidity <70%
Maintenance, repair of any breaches, cleaning of the ventilation system	Once in 6 months Repairs → immediately	Prevents entry point for contamination and improves the effect of cleaning and disinfection

- 2% Bacillocid (100 ml in 5 L of water) recommended as disinfectant.
- No dry dusting or vacuum cleaning.
- Studies show no consensus benefit of HEPA filter; central ACs and even AHU is debated in some forums, but general guidelines should be kept in mind.
- OT swab monitoring in the form of periodic cultures (pre- and post-infection)
  - Every 1 to 3 months
  - Moist swabs taken from microscope end and head end of table

- 10 cm blood agar plates kept open at head end of table for 30 minutes (colony count <10 with not even a single gram-negative bacillus or fungal colony growth)
- Standard quality disposables (irrigating fluid, dyes, viscoelastic, eyedrops) should be used with no reuse system. Inspection for clarity of solutions as well as expiry date is mandatory.
- Maintenance and rigorous checks for logs.
- Training of ophthalmic personnel, including the operating surgeon, should be a routine and recurrent exercise.

3

Optics and Refraction

3.1 TOPICS

- Refraction and retinoscopy
- Lenses

3.2 REFRACTION AND RETINOSCOPY

Definitions:

- Refractometry: The measurement of the refractive state of the eye.
- Refraction (ophthalmic definition): A process of both objective measurement (retinoscopy) and subjective verification of the refractive state of the eye.
- Refraction (optical definition): The change in the path or direction of light as it travels from one medium to another.
- Principal meridians: Meridians of maximum and minimum curvature; in ophthalmic lenses, these are 90° to each other.
- Ocular refractive status: The locus within the eye conjugate with optical infinity during minimal accommodation.
- Retinoscopy/Skiascopy: Objective method of deducing the refractive error of the eye.

What is the aim of retinoscopy?

- To illuminate the retina and locate its image in space.
- Far point is the position of the retinal image and its position in dioptric unit is refractive error.
- Punctum remotum, or far point, optically is the point conjugate with the retina during minimal accommodation.
- A small proportion of light entering the eye is reflected, and this is brought to a focus at the far point of the eye.

- The observation of the movement of this image produced by movement of the light source allows location of this far point.

What are the stages of retinoscopy?

- Illumination: Using a light source reflected via a plane or concave mirror
- Reflex: Image formation at the far point
- Projection: Location of the far point
- Point of reversal: Also called neutral point of retinoscopy; reached when the patient's far point coincides with the observer's nodal point

What are the instruments used during retinoscopy?

- Plain mirror (Priestley–Smith mirror)
- Streak Retinoscope

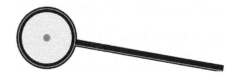

Figure 3.1 Plain mirror/Priestley–Smith mirror, usually with the bulb placed behind the patient's head

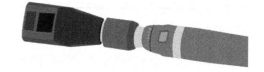

Figure 3.2 Streak retinoscope

What are the observed movements using a plane mirror during retinoscopy?

- Very accurate technique
- Against movement: Myopia of greater than working distance

DOI: 10.1201/9781003455646-3

- With movement:
  - Emmetropia
  - Myopia of less than working distance
  - Hypermetropia
  - The far point of vision is the position of an object such that its image falls on the retina in the relaxed eye, i.e., in the absence of or with minimal physiological accomodation
- Position of far point
  - Emmetrope: Infinity
  - Myope: Between examiner and patient
  - Hypermetrope: Behind the eye, carries a negative sign

How does one correct for astigmatism?

- Check the movement in principal meridians and correct with trial lenses using spheres or spherocylinder form.
- When astigmatism is suspected, check the movement in both principal meridians and calculate refraction in both.
- For automated refraction measurement for astigmatism needs three arbitrary meridians, using which mathematically astigmatism is estimated.

What are the abnormal reflexes one may encounter?

- No glow (black/mature cataract or in a vitreous hemorrhage)
- Scissoring: Keratoconus, nuclear cataract
- Speed: Very slow (high ametropia)
- Irregular: Cataract or a corneal opacity

What are the other uses of retinoscopy?

- Diagnosis of keratoconus
- Diagnosis of astigmatism
- Diagnosis of cataract based on glow (nuclear sclerosis or PSC)

What are the types of retinoscopy?

- Static retinoscopy
- Dynamic retinoscopy

What is a Jackson's cross cylinder? What are its uses and method of use?

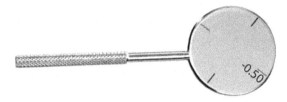

Figure 3.3 Jackson's cross cylinder

- Spherocylindrical lens in which the power of the sphere is half the power of the cylinder and is of the opposite sign; powers: +0.25 D to +2.00 D
- Uses:
  - Axis determination
  - Determination of cylinder power
  - To confirm the absence of cylinder
- Method:
  - Only of use if close to a real cylinder on retinoscopy.
  - Encourage active accommodation and use circular targets one line above the vision line on acuity charts.
  - Check cylindrical axis, then power and then again axis.
  - Change of 0.5 D in cylinder requires the addition of a 0.25 D sphere of opposite sign.

What is a stenopeic slit?

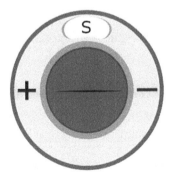

Figure 3.4 Stenopeic slit

- Restricts blur circle in one meridian.
- Subjective technique for correction of astigmatism using BVS technique.
- Best vision sphere (BVS) is a technique for subjective refraction by using the spherical equivalent. In cases of astigmatism, stenopeic slit can be used to find the BVS in the two principal

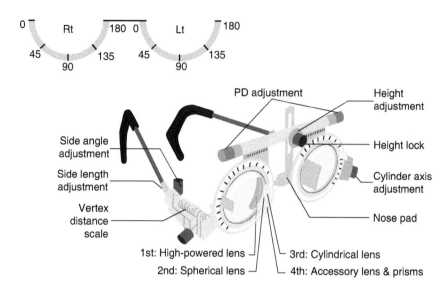

Figure 3.5 Trial frame

meridians and hence estimate the astigmatic error.

- BVS is usually estimated subjectively by either using fogging or duochrome test.

Identify and describe this instrument

- Specially designed spectacles for the assessment of refraction
- Typically consists of two connected wells for each eyepiece, separated by an adjustable bar. Usually, the trial frame has multiple adjustable knobs for controlling adjustments—this can vary depending upon the model.
  - IPD
  - Height
  - Pantoscopic tilt
  - Axis lock
  - Back Vertex Distance
  - Adjustable temple screws and nosepiece screws
- Each well has multiple sockets for the reception of various lenses, usually in the order (from patient to examiner's side).
  - Higher power spherical (especially plus) lenses, near addition (at the back)
  - Spherical Lenses for distance
  - Cylindrical lenses
  - Occluders/pinhole/Maddox rod/Bagolini lenses/stenopeic slit, prism, etc. (at the front)
- Each well further has etchings for the axis orientation, usually below the eye level.

- The left side of the examiner starts with 0° and reaches to 180° on each end of the examiner's right side.
- Each axis mark has an interval of 5°.
- Important variants:
  - Plastic based
  - Steel based
  - Pediatric trial frames
  - Clip on single-eye trial frame clip lens
  - Phoropter-based trials frame

What is an occluder?

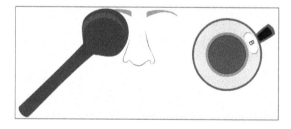

Figure 3.6 Occluder

- Opaque occluder, in the form of a disc
- Usually, black
- Available as trial frame occluder or handheld occluder; also available as patches, spectacle frame add-ons, and even contact lens occluders
- Variation in the form of Spielman occluder, for visualization of the movement of eyes through the occluder

- Usually plastic; can be metal
- Uses:
  - Diagnostic:
    - Checking uniocular vision, blocking the other eye
    - Cover: Uncover test
    - Strabismus tests: PBCT, Maddox tests, preferential looking test
  - Therapeutic:
    - Treatment of amblyopia: Full-time occlusion, part-time occlusion
    - Temporary treatment of amblyopia

What is this (pinhole)?

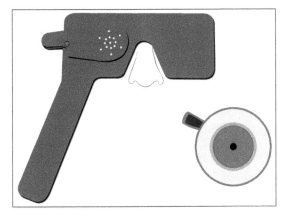

Figure 3.7 Pinhole

- Opaque occluder with a central hole, usually 0.5 mm to 1.5 mm in diameter (average 1.2 mm). Available as a trial frame pinhole or handheld one.
- Also available as multiple pinholes, useful in eccentric pupils and retinal/macular diseases.
- Useful initial test to assess if the decrease in vision is due to refractive error or other causes.
- If vision significantly improved through pinhole, then the cause is usually refractive.
- It works by increasing the depth of focus (ideally, a pinhole should allow a single ray of light to pass through, correcting any amount of refractive error; however, practically a wavefront passes through, so diffusion blur occurs).
- It can usually correct up to 4–5 D of refractive error.

- Other uses:
  - Double pinhole: Macular function test
  - Multiple pinhole spectacle for retinal surgery patients in selected cases.

How is refraction performed (objective)?

- The process of both objective measurement (e.g., retinoscopy) and subjective verification (e.g., trial frame acceptance).
- Refractometry is the measurement of the refractive state of the eye.
- Manifest refraction: A refraction without cycloplegic drops (which dilate the pupils and prevent accommodation); also known as dry refraction.
- Cycloplegic refraction: Refraction done with cycloplegic drops given to dilate the pupils and prevent accommodation; also known as wet refraction.
- Post-cycloplegic refraction: A dry refraction performed on a visit at least few days (depending upon the type of cyclopegia used) after a wet refraction. The purpose is to see how much of the full cycloplegic refraction found on the previous visit can be tolerated. Also sometimes called post-mydriatic refraction (PMT).
- The goal of refraction is to give the simplest system that satisfies the individual patient's visual needs. Comfort is more important than clarity.

What are the steps of refraction?

- Record baseline vision (binocular, uniocular with associated head posture, etc.), along with routine ophthalmological records, including refractive history.
- IPD measurement, adjust trial frame or phoropter accordingly.
- Mention back vertex distance (BVD) for higher refractive errors (>6 D SE).
- Cover test with and without correction, for distance and near, in primary gaze.
- Objective refraction: Measurement of the mathematical refractive state of the eye, at present, noting the appropriate accommodative state. The following methods can be used:
  - Retinoscopy (plain or streak)
  - Auto-refractometry (AR)
  - Corrective lenses by comparing with power of old glasses (PGP)

- Subjective refraction or clinical refraction is to determine the strength of the corrective lens that will achieve a refractive state of the eye as a whole to ensure rays of light coming from infinity will be focused onto a single point on the retina, within physiological limits of accommodation. The goal is to give the simplest system that satisfies the individual patient's visual needs. Typically, needs response and confirmation from the patient's perspective. Comfort is more important than clarity. The following methods can be used:
  - Trial frame with loose lenses.
  - Phoropter.
  - Spherical over-refraction over the patient's current glasses.
  - Refine sphere with duochrome test.
  - Cylindrical power and axis confirmation with JCC or stenopeic slit or astigmatic fan test.
  - Adjust the spherical power for one eye subjectively to obtain best possible comfortable visual acuity, using maximum plus (or minimum minus)—this is the best vision sphere (BVS).
  - Confirm power and axis of cylindrical correction, if any.
  - Record subjective refraction result and visual acuity.
  - Check spherical equivalent (SE) subjectively and record VA with this lens.
  - Repeat for the other eye.
  - Uncover both eyes and check binocular VA—this is often a line better than monocularly. If needed, use binocular balance with fogging and prism dissociation.
  - Assess near vision ability. Is there presbyopia? If so, prescribe an appropriate reading addition per the patient's needs.
  - Show the patient the prescription in a trial frame and ask to move head or walk around casually, especially if cylindrical change. Compare with previous spectacles if any.
  - Write out final prescription (including need for specific type of spectacle, centration, etc.), and explain your findings and recommendations.

Kindly explain objective refraction methods in greater detail?

- Retinoscopy (ret):
  - An objective measurement of the refractive state of the eye using an illuminated area of the retina (patient's) as an object and locating the image at the far point of the patient's eye by moving the illumination across the fundus and noting the behavior of the luminous reflex in the pupil.
  - Types: Static/dynamic and streak/spot/ spiral.
  - Principle: When light is reflected from a mirror into the eye, the direction in which light travels across the pupil will depend upon the refractive state of the eye.
- Auto-refractometry (AR):
  - Automated machines for calculating the refractive state of the eye using infrared light.
  - Types: Fully automated, semi-automated, manually operated.
  - Principle: Basic principle of retinoscopy along with the Badal optometer principle. (Badal is based on the observation that if the eye is placed at the focal point of a plus lens, the virtual image of an object located between the lens and the anterior focal point will always subtend the same visual angle.)
  - With technological advancements, many modifications are now available.
- Photorefraction:
  - Useful in those who are unable to fixate for long or patients uncooperative for sitting on the AR.
  - Uses flash photography to roughly estimate the refractive error.
  - Based on the red reflex principle and the direct dynamic retinoscopy module.
  - Not as accurate.
- Other tests for objective components of refraction (oculomotor and accommodation tests:
  - Distance heterophoria by Maddox rod
  - Measure amplitude of accommodation, monocular and binocular
  - Measure near heterophoria by Maddox wing
  - Measure near point of convergence

- Additional tests may be used if appropriate
  - Fixation disparity
  - AC/A ratio
  - Fusional reserves
  - Stereopsis

Kindly explain subjective refraction methods in greater detail.

- Basic steps of subjective refraction can be broken down into:
  - Estimate the spherical component.
  - Refine the cylinder axis and power.
  - Refine the sphere power.
  - Basic estimation of sphere is derived from the spherical equivalent (SE) calculated using the various objective refraction techniques mentioned:
    - If the circle of least confusion is in the plane of the outer limiting membrane of the retina, both principal astigmatic meridians are equally out of focus. This is usually the position of best acuity of the uncorrected astigmatic eye. The spherical lens power that achieves this is known as the spherical equivalent. (Mathematically, add one-half of the cylinder power to the sphere; algebraically, maintain the plus and minus signs.)
  - The cylindrical axis is first refined after putting the basic cylindrical lens as obtained using objective refraction techniques, using JCC.
    - A spherocylindrical lens with a plus cylinder in one axis placed perpendicular to a minus cylinder in opposite axis.
    - Generally available as 0.50 D and 1.0 D, marked on it.
    - Axis to be refined is the one found in initial estimation.
    - Straddle the axes of the JCC on either side of the axis to be refined; usually handle of JCC is in line with the axis to be estimated.
    - Generally, show target one/two Snellen less than BCVA, as JCC blurs vision.
    - JCC is flipped with the handle remaining in same position (along axis to be refined), and the patient is asked which of the two lenses is better.
    - Rotate the cylinder of the trial axis in the direction of the same sign as the position which lead to clearer vision. (Initial rotation 10°, then finer adjustment of 5°, can go up to 3–2–1).
    - Test again, making sure the handle is along the axis of the newly refined trial axis.
    - Repeat.
    - End point is when both the flips show equally blurred line.
  - Cylindrical power by JCC.
    - Now place the handle of the JCC at 45° to that of the trial axis (whose power is to be refined) or place any of the marked JCC axes along the trial axis.
    - Power to be refined is the one found in initial estimation.
    - Generally, one line higher of Snellen is used from axis estimation step.
    - JCC is flipped with the handle remaining in same position (45° to that of the trial axis already refined), and the patient is asked which of the two lenses is better.
    - If any of the position is better, make the power of the axis move toward the same in increments of 0.25 till equally blurred.
    - Example, if testing with PLUS cylinder, and JCC's PLUS cylinder placed over the trial axis gives better result, increase PLUS cylinder power by 0.25 D.
    - End point is when both the flips show equally blurred line.
    - While refining the cylinder power, an adjustment to spherical power must be made whenever the cylinder power has been modified by a half diopter. This is necessary to keep the circle of least confusion on the retina.
  - The JCC is now on axis.
- Other methods for cylindrical refinement: Stenopeic slit, astigmatic fan test, or dial test.
- Refine the final sphere.
- Show patient a series of two choices and try to elicit which is clearer or if they are the same.
- Choices given in both directions, plus and minus, refining with 0.25 D.
- Always check in plus direction first, which helps to avoid stimulating accommodation.

- End point: Patient says clearest view on the VA chart; if equal, always prefer less minus.
- This is the spherical equivalent, or this step places the circle of least confusion onto the retina.
- Other ways to refine sphere:
- Duochrome test:
  - Uses ocular chromatic aberrations; shorter-wavelength green light refracted more than red.
  - Should be used with other methods of BVS testing.
  - First impression of target clarity important.
  - Emmetropic individual: Equally bright target.
  - Myopic individual: Red more distinct.
  - Hypermetropic individual: Usually green more distinct; may accommodate to either.
  - Can be used even if the patient is color blind; simply ask which line is clearer.
  - The red-green duochrome test: If red is clearer, add minus; if green is clearer, add plus = mnemonic RAMGAP (red, add minus; green, add plus).
- Binocular balance: During monocular refraction a different state of accommodation may occur as one is being tested alone.
  - Fogging method:
    - Can be neutralized by alternate occlusion, after each eye monocular.
    - Refraction: Fog both eyes with 0.75 D.
    - Occlude each eye alternately for 0.5 seconds, adding +0.25 D to the eye.
    - With better vision till both "equalize."
    - Fog both eyes with 0.75 D. Perform one eye BVS.
    - Fog with additional +0.25 D till blurred, and then remove till clear.
    - Repeat in other eye.
  - Another method is the prism dissociation method.
    - Simultaneous dissociative prisms are used for each eye to enable visualization of subjective diplopia and comparison of each eye's image by the patient.
    - Can be discomforting, and the prisms themselves blur the image to a certain extent.

3.3 LENSES

How do you differentiate prisms from cylindrical and spherical lenses?

- Prisms cause displacement of the image.
- Cylindrical lenses cause distortion of the image.
- Spherical lenses cause neither displacement nor distortion.
- Rotation of the lens, if maintained through the principal axis, does not alter the image turn in spherical and cylindrical lenses but will alter the image in prisms rotation.
- To describe lenses, mention the shape, image type, and image change on X and Y axis movement and on rotation around the Z axis.

How do you identify a concave spherical lens?

- The center is thin and the periphery is thick.
- The object can be seen, though it appears minified.
- When the lens is moved, the object seen through it moves in the same direction as the lens because the image formed is erect.
- Rotation does not cause the image to turn if the central principal axis is maintained.

What are the uses of concave lenses?

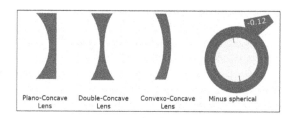

Figure 3.8 Concave spherical lens

Uses of concave lenses:
- Diagnostic:
  - To diagnose myopia during retinoscopy
  - Hruby lenses for fundus examination as a slit lamp attachment
- Therapeutic:
  - Treatment of myopia
  - Treatment of myopic astigmatism

- Low visual aids, used as part of low visual aid (LVA) telescopes
- Instruments:
  - Direct ophthalmoscope

Define myopia.

- Myopia, or short-sightedness, is a refractive state of the eye wherein parallel rays of light from infinity are focused in front of the retina with accommodation being at rest.

Explain the optics of myopia.

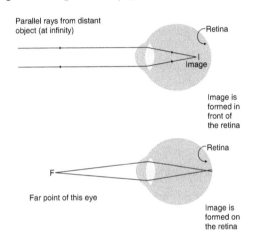

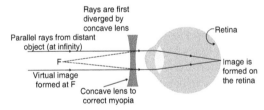

Figure 3.9 Optics of a myopic eye

- Optics of myopia:
  - In a myopic eye, the image is made up of the circle of diffusion due to a diverging beam.
  - Far point is at a finite distance, unlike in an emmetropic eye, which is at infinite distance.
  - This distance is the measure of myopia
  - Images in myopes are larger than in emmetropes as the nodal point is further away from retina.
  - Apparent convergent squint is due to a negative angle kappa, or there is a true

divergent squint because the attempt of conversion is given up and its insufficiency leads to a muscular imbalance
  - In emmetropes, angle kappa is positive, but less than 5°; therefore, it gives an impression of pseudoexotropia.
  - In myopes, there is an impression of pseudoesotropia due to the negative angle kappa.

What is far point or punctum remotum?

- It is the farthest point at which object can be seen clearly, while accommodation is within physiological limits.

What is angle alpha?

- It is the angle formed between optical axis and visual axis at the nodal point.

What is angle kappa?

- It is the angle between the visual axis and pupillary axis.

What is the classification of myopia?

- Etiological classification:
  - Axial:
    - Commonest
    - Increase in antero-posterior length of the eyeball
    - 1 mm increase in axial length increases the myopia by 3 D
  - Curvatural:
    - Increased curvature of cornea, lens, or both (e.g., keratoconus, lenticonus)
    - 1 mm increase in radius of curvature increases the myopia by 6 D
    - Positional
    - Produced by anterior displacement of crystalline lens in the eye
  - Index:
    - Increase in refractive index of crystalline lens associated with lens protein changes due to nuclear sclerosis
  - Others:
    - Myopia due to excessive accommodation
    - Myopia due to relaxed or ruptures suspensory ligament or zonules

- Clinical classification:
- Simple:
  - Has no degenerative changes in fundus
  - Does not progress after puberty
  - Myopia is up to 5–6 D
  - Developmental
  - Born with eyes with an in abnormally long axial length
  - Rare progression
- Pathological:
  - Fundus shows degenerative changes
  - Progressive
  - May increase to 15–20 D or more
  - The condition is strongly hereditary (autosomal recessive)
- Induced:
  - Also known as acquired myopia; may result from exposure to various drugs; increases in glucose levels, nuclear sclerosis, and oxygen toxicity (e.g., from diving or from oxygen, hyperbaric therapy).
  - The encircling bands in retinal surgeries may induce myopia by increasing the axial length of the eye.
- According to the degree of myopia:
  - Low myopia (<3 D)
  - Medium myopia (3–6 D)
  - High myopia (>6 D)
- According to the age of onset:
  - Congenital myopia
  - Youth-onset myopia (<20 years of age)
  - Early-adult-onset myopia (20–40 years of age)
  - Late-adul-onset myopia (>40 years of age)

What are the drugs causing myopia?

- Pilocarpine
- Phenothiazine
- Sulfa drugs
- Hydralazine
- Chlorthalidone

What are the symptoms of myopia?

- Decreased vision for distance
- Headache and eyestrain
- Black spots and floaters (muscae volitantes)
- Rarely flashes

What are the anterior segment signs one checks for in a myopic patient?

- Prominent eyes
- Semi-dilated pupils
- Deep anterior chamber (AC)
- Apparent convergent/true divergent squint

What are the other causes of a deep AC?

- Aphakia
- Myopia
- Keratoglobus
- Buphthalmos
- Keratoconus
- Posterior perforation of the globe

Why does the pupil in myopes appear semi-dilated?

- Because of the absence of stimulus to accommodation, circular fibers of the ciliary muscle tend to get atrophied.

What are the posterior segment signs of myopia?

- Posterior staphyloma
- Equatorial staphyloma
- Retinal
  - Generalized chorioretinal atrophy
  - Myopic crescent
  - Foster–Fuchs spots
  - Vitreous floaters
  - Tilted disc
  - Peripapillary atrophy
  - Angioid streaks
  - Lacquer cracks
  - Macular changes: CNVM, macular atrophy
  - Macular hole
  - Retinal holes, tears
  - Lattice degeneration
  - Retinal detachment

Why is difficult to diagnose POAG in myopes?

- Field changes are masked by degenerations in the retina.
- Disc cupping is limited by anterior displacement of lamina cribrosa.
- Indentation tonometry is inaccurate due to low scleral rigidity.

- Fixation is difficult (if there is foveal involvement due to Foster–Fuchs spots/CNVM).

What is the treatment of myopia?

- Glasses:
  - Correction with concave lenses.
  - Myopes must not be overcorrected.
    - Low myopia: Give full correction, and ask the patient to use the glasses constantly.
    - Young myopes: May give undercorrection for near.
    - High myopes: Undercorrect for distance and still weaker lenses for near.
- Give the lenses at the minimum vertex distance as:
  - It decreases image minification.
  - It decreases lens strength.
  - It decreases prismatic displacement.
- Risk of amblyopia is low in myopes.
- Myopia with squint:
- Myopia with exophoria: Give overcorrection.
- Myopia with esophoria: Give undercorrection.
- Spectacle recommendations in children (**Table 3.1**).

- Contact lenses:
  - Distortion and prismatic effect of thick concave glasses are reduced.
  - Field of vision is better.
  - Image size is less minified.
- Low vision aids (LVA):
  - For high pathological myopes.
  - Compound telescopic glasses may be used.
  - Non-visual educational aids can be used.
- Surgical options:
  - Corneal procedures (**Table 3.2**)
  - Lens procedures (**Table 3.3**)

How do you identify Spherical convex lenses?

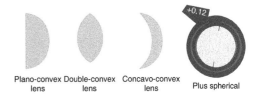

Plano-convex lens Double-convex lens Concavo-convex lens Plus spherical

Figure 3.10 Spherical convex lenses

- The central part is thick, and the periphery is thin.

Table 3.1 Spectacle Recommendations in Children

Minimum refractive correction to be prescribed in infants and young children
Source: National Consensus Guidelines, 2020

Condition	Refractive Errors in Dioptres (D)		
<1 year	1–2 years	2–3 years	
Isoametropia			
Myopia	≥ −3.0	≥ −3.0	Per refraction
Hyperopia (− deviation)	≥ +4.0	≥ +4.0	≥ +4.0
Hyperopia (with ET)	≥ +1.50	≥ +1.50	≥ +1.50
Astigmatism	≥ 3.0	≥ 2.0	≥ 2.0

Minimum refractive correction to be prescribed in infants and young children
Source: National Consensus Guidelines, 2020

Condition	Refractive Errors in Dioptres (D)		
Anisometropia (without strabismus)			
Myopia	≥ −3.0	≥ −3.0	Per refraction
Hyperopia	≥ +2.0	≥ +1.50	≥ +1.50
Astigmatism	≥ 2.50	≥ 2.0	≥ 2.0

Table 3.2 Corneal Procedures

Name of Surgery	Correction	Advantages	Disadvantages
Photorefractive keratectomy (PRK)	1–4 D	• No risk of flap complications and can be done on thin corneas	Delayed recovery, faint corneal haze
Laser-assisted in situ keratomileusis (LASIK)	2–12 D	• Less operative time, effective, better correction results	Infection, astigmatism, thinning and ectasia, glare during night driving
Laser-assisted sub-epithelial keratectomy (E-LASEK)	1–6 D	• Similar to PRK but epithelial flap not lifted • Microkeratome is used • Corrects 1–6 D	Longer visual recovery time Full visual recovery is longer than LASIK, though similar to PRK More pain and discomfort than LASIK, but less pain than PRK
Orthokeratology	1–5 D	• Hard contact lens to flatten cornea • Keratoconus treatment • Irregular astigmatism • Corrects 1–5 D	Expensive, irregular astigmatism

Table 3.3 Lens Procedures

	Advantages	Disadvantages
Fukala's operation of removing clear lens	• Can be done in very high myopes	• Accommodation is lost • RD risk increases • Irreversible
Phakic IOLs	• Reversible • No need for specialized machines • Can be done in patients with good endothelial count • Requires deep AC	• Glaucoma • Cataract • Endophthalmitis

- An object held close to it appears magnified when viewed through the lens.
- When the convex lens is moved, an object seen through it moves in the opposite direction because the image formed is inverted.

What are the uses of convex lenses?

- Diagnostic:
  - Hypermetropia during retinoscopy
  - Presbyopia
  - Malingering
- Therapeutic:
  - Correction of hypermetropia
  - Correction of presbyopia
  - Correction of aphakia
  - Low visual aids
- Instruments:
  - Direct and indirect ophthalmoscopes
  - Slit lamp
  - Ophthalmic loupe
  - Telescope
  - Operating microscope
  - +90 D, +78 D, +20 D lenses
  - Magnifying glasses

Define hypermetropia.

- Hypermetropia, or "long-sightedness," is that refractive state of the eye in which when accommodation is at rest, parallel rays of light from infinity come to a focus posterior to the light-sensitive layer of the retina.

- Optics: The far point is behind the eye, thereby producing no clear image.

Describe the optical condition of a hypermetropic eye.

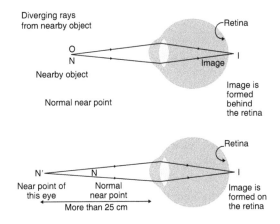

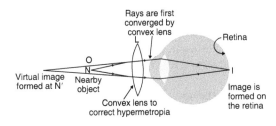

Figure 3.11 Optics of Hypermetropic Eye

- The optical condition of a hypermetropic eye:
- Image is formed behind the retina so diffusion circle on the retina is blurred.
- Image is smaller.
- Emerging rays will be divergent so they meet behind retina.
- To focus them on the retina, we will need convex lens or accommodation.

Describe the types of hypermetropia?

- Axial:
  - Length of the eyeball is small
  - 1 mm decrease in axial length produces 3 D of hypermetropia
- Pathology based on other structures:
  - Microphthalmos
  - Intraorbital space occupying lesions

- Retinal detachment
- Curvatural:
  - Flat cornea as in cornea plana
  - A 1 mm decrease in the radius of curvature produces 6 D of hypermetropia
- Index:
  - Increase in refractive index of cortex of lens (senile, diabetics)
  - Backward displacement of lens

What are the causes of pathological hypermetropia?

- Senile/acquired:
  - Curvatural: Curvature of outer lens fibers
  - Index: Acquired cortical sclerosis with dense cortex forming two converging menisci around a rarer nucleus
  - Positional: Posterior subluxation of lens
  - Consecutive: Surgically overcorrected myopia after refractive surgery or after cataract surgery
- Functional: Paralysis of accommodation associated with third-cranial-nerve palsy, internuclear ophthalmoplegia
- Secondary: Associated with retinal detachment, central serous retinopathy, orbital tumors

What are the symptoms of hypermetropia?

- Sometimes may not have any symptoms at all.
- Increased strain at evening time, eye ache, burning, dryness, increased blinking
- Conjunctival hyperemia, frontal headaches
- Frequent eye rubbing by children, hence recurrent styes, chalazion, and blepharitis
- Accommodative asthenopia due to perpetual over action of ciliary body as there is accommodation for distance and near
- Convergent squint in children: Excessive accommodation and excessive convergence
- Range of symptoms
  - Asymptomatic
  - Accommodative asthenopia
  - Blurred near vision
  - Sudden persistent blurring of vision
  - Convergent squint
  - Amblyopia

Table 3.4 Symptoms of Hypermetropia

	Distance			Near			Symptoms
	Vision	Accommodation	Convergence	Vision	Accommodation	Convergence	
Normal	N	0	0	N	+	=	None
Low HM	N	+	0	N	++	+	A±
Moderate HM	N or Mild reduction	++	0/+		+++	+	A ++, VN +, ET +
High HM		0	0		0	0	VN +, ET +

A= Asthenopia; VN = Drop in vision; ET= Esotropia
Grading: N= Normal; 0 = No symptoms; + = Mild symptoms; ++ = Very symptomatic

- School dropouts and learning disability children were found to be more in hypermetropic as compared to myopic children (**Table 3.4**)

What are the signs of hypermetropia?

- Anatomically smaller eyes
- Small corneal diameter
- Shallow AC (partly due to normal lens in small eye hence, they have an increased incidence of closed angle glaucoma)
- Retina:
  - No abnormality.
  - Bright reflex like watered silk: Fundal reflexes are heightened.
  - Optic nerve: Due to crowding of nerve fibers, optic neuritis is simulated resulting in pseudopapillitis.
  - Macula is farther away from the optic disc; therefore, the visual axis cuts cornea inside the optic axis, resulting in a positive angle kappa and an apparent divergent squint.

What are the causes of a shallow anterior chamber?

- Primary narrow-angle glaucoma
- Hypermetropia
- Anteriorly subluxated lens
- Intumescent cataract
- Postoperative shallow anterior chamber (after intraocular surgery due to wound leak or ciliochoroidal detachment)
- Malignant glaucoma

- Anterior perforations (perforating injuries or perforated corneal ulcer)
- Cornea plana

What are the complications as a result of hypermetropia?

- Accommodative convergent squint by 2–3 years
- Ametropic amblyopia, anisometropic amblyopia, or strabismic amblyopia
- Predisposition to angle-closure glaucoma

Why does the optic disc look small in hypermetropia?

- Nodal point in hypermetropes is closer to retina.

Where are the components of hypermetropia?

- Normally, a considerable amount of hypermetropia is corrected by contraction of the ciliary muscles due to its physiological tone.
- This is neutralized by various means to find the components of hypermetropia:
  - Latent hypermetropia:
    - Due to ciliary muscle tone
    - Found by maximum plus lens with which clear vision is obtained after full atropinization, subtracted by the maximum plus lens giving clear vision without atropinization (Latent = Total hypermetropia – Manifest hypermetropia)

- Decreases with age, but usually 1 D; later becomes manifest as tone of ciliary muscle decreases
- Manifest hypermetropia:
  - Amount of hypermetropia which is uncorrected by the subject's physiological tone of ciliary muscle
  - Found by maximum plus lens with which clear vision is obtained without atropine use
  - Subdivided into facultative and absolute
- Facultative hypermetropia:
  - Due to patient's accommodation
  - Found by difference between strongest and weakest plus lens with which clear vision is obtained without atropine use (Facultative = Manifest hypermetropia – Absolute hypermetropia)
  - With age, more of facultative becomes absolute as range of accommodation becomes smaller
- Absolute hypermetropia:
  - Amount of hypermetropia not overcome by patient's accommodative effort
  - Found by weakest plus lens with which clear vision is obtained without atropine use
  - Almost zero in early life; becomes all of hypermetropia beyond 65 years (apparent)
- Total hypermetropia:
  - Latent hypermetropia + Manifest hypermetropia
  - Found by the maximum plus lens with which clear vision is obtained under full atropinization (same as latent if no manifest hypermetropia)
  - Cyclopegia used: Atropine (full and complete relaxation of ciliary muscle)
- Acquired hypermetropia:
  - In old age, the refractive index of the cortex of the aging lens increases as the lens becomes more homogenous.
  - The lens acts as a single lens with less converging power than before. Hence, for emmetropic eyes at 30 years, there is approximate 0.25 D of hypermetropia at age 55 years and 1 D at 70 years.
  - In contrast, if the nucleus also increases in density, the original RI remains and may even increase, leading to the myopic shift in nuclear sclerosis leading to second sight.

What are their corrections with lenses?

- Absolute HM is the amount of hypermetropia corrected by the weakest convex lens.
- Facultative HM is the difference between the amount of hypermetropia corrected by the strongest and weakest convex lens that the patient accepts (under fogging technique).
- Total HM is the amount of hypermetropia estimated when refraction is done under atropine (strongest convex lens used for correction).
- Latent HM = Total – (Absolute + Facultative)

What is nanophthalmos?

- Nanophthalmos is a rare genetic disease, characterized by a small eye secondary to a compromised growth.
- Growth of lens is, however, normal.
- Patients typically have extreme axial hyperopia (15–20 mm axial length and 7–15 D hypermetropia) without obvious structural defects.
- Therefore, there is a high lens to eye volume.
- This can lead to a shallow AC and early angle-closure glaucoma.

What are the implications of nanophthalmos in cataract surgery?

- Increased chance of expulsive hemorrhage/uveal effusion and/or retinal detachment
- Increased incidence of shallowing of AC and cilio-choroidal detachment
- Precautions:
  - Counsel patient about nature of possible complications and risks.
  - Consider preoperative IV mannitol (1–2 mg/kg) to reduce vitreous volume, but avoid hypotony to prevent possible choroidal effusion.
  - Prefer high viscosity OVD (but avoid excess of it).
  - If the AC is very shallow, perform a vitreous tap with an automated vitrectomy cutter

(25G preferred) without infusion, but simultaneously infuse AC with viscoelastic.

- Balance IOP.
- Ensure tight incisions to avoid hypotony.
- Extra care during rhexis, as it is a possible moment of effusion, so prefer from side port using micro-rhexis forceps (23–25 G).
- Careful hydrodissection (anticipate possible zonular weakness).
- Vertical chop with lower bottle height and low flow is preferred.
- Possible need of posterior scleral window for creation of a bypass outflow route for intraocular fluid by scleral resection in cases where choroidal effusion exists and persists.
- It is important to plan decompression of vortex veins prior to any intraocular surgery.

What are the treatment modalities for hypermetropia?

- Spectacles
- Contact lens
- Surgery
- Treatment depends on:
  - Amount of error
  - Age
  - Accommodation
  - Vision
  - Presence or absence of symptoms
  - Presence or absence of squint
  - Vocation of the patient
  - Principally it is better to undercorrect the hypermetropia, as long as there is some active accommodation.

What are the indications for doing a cycloplegic refraction?

- Children <7 years of age
- Children and even adults who are accommodating on dynamic retinoscopy
- Presence of esotropia
- Precautions: Shallow anterior chambers and therefore maybe prone to angle-closure attacks

What are the methods of management of hypermetropia?

- Glasses
- Prescribing glasses for hyperopia without esotropia (**Table 3.5**)

Table 3.5 Spectacle Prescription for Children with Hypermetropia

Threshold	Age 0–1 year	Age 1–2 years	Age 2–3 years
Amount of hyperopia for which spectacles have to be prescribed	≥+6 D	≥+5 D	≥+4.5 D

Table 3.6 Spectacle Prescription for Children with Hypermetropia and Esotropia

Threshold	Age 0–1 year	Age 1–2 years	Age 2–3 years
Amount of hyperopia with esotropia for which spectacles have to be prescribed	≥−3 D	≥+2 D	≥+1.5 D

- Threshold for prescribing is +3.5 D
- Cut the plus by up to 50% but not more than 3 D
- Prescribing glasses for hyperopia with esotropia (**Table 3.6**)
  - Give the full correction (or reduce by +0.5 D).
  - Warn parents about future "worse crossing" when the glasses are removed.
- Contact lenses:
  - Cosmetically good
  - Provide an increased field of view
  - Cause less magnification
  - Eliminate aberrations and prismatic effect
- Surgery:
  - Laser procedures: Thermal laser keratoplasty, PRK, LASEK, Epi-LASIK, LASIK, LASEK
  - Miscellaneous procedures: Conductive keratoplasty
  - IOL procedures: Phakic IOLs, refractive lens exchange

Table 3.7 Change in Near Points of Accommodation with Age

Increasing near point of accom-modation with age	Age (years)	10	20	30	40	50
	Distance (cm)	7	10	14	20	40

Define presbyopia.

- Presbyopia is defined as the reduction in amplitude of accommodation with advancing age and recession of the near point, which is caused by hardening of the crystalline lens.

What is the etiology of presbyopia?

- Natural part of the aging process
- Earlier in hyperopes

What are the symptoms of presbyopia?

- The need to hold reading material at arm's length (**Table 3.7**)
- Blurred near vision
- Headache
- Fatigue
- Symptoms worse in dim light

How do you diagnose presbyopia?

- Visual acuity test for near
- Retinoscopy
- The correction is in the form of addition over the distance correction (**Table 3.8**)

What are trouble shooters in prescribing near add?

- Don't add too much plus because:
  - It constricts the near range of vision
  - It makes patients accustomed to higher magnification.
  - Beginners are never sure of their working distance.
  - Tall people hold books further away and, therefore, require less near addition.

What are the different spectacle lenses available for presbyopes?

- Convex lenses are used for the correction of presbyopia.
- Bifocals:
  - Kryptok
  - D-type lenses produce less image jump
  - Executive type
    - Larger near segment
    - Less image jump
    - Poor cosmesis
- Trifocals:
  - Have intermediate add for intermediate distance.
  - Intermediate add is calculated as half of the reading addition prescribed.
- Multifocal or progressive addition lenses (PALs): Progressives, or PALs, are lenses designed for presbyopes in which the power gradually increases from the distance zone, through a progression to the near zone.

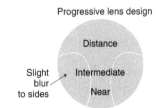

Progressive lenses have 3 fields of vision for everyday use

Figure 3.12 Progressive addition lenses (PALs)

Compare the advantages and disadvantages of these lenses (Table 3.9).

What are the advantages of PALs?

- Better vision as intermediate is clear; no jump in vision from distance to near
- Lighter/thinner
- More natural vision and comfort
- Confidence in mobility

Table 3.8 Rough Guide to Near Additions Adjusted for Age

Age	40–45	45–50	50–55	50 upward	Aphakia
Near addition	+1.00 to +1.50	+1.50 to +2.00	+2.00 to +2.50	+2.50 to +2.75	+2.75 to +3.00

Table 3.9 Comparison of Various Lenses for Presbyopic Correction

	Bifocal	Trifocal	MultiFocal (PALs)
Advantages	Economical	Intermediate vision not affected	Cosmetically better Power change from distance to near add
Disadvantages	Intermediate vision affected	Difficult to make	Need adaptation period

What are the disadvantages?

- Straight lines appear curved, and therefore requires more adaptation
- Decreased width of vision at intermediate and near produce limited lateral movement
- Increase in eye and head movement for reading comfortably

What are some things patients may complain of with PALs?

- Blurred distance or near vision
- Swimming sensation
- Reading area too small or having to look to the side to read
- Having to tilt the head too far backward/forward to read
- Having to tilt the head backward/forward for distance
- Progressive lenses are excellent, but they must be fitted with scrupulous care and precision to really work well.

What are some of the practical points to keep in mind when prescribing glasses?

- Low hyperopes, especially the young, can cope without glasses as they can easily accommodate to overcome the error.
- A +0.25 D and + 0.5 D (and perhaps even + 0.75 D) may not be prescribed.
- But low hyperopes can develop symptoms of asthenopia in their late 30s as accommodation weakness begins.
- Low myopes can manage even without reading glasses sometimes even in their late 40s; however, per need and symptoms, reading glasses should be prescribed.
- Remember that a person who does not read does not need reading glasses but may need glasses for sewing, knitting, and other odd jobs.

- Do not encourage people to have bifocals if their distance prescription is small.
- If you obtain less than one line improvement in vision, there is no real benefit in prescribing new glasses.
- Aim for 6/9 or better.

What are some instructions you would give first-time users?

- Head straight ahead for distance viewing.
- While they are climbing stairs, they must be warned to look through the distance segment.
- Reading material must be held at a correct distance.
- For reading, one must rotate their eyes and not their heads.
- In case a higher near addition is given, the working distance is reduced, and the patient should be instructed about using the same.
- Ask patients to regularly check if spectacle frame is bent or tilted, especially patients with astigmatism and those using progressive glasses.

Mention some other methods of presbyopia correction?

- Contact lenses:
  - For those who are already using contact lenses.
  - Mono-vision contact lens fitting can be used where the dominant eye is corrected for far and non-dominant eye for near.
  - Nowadays multifocal contact lenses are also available.
    - They are available in soft/RGP/hybrid materials/silicone hydrogel.
    - Types of multifocal contact lenses are simultaneous vision designs and segmented designs.

- Surgery:
  - Monovision LASIK/PRK
  - Intracorneal ring segments
  - Refractive lens exchange
  - Corneal inlays and onlays

Describe cylindrical, convex, and concave lenses.

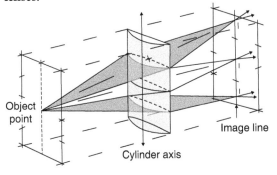

Figure 3.13 Cylindrical lenses

- An object appears distorted when a cylindrical lens is rotated around its optical axis.
- When moved up and down or sideways, the object will move with the lens (concave cylinder) and opposite to the lens (convex cylinder) only in one direction.

What are the uses of cylindrical lenses?

- Diagnostic: To diagnose astigmatism during retinoscopy
- Therapeutic: To treat astigmatic refractive errors

Define astigmatism.

- It is that condition of refraction wherein a point focus of light cannot be formed on the retina.

What is Sturm's conoid?

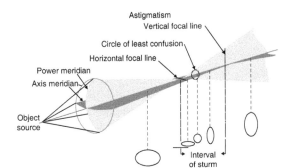

Figure 3.14 Sturm's conoid

- Sturm's conoid is the geometric configuration of light rays emanating from single point source and refracted by spherocylindrical lens.
- The parallel rays of light are not focused on a point but form two focal lines.
- The configuration of rays refracted through astigmatic surface is called Sturm's conoid.
- The distance between two focal lines is known as the focal interval of Sturm.
- The length of this focal interval is a measure of degree of astigmatism.

What is the incidence of astigmatism?

- In infants: About 50% full-term infants in first year of life have astigmatism of over 1 D.
- In adults: Incidence decreases as the child grows, and by adulthood, 15% have >1 D and only 2% have >3 D.

What is the classification of astigmatism based on etiology?

Classification of astigmatism

- Curvatural:
  - Cornea:
    - Normally vertical curve is more than horizontal due to constant pressure of the eyelid (physiological/direct/with the rule astigmatism)
    - Keratoconus
    - Trauma
    - Postsurgical
    - Scarring following inflammation
    - Induced astigmatism due to pressure of lid swelling
  - Lens:
    - Lenticonus
    - Minor variation due to change in lens curvature
  - Retina: Due to oblique placement of macula
- Centering: If the placement of lens is out of line in the optical system
- Index: Inequality in the refractive index of the different meridians in a cataractous lens

What are the clinical types of astigmatism?

- Regular astigmatism:
  - With the rule: Where vertical curvature is greater than the horizontal curvature.

The stronger refracting meridian is vertical, and the weaker meridian is horizontal. The minus cylinder axis is at about 180°.

- Against the rule: Where the horizontal curvature is greater than the vertical curvature. The stronger refracting meridian is horizontal, and the weaker meridian is vertical. The minus cylinder axis is at about 90°.
- Oblique astigmatism: When greatest and least curvature are at right angles to each other, but not actually vertical or horizontal, then it is called oblique astigmatism.
  - Symmetrical: E.g., 30° in both eyes.
  - Complementary: E.g., 30° in 1 eye, 150° in opposite eye.
- Bi-oblique astigmatism: When greatest and least curvature are not at right angles to each other, then it is called bi-oblique astigmatism (uncommon).
- Irregular astigmatism:
  - Irregularity of curvatures in various meridians is so different that it does not follow any particular geometrical pattern.
  - E.g., Scarred corneas, keratoconus, lenticonus, incipient cataract.

How do you classify astigmatism based on the axis of the principal meridian?

- Regular astigmatism: Principal meridians are perpendicular.
  - "With the rule" where the stronger refracting meridian is vertical and the weaker horizontal, the minus cylinder axis is at about 180°.
  - "Against the rule" where the stronger meridian is in the horizontal, the minus cylinder axis is at about 90°.
  - Oblique astigmatism where the axes are around 45° and 135°.
- Irregular astigmatism: Principal meridians are not perpendicular.

How do you classify astigmatism based on focus of the principal meridians?

- Simple: When one meridian is emmetropic and other is either hypermetropic or myopic

- Simple hypermetropic astigmatism
- Simple myopic astigmatism
- Compound: When neither of the 2 foci lie on the retina
  - Compound hypermetropia: Both foci are in front of the retina
  - Compound myopia: Both foci are behind the retina
- Mixed: When one meridian is myopic and other is hypermetropic

What are the symptoms of astigmatism?

- Blurred vision (tailed-off appearance, circle appears oval)
- Asthenopic symptoms: Eye strain, headache
- Posturing, head turn, head tilt
- Reading material may be held close to eye
- Burning and itching sensation low astigmatic errors

How does one diagnose astigmatism?

- Refraction
- Keratometry
- Astigmatic fan and Jackson cross cylinder (for regular astigmatism)
- Placido disc (for irregular astigmatism)
- Topography

What are the non-surgical treatment options for astigmatism?

- Optical treatment: Cylindrical lenses in form of spectacles
- Hard contact lens: 2–3 D of regular astigmatism
- Higher degrees of astigmatism: Toric contact lenses

What are some general guidelines for the treatment of astigmatism?

- Regular astigmatism:
  - Small astigmatism (0.5 D or less): Treated only if asthenopia symptoms are present or there is a deterioration of vision.
  - High astigmatism: Correct cylindrical error fully. If not accepting the complete correction, the refractive error should be undercorrected until the patient is accustomed to cylinder.
  - Change in axis of astigmatic correction: Don't change unless necessary. A change in axis is poorly tolerated and should be done cautiously.

- New astigmatic correction may produce intolerable distortion, even if measurable visual acuity is improved. Thus, a period of adjustment is advised.
- Bi-oblique, mixed, and high astigmatism are better treated by contact lenses.
- Spherical component should be prescribed per guidelines.
- Irregular astigmatism:
  - Optical treatment: Rigid gas permeable contact lenses
  - Surgical treatment: Depending on the extent of corneal scarring: Phototherapeutic keratectomy (PTK), lamellar corneal surgeries, full-thickness penetrating keratoplasty (PK)

Define aphakia.

- Aphakia is the absence of crystalline lens from its normal situation.

What are the causes of aphakia?

- Commonest: Postsurgical (after crystalline lens removal)
- Traumatic lens extrusion
- Congenital anomaly
- Posterior dislocation into the vitreous

What are the types of aphakia?

- Congenital aphakia
- Acquired aphakia
  - Trauma
  - Surgical removal (couching)

What are the symptoms of aphakia?

- Decreased vision for distance due to increase in hypermetropia
- Decreased vision for near due to loss of accommodation

What are the signs of uncomplicated aphakia?

- Anterior chamber is deep.
- Anterior chamber may be shallow in the following circumstances:
  - Peripheral anterior synechiae
  - Positive vitreous pressure
  - Pupillary block glaucoma
  - Iris bombé
  - Choroidal detachment

- Iridodonesis: Absent if synechiae or iris atrophy is present
- Jet-black pupil (except if there is an exudative membrane)
- Scar of surgery (except if the conjunctival flap after a well-operated and sutured case shows minimal scarring)
- Iridectomy: May or may not be present

What are the optical changes in the eye due to the absence of the crystalline lens?

- Eye becomes hypermetropic (since the crystalline lens contributes +18 D)
- Astigmatism (in post-op cases, usually against the rule, i.e., vertical meridian is flatter)
- Absence of accommodation
- Colors differ: Since normal lens absorbs certain wavelengths of light

How does one correct aphakia?

- Glasses
- Contact lenses
- Secondary IOL

What are the problems with prescribing aphakic glasses?

- Are the simplest and easiest solution.
- Although normal human lens contributes +18 D, a lens of +10 D outside the eye corrects the refractive error in emmetropes.
- Problems with glasses:
  - They are thick, heavy convex lenses.
  - Size of image is increased by 25–30%.
  - If the other eye has good vision, attempts for binocular vision result in diplopia.
  - The field of vision is reduced.
  - Straight lines appear curved, called the pin cushion effect.
  - There is false spatial orientation; hence, coordination of finer movements is affected (e.g., sharpening of pencil, placing a key in a lock).

What is jack-in-the-box phenomenon, or roving ring scotoma?

- The jack-in-the-box phenomenon, or roving ring scotoma, is due to the prismatic effects at the edges of the lens. It is due to the prismatic errors resulting from the displaced optical centers of lenses. It results in reduced visual fields and poor eccentric visual acuity.

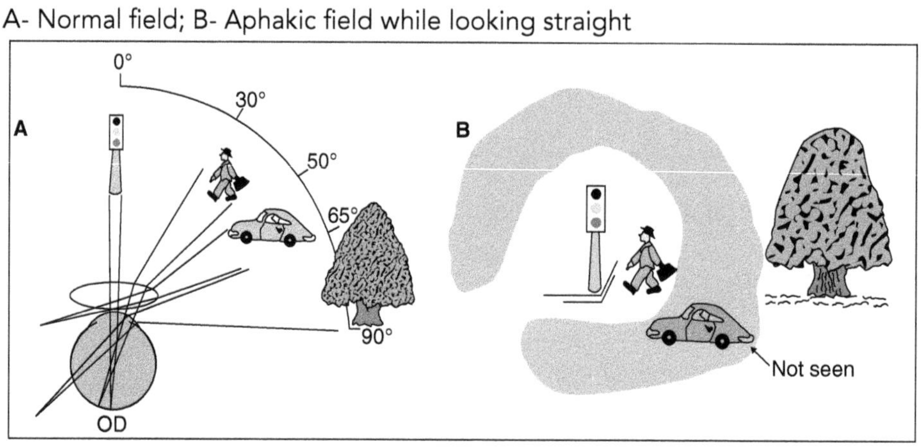

A- Normal field; B- Aphakic field while looking straight

Figure 3.15 Jack-in-the-box phenomenon

- In aphakic patients, due to high convex lens, this optical phenomenon occurs.
- In different degrees, in an aphakic spectacle-wearing person, this field-of-vision change occurs.
  - 0–50°: Refracted rays of light enter the eye.
  - 50–65°: Rays are refracted but do not enter the eye.
  - 65–90°: Unrefracted rays of light.
- The rays between 50° and 65° are bent and do not enter the eye; therefore, optical scotoma is produced in the absence of any organic disease (in increased convex lenses in aphakia).

- View seen by the patient:
  - Shaded area: Ring scotoma (optically blind area).
  - Rays 30–50°: Fail to enter eye.
  - Rays 50–90°: Unrefracted because they fail to enter the spectacle glass.
  - Patient has the signal in front, when the patient tries to look at a person in his 30° view the man disappears, when the patient looks further away, man reappears as he goes beyond the scotoma (65–90°).
  - When gaze returns centrally, a person reappears (jack-in-the-box or roving ring scotoma).

What are the advantages and disadvantages of any other methods to correct aphakia?

- Contact lenses

- Advantages:
  - Better alternative in uniocular aphakia
  - Magnification: 7%
  - No ring scotoma, hence no jack-in-the-box phenomenon
  - No peripheral field defects
  - No pincushion defects
- Disadvantages:
  - Insertion and removal require dexterity and good vision in other eye
  - Hygiene
  - Cost
- Secondary IOLs: An IOL is placed inside the eye as a secondary procedure
  - Advantages:
    - It overcomes optical disadvantages of glasses.
    - Insertion and removal difficulties with contact lens are avoided.
  - Disadvantages:
    - Technique may be complex and is costly.
    - If removal is necessary, then it entails another surgery.

How does the presence of silicone oil in the eye affect the refractive error of that eye?

- The resultant refraction is dependent on the shape of the silicone oil bubble inside the eye and influence of posture.
- In aphakia, the oil surface is convex, resulting in a positive lens; thus, aphakic

- silicone-oil-filled eye become less hyperopic; i.e., there is myopic shift.
- In phakic eyes, the oil surface is concave as determined by the shape of the back surface of the crystalline lens, resulting in a negative lens.
- Thus, phakic eyes become more hyperopic.
- In pseudophakia, with a biconvex IOL, there is a hyperopic shift within the eye.

What is ametropia?

- It is defined as a state of refraction, when a parallel ray of light coming from infinity is focused either in front or behind the retina, in one or both the meridians, with accommodation at rest.

What is anisometropia, and what are its types?

- Anisometropia is a condition wherein refraction of both eyes is unequal.
- Types: Axial and curvatural

How does one diagnose anisometropia?

- Refraction
- Ultrasound: For axial anisometropia
- Keratometry: For curvatural anisometropia

What are its clinical features?

- Small amounts of astigmatism are very common.
- Large amounts can occur due to:
  - Congenital difference in refraction
  - Traumatic
  - Surgical causes
  - Pathological conditions of the eye, such as keratoconus, keratoplasty, or aphakia
- One eye maybe emmetropic and the other hypermetropic/myopic/astigmatic, or both eyes may be ametropic.
- Vision may be:
  - Binocular
  - Alternating
  - Uniocular
  - Diplopia after spectacle correction
- Each 0.25 D difference in refraction of both eyes cause 0.5% difference in size of image and a difference of 5% is usually the tolerable limit.

- Hence, with higher grades of error fusion of images is difficult and either alternating or uniocular vision can occur, depending on vision in each eye which can result in amblyopia ex anopsia and eventually a squint (binocular vision is tested by Worth's four-dot test or a FRIEND test).
- Binocular vision is the usual result, reported even in difference of up to −6 D of refractive error between the two eyes.

What is the treatment of anisometropia?

- Optical correction.
- Mild or moderate anisometropia requires a full correction (it must be given at the anterior focal plane—15.7 mm in front of cornea to minimize image size disparity).
- Contact lens:
  - Image size disparity is reduced.
  - Prismatic effect in high refractive glasses is not present.
- Surgical treatment: Laser/surgical

What is aniseikonia?

- It is a condition wherein the size and shape of the images between the two eyes are unequal.

What are its types?

- Optical: Due to difference in dioptric condition of the two eyes, i.e., ametropia.
- Anatomical: Because of difference in the distribution of retinal elements. If widely spaced, this can cause micropsia (since few photoreceptors are stimulated).
- Physiological in small amounts, which helps in developing stereopsis. Binocular vision is present if aniseikonia does not exceed 5%.
- Symmetric: When image size in one eye is larger than other in all directions/in one meridian.
- Asymmetric: When image is distorted, progressively larger/smaller in one eye.

What are the symptoms and how does one diagnose and treat this condition?

- Symptoms: Due to basic defect
- Diagnosis: Standard or space eikonometer, which diagnoses size disparity
- Treatment: By iseikonic lenses

What are prisms?

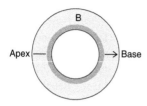

Figure 3.16 Prism

- Definition: Transparent material with 2 refractive surfaces inclined to each other.
- Refracting angle is the angle between 2 surfaces.
- Light is deviated toward the base, and the image displaced toward the apex.
- Convex lens: 2 prisms with base against each other.
- Concave lens: 2 prisms with apex against each other.

What is Prentice's rule?

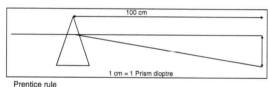

Figure 3.17 Prentice's rule

- Prism diopter: 1 prism diopter is equal to the displacement in centimeters of light ray passing through prism measured 100 cm from prism.
- Prentice's rule: $P = d \times F$, where prism power of a lens (P) at any point on the lens is equal to the distance of the point from the optic axis in cm (d) multiplied by the power of lens in diopters (F).
- Clinical implications:
  - In squint measurement of angle of deviation
  - Minus lenses: Increase angle of deviation
  - Plus lenses: Decrease angle of deviation

What are the uses of prisms?

- Diagnostic:
  - Squint:
    - Tropias: Prism cover test/Krimsky test
    - Phorias: Prism cover test/Maddox rod
    - Cyclo Maddox double rod + prism (to measure cyclodeviation)
    - 4 prism base out: Diagnose microtropia
  - Fusional reserve
- Therapeutic:
  - Exercise: Convergence insufficiency
  - Relieving
    - Postsurgical squint
    - Diplopia
- Recovering acquired a sixth-nerve palsy
- Progressive pathology like CPEO, myasthenia, and thyroid eye disease
  - Patient refusing/not fit for surgery
  - Convergence insufficiency: Organic, adult
  - Phorias, which are symptomatic
- Instruments
  - Applanation tonometer
  - Slit lamp: Porro prism
  - Laser interferometry: Dove
  - Haidinger's brush: Nicolle
  - Rotary refractometer: Risley
  - Keratometer
  - Operating microscope
  - Synaptophore
  - Indirect ophthalmoscope has reflecting prisms in eyepieces
  - Koeppe's gonio lens

What are Fresnel prisms?

- Thin strips of polyvinyl chloride molded to form prisms

Figure 3.18 Fresnel prism

- Advantages:
  - Can be stuck to glass with water
  - Lightweight
  - Cosmetically acceptable
  - Can give higher prismatic correction
- Disadvantage: Decrease in vision (because of light scatter)
- Example: 3M Press-On

How should you prescribe prisms?

- In case of a vertical squint, prescribe the full correction.
- In a horizontal squint, prescribe 50% of the full correction equally divided between the two eyes.

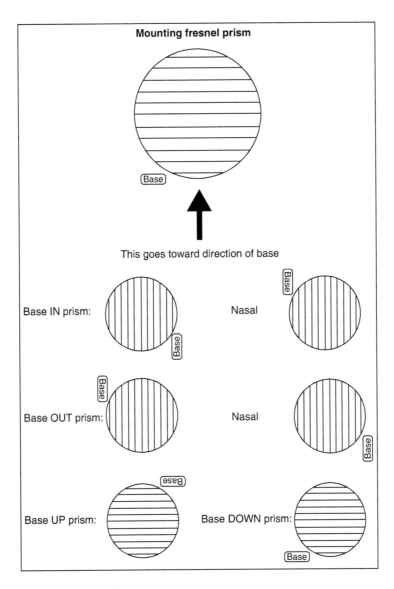

Figure 3.19 Fresnel prism prescription

4

Cornea

4.1 TOPICS

- Instruments used in full-thickness keratoplasty
- FAQs on keratoplasty
- Instruments used for lamellar corneal surgeries
- FAQs on lamellar corneal surgeries
- Keratoprosthesis
- FAQs on keratoprosthesis
- LASIK instruments
- FAQs on LASIK
- LASEK/PRK instruments
- FAQs on PRK/LASEK
- Aberrations
- Phakic IOLs and instruments
- FAQs on phakic IOLs
- Corneal collagen cross-linking with riboflavin (C3R)
- Intracorneal ring segments (ICRs)

4.2 INSTRUMENTS USED IN FULL-THICKNESS KERATOPLASTY

What are the instruments used for a penetrating keratoplasty?

- Barraquer wire speculum
- Calipers
- Teflon block
- Trephine/endothelial punch
- Flieringa ring
- No. 15 blade
- Radial marker
- Trephine
- Castroviejo corneo-scleral scissors (left and right)
- Patton's spatula and spoon

- Pollack forceps
- Portable keratometer

Identify and describe the Flieringa scleral fixation rings.

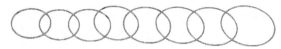

- These are the Flieringa scleral fixation rings.
- Sutured to the sclera before starting the graft procedure.
- It prevents the collapse of the globe and thus prolapse of ocular contents and prevents distortion of the corneal rim.
- Four scleral sutures are used to secure the ring to the sclera anterior to the rectus insertion.
- Available as a set of 8 rings, sizes 14–22 mm.
- Sutured to sclera with 7-0 Vicryl before surgery.
- Maintains rigidity of the recipient's globe after trephination.

What are its uses?

- In cases with low scleral rigidity like in:
  - High myopes
  - Pediatric cataract
  - Vitrectomized eye
  - Penetrating Keratoplasty surgery

What are its disadvantages of the Flieringa scleral fixation ring?

- Can distort the eyeball and induce astigmatism if fixation to the globe is inadequate.

DOI: 10.1201/9781003455646-4

- Can induce subconjunctival hemorrhage.
- Can cause oval cut in keratoplasty.
- High astigmatism
- Can reduce working space during suturing.

What are the uses of trephines?

- These are sharp blades to create circular incision.
- Corneal trephines are used in:
  - Penetrating keratoplasty (PKP)
  - Tattooing
  - Lamellar keratectomy
  - Keratoprosthesis (K-Pro)
- Skin punch:
  - 3 mm diameter trephine
  - Useful in DMEK/DSEK surgery before applying orientation stamp

What are the types of trephines?

- Handheld trephine
- Suction (Hessburg–Barron suction trephine)
- Guided trephines (Krumeich guided trephine system)
- Motor (Mikro–Keratron)
- Laser trephination (using a femtosecond laser)
- Depending on sterilization, they can be disposable (single-use) or reusable of stainless steel that can be autoclaved.

Identify and describe the handheld corneal trephines.

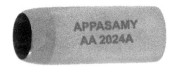

- Handheld corneal trephines
- Most used trephine
- Available in sizes from 6 to 16 mm in diameter
- Can be attached to a handle or to an endothelial punch for greater stability and control
- Donor trephination done with endothelial side up

Describe the Hessburg–Barron vacuum corneal trephine.

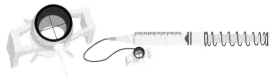

- It is a suction fixation corneal trephine used for controlled complete or partial trephination of the host.
- It has cross-hairs for centration over the host cornea.
- It rotates 250 μm in depth with each 360° rotation.
- The sizes that are available are from 6 to 9 mm with 0.25 mm increments.

What are the advantages and disadvantages of suction trephines?

- Advantages:
  - Consistency and predictability of the depth of the cut
  - Can be used in perforated eyes.
  - Can be used in eyes with low pressure.
  - Easy centration due to cross hair
- Disadvantages:
  - Has a tendency to undercut, if there is loss of suction there may be an asymmetrical cut
  - May cause endothelial cell damage
  - Requires a trained assistant and an experienced surgeon
  - Expensive
  - Useful only for recipient cornea as a separate trephination system is needed for donor buttons

Describe the Barron vacuum punch.

- It is a solid stainless-steel blade which is permanently mounted in a nylon housing.
- The base of the punch features a circular groove for aspirating the epithelial side of the cornea, immobilizing it for cutting the button.
- The blade is placed on the vacuum fixed donor button and pressed with the thumb to yield a sharply cut corneal button.

Describe the endothelial punch.

- Donor cornea is placed endothelial side up on a cutting block.
- A disposable trephine to cut an appropriately sized graft is fixed at the bottom end of the stand.
- Advantages:
  - Yields sharp vertical cuts without beveling and ensures a stable, non-slippery base for the cutting block.

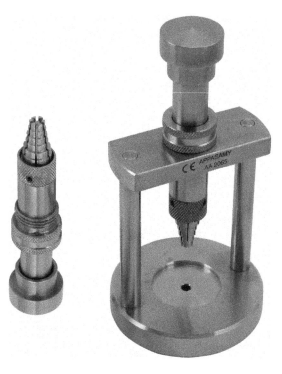

- Prevents oval or elliptical trephination that may happen if donor cornea slips during trephination

Identify the following:

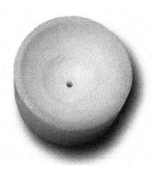

- This is a Lieberman cornea cutting block.
- It is a Teflon-based block with a central hole used for cutting the cornea during DALK, DSEK, or PKP procedures.
- The central hole serves two functions:
  - Release air/fluid trapped below the graft

- Permit accurate positioning and centration of the graft before and during trephination

Identify and describe the Paton spatula and spoon.

- This is a Paton spatula and spoon.
- Flat spatula at one end
- Curved 6 mm teardrop-shaped spoon with three long openings at the other end
- Uses:
  - The spoon end is for holding the corneal button during transfer of the graft from the Teflon block to host in keratoplasty.
  - The flat spatula is used for iris repositioning and to break synechia.

Identify and describe the Pollack forceps.

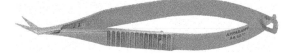

- They are fine forceps.
- 2 × 2 teeth separated by 1 mm (1.2, 1.5 mm in some models)
- Pierse-type tips
- Can be confused with Colibri forceps
- Uses:
  - These fixation forceps are used during suturing in a keratoplasty procedure.
  - Fine teeth prevent injury and provide a firm grip.

Identify and describe the Castroviejo keratoplasty scissors.

- Spring scissors with angled blades
- Inner blade is 1 mm longer than the outer blade
- Used for cutting host cornea after trephination
- Available in two sizes and with blunt tip or sharp tip
- The blunt tip is useful in DALK surgery to prevent inadvertent injury to the host endothelium.

Identify the following:

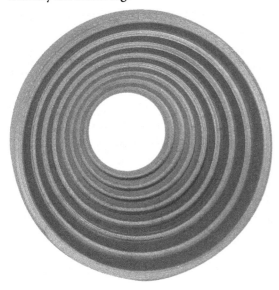

- This is the Maloney intraoperative keratometer.
- It is conical structure with an atraumatic rim that projects a series of rings onto the cornea (like a Placido disc during topography) upon illumination.
- The toricity of the cornea may be surmised from the ellipticity of the reflection, the short axis of the ellipse marks the steep meridian.
- The maximum diameter is 31 mm and height is 21.5 mm.
- Uses:
  - During keratoplasty, to find suture induced astigmatism intraoperatively and adjust tension on the sutures
  - Preoperatively before the start of phacoemulsification to identify the steep axis

Identify the following:

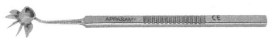

- This is an Osher–Neumann radial marker.
- Central 4.5 mm ring
- 8 or 16 blades
- Fixed round cross-serrated handle

- It marks radial lines 4 mm long and must be used with a skin-marking pen.
- Uses:
  - Helps orient the sutures during keratoplasty surgery, when placed before trephination
  - Previously used in radial keratotomy (RK) surgery
  - Advantages: Inner ring helps in centration; blunt blades allow minimal marking pressure.

What are the various types and uses of corneal markers?

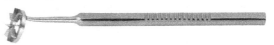

- The corneal marker is stained with a gentian violet pen and kept on host cornea before trephination.
- Eight arms act as a guide for interrupted sutures (Anis marker).
- Radial marker, 4, 6, 8, and 12 blades (Osher–Neumann).

Describe surgical marking pens and their uses?

- Gentian violet ink is used in pens for preoperative marking.
- It temporarily stains the cornea without being washed out.
- A ruler (plastic) that will not tear or smear upon contact with liquids may be included with the pen. Alternatively, a millimeter scale ruler may be printed on the pen's barrel for quick measuring.
- Uses in keratoplasty surgery:
  - Geometric center of the cornea is determined by use of an iris repositor, after which a dimple is created on the same. It is best to dry the surface completely before marking to prevent smudging of the ink. The ultrafine tip is then used to mark the center to guide accurate centration of the trephine.
  - The broad tip may be used to place light marks on the trephine edges to ensure centration.

- A radial keratotomy marker may be used to guide suture marks over the recipient bed before attempting to complete the trephination.

4.3 FAQs ON KERATOPLASTY

What are the types of grafts that you know of?

- Based on thickness:
  - Full-thickness, or penetrating, keratoplasty
  - Partial-thickness, or lamellar, keratoplasty
- Anterior:
  - Anterior lamellar keratoplasty
  - Deep anterior lamellar keratoplasty (DALK)
- Posterior:
  - Posterior lamellar keratoplasty
  - Deep lamellar endothelial keratoplasty (DLEK)
  - Descemet's stripping endothelial keratoplasty (DSEK)
  - Descemet's stripping automated endothelial keratoplasty (DSAEK)
  - Descemet's membrane endothelial keratoplasty (DMEK)
  - Femtosecond-laser-enabled endothelial keratoplasty (FLEK)
- Based on the source:
  - Xenograft: Graft from different species
  - Allograft: From the same species
  - Autograft: From the same person
- Based on indications:
  - Optical:
    - Corneal scars
    - Pseudophakic/aphakic bullous keratopathy (PBK/ABK)
    - Keratoconus
    - Corneal degeneration
    - Graft failure
    - Fuchs endothelial dystrophy
  - Tectonic:
    - Ectasia
    - Keratoglobus
    - Keratoconus
    - Corneal perforations
  - Cosmetic
  - Refractive
  - Therapeutic:
    - Microbial keratitis

- Temporary keratoprosthesis during combined vitreoretinal surgeries with corneal transplant.

What are the contraindications of donor selection?

- Rabies
- Leukemia/lymphoma
- Disseminated intraocular tumors
- CNS infectious diseases, such as Creutzfeldt–Jakob disease, subacute sclerosing panencephalitis (SSPE), and progressive multifocal leuko-encephalopathy (PML)
- Death due to unknown cause
- Systemic diseases like HIV, hepatitis B and C, syphilis, septicemia

What are the contraindications of keratoplasty?

- No perception of light
- Grade 4 chemical burns
- Severe dry eye

What are the complications of keratoplasty?

- Intraoperative:
  - Reversal of host and donor trephines
  - Eccentric trephination
  - Damaged donor button
  - Inversion of donor graft
  - Suprachoroidal bleed
  - Non radial suturing or at inappropriate depth leading to wound leaks
- Postoperative (early):
  - Shallow AC and wound leak
  - Graft rejection
  - Primary graft failure
  - Microbial keratitis
  - Endophthalmitis
  - Increased IOP and pupillary block
- Postoperative (late):
  - Graft rejection
  - Urrets–Zavalia syndrome
  - Glaucoma
  - Astigmatism

Which are diseases commonly reported to recur in the graft?

- Stromal dystrophies:
  - Granular dystrophy
  - Macular dystrophy
  - Lattice dystrophy

- Reis buckler dystrophy
- Schnyder crystalline corneal dystrophy
- Herpetic eye disease

Classify the diseases according to prognosis following a PK?

- Best prognosis:
  - Keratoconus
  - Early Fuchs endothelial dystrophy
  - Lattice and granular stromal dystrophy
  - Avascular corneal scars
- Worst prognosis:
  - Ocular pemphigoid
  - Stevens–Johnson syndrome
  - Severe chemical burns
  - Severe dry eyes

What are the considerations of graft size in keratoplasty?

- The size of the graft depends on diameter of recipient tissue that is cut.
- If the diameter of the recipient bed size is more than 9 mm or less than 7 mm, the graft should be oversized by more than 1 mm.
- If the diameter of the recipient bed size is 7–9 mm, the graft should be more than 0.5 mm in aphakic patients and more than 0.25 mm in pseudophakic and phakic patients.
- Generally, a graft-host disparity of more than 0.5 mm is used.
- In keratoconus (KC), the graft is either oversized by 0.25 mm or kept of the same size as the host to compensate for the patient's myopia.
- In pediatric patients, oversize the graft by 1 mm.

What are the disadvantages of a large and small graft?

- Large graft:
  - Increase in vascularization and subsequent higher chances of rejection
  - Increase in IOP
- Small graft: Increase in tissue tension causes an increase in astigmatism

What is graft failure vs. graft rejection and give their subtypes?

- Primary graft failure:
  - Immediately after penetrating keratoplasty
  - Corneal edema with large folds

- No period of clear cornea
- Due to faulty donor tissue with poor endothelial cell count or poor surgical handling, damaging the donor endothelium
- Secondary graft failure:
  - Clear graft that opacifies without inflammation due to decrease in endothelial cell count over time possibly due to repeated bouts of corneal rejection
- Graft rejection:
  - Due to an immunological process
  - The graft that was clear for the period of 2 weeks gets edematous and inflamed
  - Types:
    - Epithelial: Krachmer line
    - Stromal: Krachmer dots
  - Endothelial: Khodadoust line

How do you treat endothelial rejection?

- Topical 1% prednisolone acetate eyedrops or 0.05% difluprednate
- Oral prednisolone acetate, 1 mg/kg body weight
- Single-pulse or three-pulse intravenous dose of 500 mg of IV methyl prednisolone
- Subconjunctival dexamethasone 0.5 mg or subconjunctival betamethasone 3 mg
- Calcineurin inhibitors, including cyclosporine A (CsA) and tacrolimus (FF-506), are viable options for patients in whom corticosteroids are contraindicated.

What are the high-risk factors for graft rejection?

- Two or more regrafts
- Young age
- Corneal vascularization
- Active inflammation at the time of surgery
- Large grafts
- Eccentric grafts
- Therapeutic keratoplasties
- Other conditions: Uveitis, atopic dermatitis, eczema, herpes simplex keratitis
- A collaborative corneal transplant study (CCTS) for prediction of risk factors for graft rejection found that there was no significance in HLA matching of the donor and the recipient; however, ABO compatibility was found to be more useful.

Describe the various corneal storage media.

- Moist chamber:
  - Storage of whole globe at 4°C
  - Duration: 24 hours
  - Simple method
  - Disadvantage: Stromal edema
- McCarey–Kaufman medium (MK medium)
  - Tissue culture medium (Tc-199), dextran (5%)
  - Buffer: HEPES
  - Antibiotics: Penicillin, gentamicin
  - Duration of storage: 96 hours
- K-Sol
  - Purified chondroitin sulfate
  - Tissue culture medium (Tc-199)
  - Duration: 7–10 days in 4°C
- Dexol
  - MEM base medium
  - 1.35% chondroitin sulfate
  - 1% dextran
  - HEPES buffer
  - Gentamicin
  - 0.1 mM non-essential amino acids
  - Sodium bicarbonate
  - 1 mM sodium pyruvate
  - Additional antioxidants
  - Duration: 7–10 days in 4°C
- Optisol
  - Hybrid of Tc-199 and MEM
  - 2.5% chondroitin sulfate
  - 1% dextran
  - HEPES buffer
  - Gentamicin
  - 0.1 mM non-essential amino acids
  - Sodium bicarbonate
  - 1 mM sodium pyruvate
  - Additional antioxidants
  - Ascorbic acid, vitamin B12, ATP precursor
  - Duration: 7–10 days in 4°C
- Long-term organ culture storage system
  - Defined fetal bovine serum 10%
  - Chondroitin sulfate 1.35%
  - L-glutamine 2 mM
  - Sodium pyruvate 1 mM
  - Non-essential amino acids
  - Mercaptoethanol
  - Gentamicin
  - Duration: 35 days

4.4 INSTRUMENTS USED FOR LAMELLAR CORNEAL SURGERIES

What are the instruments used for DALK?

- Wire speculum
- Calipers
- Trephine
- DALK dissector to create a stromal pocket
- DALK cannula to inject air to make a big bubble
- No. 15 blade
- Pollack forceps
- Keratometer
- Kelman–McPherson forceps

Identify and describe the Tooke knife.

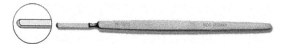

- Straight blade with curved cutting edge
- Blade is 3 mm × 18 mm in size.
- For initiation and pocket creation during lamellar dissection

Identify and describe the Paufique knife.

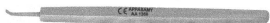

- Has an angled tip with curved cutting edge
- Outlines the graft and helps in pocket formation and dissection
- Alternative instruments
  - Crescent knife
  - No. 15 blade

Identify and describe the DALK cannula.

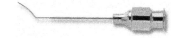

- Tan DALK cannula
  - It is used to create an ideal big bubble.
  - The tip is blunt and smooth to prevent inadvertent perforation.

- The curved shaft is useful for easy tunnelling through deep stroma.

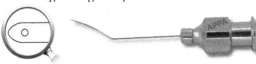

- Rosenwaser DALK cannula
  - It has a "cobra-shaped" head and air opening on the underside.
  - The broad head seals the channel, aiding in the pneumatic dissection of the stroma from the underlying Descemet's membrane during big bubble DALK.
  - The 0.2 mm posterior port allows air injection in a controlled fashion.

Identify the following:

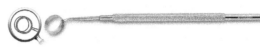

- This is a DALK dissector.
- The tip of this instrument is used to dissect to the interface plane and continue along it during dissection of the stroma.
- It has a flattened, vaulted spatula with a blunt beveled tip.

What are the uses of lamellar dissectors?

- DALK surgery
- Dermoid excision
- Trabeculectomy
- SICS
- Pterygium excision
- OSSN excision
- Scleral buckle (implant placement)

What are the instruments used in DSEK?

- Wire speculum
- No. 15 blade
- Crescent blade and keratome blade
- DSEK marker and skin marker pen
- AC maintainer
- Reverse Sinskey hook
- Artificial anterior chamber
- Trephine
- Busin glide

Identify the following:

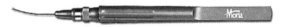

- This is a DSEK reverse Sinskey hook.
- The 0.22 mm pointed tip is directed upward.
- This is used for atraumatic scoring of the Descemet's membrane during endothelial keratoplasty.

What is the use of the DSEK corneal marker?

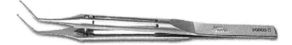

- This is a DSEK corneal marker.
- Sizes are 8 and 9 mm.
- This marks the area to be stripped on the host cornea.

What are the uses of the DSEK spatula?

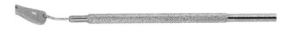

- It is available in 45° and 90° angle tip model in both irrigating and non-irrigating versions.
- It is used to strip the Descemet's membrane of the recipient.

What is the use of the Ogawa DSEK forceps?

- The tips of the forceps remain separated when the handles are closed, to minimize injury to the folded donor tissue during DSEK surgery.
- The folded graft is then easily released into the anterior chamber.

Identify and describe the Busin glide in DSEK surgery.

- This helps unfold the graft and helps in the centration of the donor corneal button.
- It minimizes graft manipulation and endothelial cell loss.
- The donor lamella is loaded endothelial side up into the glide and the glide is inserted into the eye via 3.2 mm incision.

Identify and describe uses of the Busin forceps in DSEK surgery.

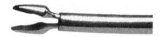

- Micro incision forceps with 20G diameter
- It helps to position the graft in the glide and pull it in the anterior chamber of the host.

Identify the following:

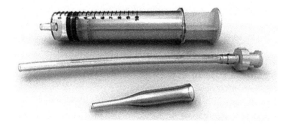

- This is a DMEK injector set.
- DMEK injector set which contains: Single-use DMEK cartridge, tubing, standard single-use syringe.
- Fine oval tip with rounded larger opening of the cartridge that is attached to a disposable syringe along with a piece of silicon tubing.
- Uses:
  - For contactless intake of the graft into the cartridge and gentle injection into the anterior chamber
  - Safe and easy intake of graft
  - Small incision size (fine oval opening)

4.5 FAQs ON LAMELLAR CORNEAL SURGERIES

What are the indications of doing DALK surgery?

- Optical:
  - Corneal ectasia
  - Keratoconus/pellucid marginal degeneration

  - Post-refractive surgery keratectasia
  - Corneal scars
  - Corneal anterior stromal dystrophies: Except macular stromal dystrophy (as endothelium may be involved)
  - Ocular surface disease
  - Corneal degeneration such as in patients with Salzmann's nodular degeneration, spheroidal degeneration, and band-shaped keratopathy
  - Corneal scarring due to dermoid
  - Lipid keratopathy
- Tectonic:
  - Descemetocele
  - Sterile Mooren's ulcer

What are the techniques of DALK?

- Anwar's big bubble technique
  - Developed by Anwar and Teichman. It utilizes the naturally occurring virtual space between the DM and posterior stroma.
  - 300 to 400 μm deep trephination is performed first.
  - Next, a 30G needle, bent to 40°, is advanced with the bevel facing down and air is injected forcibly. (This causes whitening of the peripheral stroma as a large air bubble enters the pre-DM plane.)
  - Blunt scissors can be used to cut the stroma into quadrants and excise it within the trephination.
  - Once DM is borne, the donor button can be sutured in place
- Melles technique: Technique utilizes an air bubble in the anterior chamber to create a mirror image of the dissector blade. This serves as an indicator of stromal depth. The exposed DM can be recognized by its glossy smooth appearance.

What are the complications of DALK surgery?

- Formation of double (pseudo) anterior chamber
- Corneal stromal graft rejection
- Interface haze
- Graft dehiscence
- Descemet's membrane folds
- Interface keratitis
- Urrets–Zavalia syndrome
- Suture-related complications

What are the advantages and disadvantages of anterior lamellar over penetrating keratoplasty?

- Advantages:
  - It is an extraocular procedure and hence is devoid of intraocular complications, like hyphema, endophthalmitis.
  - A large graft can be placed.
  - Less chances of rejection.
  - Tissue with low endothelial count is used.
  - Less stringent donor selection.
  - Faster recovery.
  - Better wound strength.
- Disadvantages:
  - The procedure is technically more demanding.
  - Visual acuity can be impaired due to uneven dissection of recipient or donor corneal tissue and interface scarring.
  - Particulate debris trapped in lamellar interface.
  - Mechanical folds in the posterior layer over the visual axis due to flattening of this layer especially in keratoconus.
  - Vascularization and opacification at the interface.

What are the indications of DSEK?

- Bullous keratopathy
- Failed penetrating keratoplasty due to endothelial dysfunction
- Fuchs endothelial dystrophy
- CHED (congenital hereditary endothelial dystrophy)

What are the relative contraindications of DSEK?

- Stromal scarring
- ACIOL

- Anterior segment disorganization
- Filtering bleb

What are the advantages of DSEK over PKP?

- Recipient cornea is structurally intact.
- No suture-related complications.
- Risk of expulsive hemorrhage is minimal.
- Obviates complex recipient trephination and dissection technique.
- Better visual outcome.

What is the difference between DSEK, DSAEK, and FLEK? (Table 4.1)

- DSEK: Donor dissection is done using a manual artificial anterior chamber.
- DSAEK: Donor dissection is done using an automated microkeratome.
- FLEK: Donor tissue is cut with a femtosecond laser.

What are the prerequisites for a DSEK donor tissue?

- Large scleral rim of more than 16 mm
- High endothelial count
- Short preservation time

What is the technique involved in performing a DSEK surgery?

- Donor preparation:
  - Artificial chamber filled with BSS/Cornisol/Eusol C, and tissue carefully mounted on it and fixed, ensuring no leak.
  - Donor corneal epithelium may or may not be debrided.
  - Corneal thickness is measured by pachymetry.
  - IOP maintained at about 40–50 mmHg.

Table 4.1 Differences between DSEK, DSAEK, and FLEK

Terminology	DSEK	DSAEK	FLEK
Donor Dissection	Manual	Microkeratome	Femtosecond
Thickness	Variable	Dependable	Precise
Interface	Less smooth	Smoother	Less smooth (because of applanation force which in turn folds the posterior stroma)
Cost	Cost-effective	Expensive	Very expensive
Operative time	More	Less	Less

- 4 mm wide vertical incision at limbus of preset depth of 350–400 μm is made using a guarded blade.
- DSEK: Manual lamellar dissection done with a crescent blade and Melle's dissector ensuring to stay in the same plane, from limbus to limbus.
- DSAEK: A 300/350 micron microkeratome blade is used to cut ~9 mm diameter of anterior stromal cap and after the pass, the cap is replaced over the corneal mount.
- The center of the dissection and its margins are marked with a marker pen on the epithelial side.
- The tissue is carefully dismounted and placed endothelium side up on a donor vacuum trephine.
- The center of dissection must coincide with the center of the base.
- The donor is punched and transferred back into preservation medium.
- Descemet's stripping:
  - Descemet's stripping performed under air/ sodium hyaluronate or anterior chamber maintainer from the side port leaving a 2 mm rim near the limbus.
  - Scleral tunnel made.
- Insertion technique of the endothelial graft:
  - Protection of endothelium during insertion.
  - Use small amount of viscoelastic when tissue is folded (or over the Sheet's glide) to minimize endothelium to endothelium touch.
  - Various instruments used for insertion:
    - Forceps: Kelman, Utrata, Goosey
    - Multi-sided spatula (Rosenwasser)
    - IOL cassette
    - Sheets Glide (AC glide)
    - Suture pull
  - Donor size of 8.25 mm inserted with forceps or over a Sheets glide, Macaluso or Busin glide and unfolded slowly with air and BSS.
  - Scleral tunnel and side port sutured with 10-0 Nylon.
  - Interface fluid removed.
  - 75% air bubble left at end of surgery.
- Postoperative care:
  - Admitted for 24 hours.
  - Strict supine position for 2 hours.
  - Semi-supine position for next 24 hours.
  - Sustained release acetazolamide orally.

What are the complications related to DSEK surgery?

- Donor-related:
  - Thick donor
  - Thin donor
  - Incomplete dissection, irregular donor thickness
  - Anterior/posterior perforation
- Recipient-related:
  - Difficulty in Descemet's stripping
  - Hypotony (in vitrectomized eye)
- Postoperative:
  - Dislocation of graft (1%)
  - Primary graft failure (5–10%)
  - Pupillary Block (15%)
  - Interface haze

What are the causes of donor dislocation?

- Recipient posterior surface irregularity
- Viscoelastic material in the interface
- Geometric mismatch of the donor and the recipient
- Strands of stripped Descemet's membrane prevent apposition
- Fluid trapped in interface
- Eye rubbing
- Wound leak
- Soft eye
- Iatrogenic
- Non-viable donor

What is DMEK surgery? What are its advantages over DSEK?

- Descemet membrane endothelial kerato-plasty (DMEK): Partial-thickness cornea transplant procedure with selective removal of the patient's Descemet's membrane and endothelium followed by only donor DM and endothelium being transplanted, in contrast to posterior stroma, DM, and endothelium used in DSEK.
- The graft tissue is merely 10–15 μm thick.
- Modifications:
  - Descemet's membrane automated endo-thelial keratoplasty (DMAEK): The rim of stroma was left at the periphery of the donor tissue. It utilizes a microkeratome or

femtosecond laser for the initial posterior lamellar dissection.

- Descemet's membrane endothelial keratoplasty with a stromal rim (DMEK-S): The rim of stroma is left at the periphery of the donor tissue, but the donor tissue is prepared manually.
- Indications for DMEK are like those for DSEK.
- Advantages:
  - Faster visual rehabilitation
  - Better final visual acuity due to minimal optical interface effects
  - Lower risk of allograft rejection due to less transplanted tissue
  - Less long-term reliance on topical steroids and their inherent side effects
- Disadvantages:
  - Scrolling properties of the graft make the graft tissue difficult to handle (tends to scroll with the endothelium inward)
  - Technically more challenging
  - Greater chances of re-bubble procedure due to higher number of graft edge lift compared to DSEK

4.6 KERATOPROSTHESIS

Identify keratoprosthesis (K-Pro).

4.7 FAQs ON KERATOPROSTHESIS

What is a keratoprosthesis (K-Pro) and what are its components?

- Keratoprosthesis, or prosthokeratoplasty, is the replacement of an opaque cornea with an artificial cornea.

- Optic: Forms the central part for viewing, it is a cylinder made of polymethyl methacrylate (PMMA).
- Haptic: Determines the type of the prosthesis and is of the following types:
  - Biocompatible, which is usually a PMMA skirt with the corneal graft as in the Boston type 1 and 2 K-Pro.
  - Bio-integrated, in the Dacron mesh that forms the skirt around the PMMA optic in the Pintucci K-Pro.
  - Biological, in the form of tooth or the bone that forms an autologous biological tissue that supports the optical cylinder in the osteo-odonto- and the osteo-K-Pro, respectively.
- Supporting cover tissue:
  - Type 1 K-Pro: Bandage contact lens (BCL) prevents the carrier graft desiccation.
  - Type 2 K-Pro: Skin in the Boston type 2 and the buccal mucosa for the osteo-odonto-keratoprosthesis.

What are the types of temporary keratoprosthesis (TKP)?

- Eckardt's TKP
- Landers–Foulks TKP
- Features of temporary keratoprosthesis:
  - Used for intraoperative replacement of a diseased cornea when insufficient view through injured cornea precludes retinal surgery
  - Made of PMMA
  - Provides outstanding optics for intra operative visualization of posterior segment

What are the types of permanent keratoprosthesis?

- Currently there are three types of keratoprosthesis in use in India

A)   B)

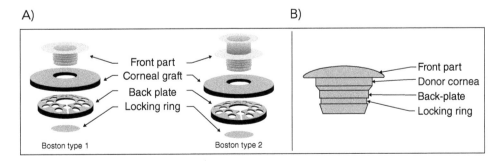

Figure 4.24 A) Boston keratoprosthesis; B) Aurokeratoprosthesis

- Boston type 1 keratoprosthesis/Auro keratoprosthesis
- Boston type 2 keratoprosthesis
- MOOKP: Modified osteo-odonto-keratoprosthesis/tibial keratoprosthesis

What are the indications of this procedure?

- Type 1 Boston keratoprosthesis
  - Good prognosis:
    - Multiple failed grafts
    - Aniridia
    - Herpetic keratitis
    - Silicone-oil-filled eyes
    Wet surface
  - Guarded prognosis:
    - Pediatric corneal conditions
    - Chemical injuries
  - Very guarded prognosis:
    - Stevens–Johnson syndrome (SJS)/ocular cicatricial pemphigoid (OCP)
    - Severe chemical injuries
- Type 2 Boston keratoprosthesis
  - SJS/OCP/mucous membrane pemphigoid
  - Severe chemical injuries
  - Severely keratinized surface
    - Bone dry ocular surface

What are the contraindications of this procedure?

- Functional vision in the other eye
- Successful keratoprosthesis in the other eye
- No light perception
- Posterior segment pathology that limits visual potential
- Uncontrolled secondary glaucoma
- Specific to MOOKP
  - Edentulous
  - Poor dental hygiene
  - Unfit for GA
- Specific for Boston type 2: Absent eyelids

What are the indications and prerequisites for each type of keratoprosthesis?

- Boston keratoprosthesis type 1/Auro keratoprosthesis
  - Eyes with adequate tears, good blink, no exposure
  - Preferably without an underlying systemic immune condition like Stevens–Johnson

syndrome or ocular cicatricial pemphigoid (OCP)
  - Preferred indications are failed grafts or chemical injuries with limbal stem cell deficiency but well-formed fornices in an adequately wet eye
- Modified osteo-odonto-Kkratoprosthesis (MOOKP)
  - Eyes with severe ocular surface damage associated with dryness and/or keratinization usually noted in patients with an underlying systemic immune condition like SJS or OCP.
  - Main prerequisites for a successful outcome of the MOOKP procedure is good dental hygiene that must be ascertained in consultation with the maxillofacial surgeon.
  - MOOKP can also be performed in eyes where a Boston type 1 K-Pro is primarily indicated; however, considering the challenging nature of the MOOKP surgery and the need for a multidisciplinary approach, the Boston type 1 K-Pro can be preferred in these eyes if the patient is willing for the postoperative care and regular follow-ups.
  - In patients with poor dental hygiene that precludes performing the MOOKP surgery, other options, such as the tibial bone or Pintucci K-Pro, might be required for visual rehabilitation.

What are the prerequisites prior to doing a keratoprosthesis?

- Presence of PL and accurate PR in the eye to be operated.
- USG shows normal posterior segment.
- IOP under control (since it is impossible to measure later.) If high, oral anti-glaucoma medication or cyclocryotherapy is considered before K-Pro.

What are the complications of this procedure?

- Boston keratoprosthesis
  - Intraoperative:
    - Blood trickling into the vitreous cavity
    - Decentered central opening in the carrier graft
  - Postoperative:
    - Retro prosthetic membrane
    - Glaucoma

- Infection
- Rim leaks and sterile melts
- Low grade anterior segment inflammation
- MOOKP
  - Intraoperative:
    - Blood loss during harvesting the tooth
    - Inadvertent entry into the maxillary sinus
    - Decentered corneal opening during stage 2 of the procedure
    - Risk of suprachoroidal hemorrhage exists during the preparatory stage as well the second stage
  - Postoperative:
    - Glaucoma
    - Lamina resorption
    - Endophthalmitis

4.8 LASIK INSTRUMENTS

Identify the speculum.

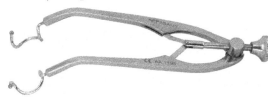

- This is the Castroviejo LASIK speculum.

Identify the instrument.

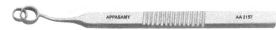

- This is a LASIK marker.
- Use: To mark the cornea prior to making flap so that repositioning the flap at the end is accurate (especially if in cases of a free cap).

Identify the instrument.

- Fukasaku LASIK spatula
- Has a rounded anterior surface and flat posterior surface that is slightly convex to conform to the curvature of the cornea
- A semi-sharp tip locates and lifts the flap edge, as well as dissects under the flap with minimal vector forces

- Uses:
  - Used to manipulate and lift LASIK flap
  - Broad end protects hinge
  - Ideal for enhancements/retreatments

Identify the instrument.

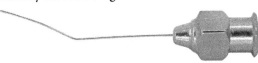

- LASIK Flap Lifter
- Combines a 45° angled Sinskey hook with a thin hook with a conical edge

Identify the following:

- LASIK irrigating cannula (3 port and 6 port)
- 45° angled
- Can be 23G or 25G
- With a cannula with 3 or 6 ports
- Uses
  - To wash particles and remove debris from the corneal flap surfaces.
  - 25G permits easy entry under the flap.
  - Cross-section permits sideways entry into the flap without dragging the epithelium into the interface.

Identify and describe the instrument.

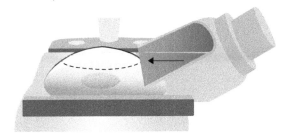

- Microkeratome
- Instrument to perform lamellar corneal dissection of known corneal diameter and depth

What are the parts?

- Suction ring
- Microkeratome head

- Handle
- Footplate
- Console
- Suction ring
  - Holds the eye
  - Inner diameter determines the flap diameter (higher the vacuum, thicker the flap)

What are the types of microkeratomes?

- Depending on cutting mechanism:
  - Linear cutting had 0° plane and fixed thickness
  - Pivotal rotation cutting
  - Pendulum-like cutting by:
    - Epikeratomes
    - Hydrokeratome
- Depending on basis of blade angulation:
  - Originally was 0°, now 25° to 30°, which allows positive lenticule
  - Advance rate: Rate at which the flap is created determines the quality of flap
  - Oscillatory rate of blade: The higher the oscillation rate, the smoother is the flap
- Depending on market availability **(Table 4.2)**

4.9 FAQs ON LASIK

What is the preoperative evaluation for refractive surgery?

- Refraction
- Slit-lamp examination rules out dry eye, glaucoma, blepharitis, meibomitis, active keratitis, keratoconus, corneal vascularization (>1 mm requires smaller suction ring)
- Pupil: Diameter measurement especially mesopic and scotopic (by a ruler, pupillometer, topography). This is important because functional optical zone should be more than mesopic area to avoid glare (functional optical zone is 25% less than the total ablation zone)
- Fundus evaluation (Prophylactic cryo/laser for lattice or HST)
- Keratometry
- Pachymetry
- Corneal topography

What are the general prerequisites for LASIK?

- Age >18 years
- Stable refraction (at least 2 stable readings over a period of 1 year)
- Myopia: −1 D to −8D
- Hyperopia: <6 D

Table 4.2 Market Availability of Microkeratomes

Name	Flap (mm)	Depth (mm)	Blade Angle (°)	Oscillation (RPM)	Hinge	Miscellaneous
(1) Hansatome	8.5, 9.5	160, 180, 200	25°	4000 to 20,000 rpm	Both	Commonly used
						In deep-set eyes and narrow palpebral aperture
						May cut skin or lashes
(2) Amadeus II	8.5, 9.0, 9.5, 10.0	140, 160	25°	4000 to 20,000 rpm	Nasal	Epi-LASEK capability and pre-assembled
(3) BD K-4000		130, 160, 180	26°	12,000 rpm		Creates thicker flap, risky in thin corneas
(4) Moria	Up to 10.5	140, 160, 180	30°			
(5) Nidek MK-2000	8.5, 9.0, 9.5		25°	9000 rpm	Nasal	
(6) Carriazo	9.0, 10.0	110, 130, 150, 170			360° free choice	Small suction ring allows use in all types of eyes

- Astigmatism: <6 D
- Central Corneal Thickness: >500 μm
- Corneas with K values between 40 D and 46 D
- Clear crystalline lens

What are the contraindications for LASIK?

- Absolute
- Age <18 years
- Unstable refraction
- Corneal pathology
  - Keratoconus
  - Pachymetry <500 μm
  - Residual stromal bed >300 μm
  - HSV keratitis
- Glaucoma
- Systemic conditions:
  - Chronic immunosuppression
  - Steroid use
  - Connective tissue disorder
  Pregnancy
- Relative:
  - Dry eye
  - Blepharitis
  - Chronic eye rubbing
  - Ocular surface diseases
  - Corneal pathology:
    - Deep-set eyes
    - Flat cornea <40 D
    - Steep cornea >46 D
  - Systemic
  - Diabetes mellitus

What are the types of flaps? (Table 4.3)

What are the complications of LASIK? (Table 4.4 and Table 4.5)

What is femtosecond LASIK?

- Intrastromal laser ablation device (alternative to microkeratome)

What is the principle?

- Photo disruption
- They operate at near-infrared wavelengths similar to Nd:YAG lasers but at pulse durations of less than 1 picosecond (ps).
- High pulse repetition rates from 10 s of kHz to even MHz are used to create continuous cut planes inside the tissue by placing pulses close to each other.
- The lower pulse energy leads to a reduction of the mechanical side effects of optical breakdown.
- The energy of femtosecond lasers with wavelengths in the 1030–1060 nm range is transmitted through all transparent structures of the eye, but opaque material scatters the laser radiation and thus reduces the amount of energy.

What is the mechanism of action?

- Photo disruption
- Computer-controlled optical delivery
- Multiple pulses at precise intrastromal locations
- Focal plasma formation breaks bonds with vaporization and disruption of tissue
- 2 μm cavitation bubble
- Uses:
  - Creation of corneal flaps
  - Lamellar resection
  - Incisions

What are the advantages of femtosecond LASIK?

- Precision of cuts
- No suction ring or automated microkeratomes related complications (epithelial ingrowth, folds, buttonholes)

Table 4.3 Types of LASIK Flaps

Nasal	Superior
Physiologically better as corneal nerves preserved better	Corneal nerves resected
No such advantages	Better position due to gravitational effect and upper lid position and blinking
Increased risk of displacement due to upper lid movement	

Table 4.4 Intraoperative Complications of LASIK Surgery

Complication	Cause	Management
Thin flap and buttonhole	Suction inadequate Steep cornea Poor microkeratome blade quality	Reposition flap Recut after 3 months
Free corneal cap	Flat cornea (<41 D) Failure of microkeratome	Keep flap moist Increase the drying time Place BCL over the eye
Incomplete flap	Failure of microkeratome Loss of suction	If hinge in periphery: ablate with reduced optic zone If central: Recut after 3 months/surface ablation
Flap subluxation or dislocation	Eye squeezing, rubbing or trauma	Relift the flap Wash the under surface Reposition the flap Prolong the drying time
Flap striae	Flap desiccation Flap misalignment	Relift and reposition Stretch and smooth tear Prolonged drying time No treatment if peripheral or visually not significant
Corneal epithelial defect	Excess topical anesthesia Trauma Drying of flap	Lubricants Antibiotics

Table 4.5 Postoperative Complications of LASIK Surgery

Complication	Cause	Prevention	Management
1. Interface			
(a) Debris	Debris from air, instruments, tear film	Particulate-free environment	Close follow-up
	Blood from limbus or vascularization	Clean instruments	Prophylactic topical steroids In recalcitrant cases, remove debris, refloat, wash, remove debris, reposition
(b) Interface keratitis	Betadine	Particle-free environment	Treat epithelial defect

Table 4.5 *(Continued)* Postoperative Complications of LASIK Surgery

Complication	Cause	Prevention	Management
(Sands of Sahara)	BSS	Clean Instruments	Topical steroids for 4–8 weeks
Diagnosis: Dust-like material at interface	Lid contamination		If excessive debris, refloat and reposition
	Instrument contamination		
	Topical medication		
	Toxins (endo, exo from bacteria)		
	Metallic debris		
(c) Interface haze	More with large ablation		Topical steroids
(Rare with LASIK)	Excessive intrastromal edema		
2. Epithelial complications			
(a) Epithelial defect	Topical anesthesia		Lubricants
	Markers		Antibiotics
	Suction ring		NSAIDS
	Microkeratome		Small defect: Medical management with lubricants and antibiotics
	Dehydration		Large defect: BCL, careful follow-up for epithelial ingrowth
	Micro trauma due to instruments		
	Predisposing factors:		
	Anterior basement membrane dystrophy		
	Recurrent corneal erosions		
	Dry eye		
(b) Epithelial ingrowth—1%	Growth of epithelium underneath the flap (most common)	Treatment of epithelial defect	Indications of treatment:
			Grade 3 ingrowth
Diagnosis:	Isolated nests (less common)		Elevate the flap
Clinically: Whitish gray material	Through the epithelial defect (least common)		Mechanically remove the epithelial sheet on the bed and undersurface of the flap

(Continued)

Table 4.5 *(Continued)* Postoperative Complications of LASIK Surgery

Complication	Cause	Prevention	Management
Under retro illumination: Margins of ingrown flap	Identify the tract		
Identify the tract			Laser removal Nd:YAG
Fluorescein: Pooling			
Topography: Surface irregularity			
Effect: Irregular astigmatism, Corneal melt			
3. FLAP complications			
(a) Folds	Large ablation depth	Proper repositioning of flap	Indicated if fold crosses visual axis or astigmatism
	Poor repositioning of the flap:	Avoid rubbing	Pre-op dilate to diagnose on retro illumination
	Horizontal folds in nasal hinge	Protective shield during sleep	Elevate flap and wash with BSS then reposition properly
	Vertical folds in superior hinge		
4. Stromal complications:			
(a) Stromal melt	Lack of O_2 to subepithelial layer		Elevate flap and remove epithelial ingrowth
Diagnosis:	Dry eyes		Bandage CL
Loss of transparency			Antibiotics
Loss of tissue			Tear substitutes
Ulceration			Rarely lamellar PKP
Infection			
(b) Infection (rare)	Untreated epithelial defect	Strict asepsis	Antibiotic
Organism: Staph		Treat epithelial defect	Lift flap and wash
		Prophylactic antibiotics	Rarely remove flap and PKP

- Flaps as thin as 100 mm can be made; therefore, LASIK possible in thinner, flatter corneas with higher degree of myopia
- Decreased epithelial ingrowth
- High-power treatment (myopia and hypermetropia)
- Customized parameters possible
- Prominent orbit rim/small eyes

What are the disadvantages?

- Costly
- Additional laser to be maintained

What are the laser delivery systems for refractive surgery?

Laser Delivery Systems (**Table 4.6**)

Table: 4.6 Laser Delivery Systems

Factors	Broad Beam	Scanning Slit	Flying Spot
1. Energy output required	More	Intermediate	Small
2. Beam uniformity	Highly required	Improved	Complex ablation pattern possible
3. Central islands	More	Less	Least
4. Maintenance	More	Less	Least
5. Acoustic shock wave	More	Less	Less
Eye tracking	Not required	Required	Required
Time	Shorter	Longer	Longest
Optic Zone limitation for PRK/PTK		No	No

What is the difference between lifting an old flap and recutting a new flap?

- Lifting the original flap
  - Advantages: No microkeratome required
  - Disadvantages:
    - Epithelial ingrowth: Increased chances
    - Epithelial defect: Increased chances
    - Rehabilitation: Longer
- Recutting a new flap
  - Advantages:
    - Decreased incidences of epithelial defect, epithelial ingrowth
    - Less pain
    - Early rehabilitation
  - Disadvantages:
    - Increased chance of thin flap, free flap, or perforated flap

What is radial keratotomy (RK)?

- Principle: Radial incisions in the paracentral cornea up to 90% depth leading to flattening of the central cornea

What are the complications of RK?

- Low BCVA
- Bacterial keratitis
- Corneal scarring
- Irregular astigmatism
- Epithelial erosions
- Long term instability
- Hyperopic shift of >1 D
- Diurnal fluctuation

- Undercorrection
- Overcorrection
- Star burst
- Corneal perforation

What is the PERK study?

- Prospective Evaluation of RK study
  - An eight-incision RK was done.
  - In repeat surgery, 8 more incisions were added.
  - Ten years later showed that:
    - Patients with 20/20—53%
    - Patients with 20/40—85%
    - 30% reported use of spectacles or contact lens for distant correction

What were the surgical techniques?

- Russian: Centripetal
- American: Centrifugal (safer, avoids inadvertent cut in central)
- Combination (Bidirectional)

4.10 LASEK/PRK INSTRUMENTS

Identify the following instrument.

- This is a LASEK trephine
- 270° semi-sharp edge with 90° cut out for flap hinge

- Alcohol retaining well
- Uses:
  - To cut through the epithelium during LASEK surgery.
  - The edge has a 90° hinge to create the epithelial flap.
  - Alcohol well is used to assist with loosening the epithelium.

Identify the following instrument.

- This is a LASEK Epithelial Micro Hoe.
- It features a delicate, 2 mm wide semicircular tip with a beveled edge to assist in finding and lifting the perimeter of the epithelial flap.
- Use: For lifting the precut margin of the epithelial flap.

Identify the following instrument.

- This is a LASEK epithelial detaching spatula.
- Use: Hockey-knife-shaped spatula with sharp anterior part to detach epithelium at the incision of the trephine.

Identify the following instrument.

- This is a LASEK epithelial flap spatula
- Use: Epithelial flap repositioning spatula

Identify the following instrument.

- Hockey knife
- Use: Can be used to remove epithelium prior to PRK surgery

Identify the instrument.

- Pettigrove PRK scraper and marker
- 6.5 mm marker and spatula at the other end
- Use: For marking and removing the epithelium prior to PRK surgery

4.11 FAQs ON PRK/LASEK

What are the indications of photorefractive keratectomy (PRK)?

- Correction of myopia: −1 to −6 D
  - Hyperopia: −4 D
  - Astigmatism: 3 D
- Treatment of epithelial dystrophy
- Treatment of recurrent epithelial erosions
- Treatment of superficial corneal opacity

What is the mechanism of action?

- Photoablation of the cornea to produce corneal flattening. The excimer laser alters the refractive state of the eye by removing tissue from the anterior cornea through a process known as photoablative decomposition. This process uses ultraviolet energy from the excimer laser to disrupt chemical bonds in the cornea without causing any thermal damage to surrounding tissue. The modified anterior corneal surface enables light to be focused on the retina, thereby reducing or eliminating the dependence on glasses and contact lenses.
- Diameter and depth of ablation determines depth of correction.

What is the technique of PRK?

- Preoperative
  - Accurate refraction
  - Planning and programming
- Technique
  - Topical anesthesia
  - Speculum
  - Corneal marking
  - Epithelial debridement:
    - From periphery to center
    - Area of debridement should be greater than the area of laser

- Methods:
  - Mechanical: Blade, spatula, brush
  - Chemical: 20% alcohol
- Excess stromal dehydration will cause overcorrection.
- Laser ablation zone should be free of epithelial debris and fluid.
- Post-op topical steroids for 1–3 months to prevent excessive haze.
- Anti-fibrotic agents maybe used after the procedure.

What are the complications of PRK?

- Corneal haze especially in deeper ablation (because local fibroblastic keratocytes cause collagen synthesis)
- Infection

What are the contraindications of PRK?

- Collagen vascular disorders
- Tendency to keloid
- Previous herpetic eye disease
- Diabetes mellitus

What are the reasons for selection of PRK over LASIK?

- Deep-set eyes
- Narrow palpebral fissure
- Epithelial basement dystrophy
- Suspicious corneal topography not suitable for LASIK
- As an additional procedure in surgeries such as: Topography guided PRK and cross-linking in keratoconus patients

What are the advantages of PRK?

- Therapeutic value in epithelial basement membrane dystrophy
- LASIK flap complication avoided
- With wavefront guided technique, LASIK flap related abrasions avoided.
- Thinner corneas
- Higher refractive errors

What is LASEK?

- Goal: Preserve the epithelium instead of debriding as in PRK

What are the advantages and disadvantages of LASEK over PRK and LASIK?

- Advantages over PRK:
  - Less pain
  - Less chances of post-operative haze
  - To increase speed of recovery of BCVA
- Advantages over LASIK
  - Flap-related complications avoided
  - Microkeratome related complications avoided
  - Safer
  - Less dry eye
  - Much thicker post-stromal bed with better biomechanical stability
- Disadvantages over LASIK:
  - Longer visual recovery time
  - More pain and discomfort
  - Needs BCL for 3–4 days
  - Use of topical steroids for 3–4 weeks

What are the indications and contraindications of LASEK?

- Indications:
  - Thin corneal pachymetry
  - Epithelial irregularities
  - LASIK complication in the other eye
  - Steep corneas
- Contraindications
  - Keratoconus
  - Glaucoma
  - Hyperopia and hyperopic astigmatism

What are the techniques of LASEK?

- Anesthetize the cornea.
- Cornea is marked with a 3 mm circle in the periphery.
- Alcohol reservoir with 20% alcohol placed.
- Epithelial margin is delineated.
- Epithelial flap is removed.
- Laser beam centration by aiming beam centered on pupil or by tracking mechanism.
- Laser applied with excimer laser.
- To decrease haze: Mitomycin 0.02% or 0.2 mg/ml can be placed on ablated zone for 30 seconds to up to 2 minutes.
- Refloat epithelial flap with chilled BSS.
- Replace epithelial flap and realign it with the margins.

Differentiate PRK, LASIK, and LASEK (Table 4.7).

Table 4.7 Differences between PRK, LASIK, and LASEK

Factor	PRK	LASEK	LASIK
Refractive correction	Low to moderately high	Same	Same
Thin cornea	Usually done	Usually done	Not done
Wide pupil	Usually done	Usually done	Not done
Post-op pain	++	++	+
Post-op steroids	3 weeks to several months	Same	1–2 weeks
Post-op dry eye	1–4 weeks	1–4 weeks	>12 months
Post-op vision recovery	3–7 days	Same	1 day
Post-op refractive stability	3 weeks to several months	Same	1–6 weeks
Complications	Haze/scarring	Same	<1%
Risk of scarring	1–2%	Less than PRK	<1%

4.12 ABERRATIONS

What is an optical aberration?

- Aberrations are deviations from an ideal optical system of the human eye.

How are they classified? (Table 4.8)

Table 4.8 Classification of Aberrations

Lower-Order Aberrations	Higher-Order Aberrations
Myopia	Spherical aberration
Hypermetropia	Chromatic aberration
Astigmatism	Coma

What is wavefront technology and its principle?

- Wavefront technology: It is used to diagnose and measure aberrations.
- Principle:
  - Narrow laser beam is focused on retina to make a point source of light.
  - The exited light from eye undergoing aberration is detected by a series of lenses.
  - Analyzing direction of this light beam gives wavefront deformation.
  - Shape of the wavefront is presented as Zernike polynomial.

What are the various aberrometers used?

- Shack–Hartmann
- Tscherning aberroscope with Dresden
- Ray tracing

What are the advantages of using wavefront technology?

- Customized LASIK per patient's aberrations possible
- Better contrast
- Less glare and halos

What are the limitations and difficulties in wavefront-guided LASIK?

- Factors affecting wavefront-guided LASIK:
  - Exact centration during aberrometry and LASIK required
  - Age: Aberration changes with age (and with increasing age advantage decreases)
  - Entire eye aberrations change with accommodation.

4.13 PHAKIC IOLs AND INSTRUMENTS

Identify and describe the instrument.

- ICL lens cartridge loading forceps
- 20 G
- Jaws feature a series of concave and convex surfaces.

Identify and describe the instrument.

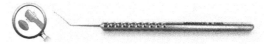

- This is the Pallikaris ICL manipulator.

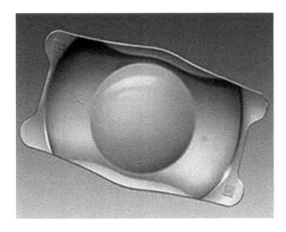

Figure 4.39 Phakic IOL

- Oval-shaped tip
- Use: Manipulates inferior and superior haptic of lens to place under the iris

Name a commonly used phakic IOL

- Visian ICL (STAAR Surgical, USA)

4.14 FAQs ON PHAKIC IOLs

What are the indications?

- Myopia: >12 D
- Hypermetropia: >4 D
- Corneal thickness: <480 μm
- Post-LASIK corneal thickness: Likely to be <280 μm

What are the contraindications?

- Narrow-angle glaucoma
- Corneal endothelial count: <2000 mm²
- Patient: <18 years
- AC depth: < 3.2 mm from epithelium, <2.8 mm from endothelium

What are the limitations of LASIK in high refractive error?

- Significant residual error
- Iatrogenic keratectasia

- Loss of BCVA
- Introduction of higher-order aberration and decrease in mesopic vision and contrast

What does the preoperative assessment include?

- Anterior chamber depth (ACD)
  - Measurement is important since it must be verified that there is sufficient space for implanting a phakic IOL (PIOL).
  - Used in the formula to calculate lens power
  - Determined by biometry (Optical)
- White-to-white diameter (WTW)
  - Calculation of lens length for angle fixated and posterior chamber PIOL's depend on the horizontal white to white corneal diameter.
  - White-to-white limbal measurement is not accurate enough because of the amount of scleral tissue overriding on the cornea is quite variable.

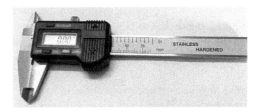

Figure 4.40 Digital Caliper

  - Measured using a digital caliper or optical biometer.
  - In iris fixated lenses, one size fits all eyes.
- Keratometric measurements
- Ultrasound Biomicroscopy (UBM)

What are the prerequisites?

- Stable manifest refraction
- Ametropia not correctable with excimer laser
- ACD ≥2.8 mm/≥3.2 mm
- Irido-corneal angle aperture: ≥ 30° (Shaffer grade 3 and 4)
- Endothelial cell count: ≥2500 cells/mm² at 20 years
- No ocular pathology

What are the advantages of phakic IOLs in high refractive errors?

- Non-optical
  - Excellent accuracy in refractive correction
  - Accommodation preserved (vs. refractive lens exchange)
  - Cornea preserved (vs. LASIK/PRK)
  - Reversible
  - Predictable
  - Rapid vision recovery
  - Cost of equipment saved
  - Technique is familiar to most cataract surgeons
- Optical: Clear vision

What are the disadvantages of phakic IOLs?

- Potential risks of an intraocular procedure (endophthalmitis)
- Non foldable models require large incision
- Low vault may damage the lens leading to iatrogenic anterior subcapsular cataract formation
- High vault can result in an increase in intra-ocular pressure, pigment dispersion, pupillary block, endothelial cell loss, pupil distortion
- Implantation in hyperopic patients can be followed by loss of BCVA due to loss of magnification effect of glasses
- May also cause pupil ovalization, induced astigmatism, chronic uveitis, pupillary block, pigment dispersion

What are the types of Phakic IOLs?

- Angle-supported anterior chamber PIOLs includes phakic IOLs with 3-point or 4-point fixation in the AC angle.
- Iris-fixated PIOLs have 2 diametrically opposed claw haptics that fixate the lens on the iris by enclavation of mid-peripheral iris stroma.
- Posterior chamber PIOLs are implanted posterior to the iris and in front of the crystalline lens in the sulcus.

4.15 CORNEAL COLLAGEN CROSS-LINKING WITH RIBOFLAVIN (C3R)

What is this solution?

- Riboflavin solution
- Vitamin B2
- Molecular weight of 376.37 g/mol
- It has three light absorption peaks: 270 nm, 366 nm, and 445 nm.
- 366 nm provides the greatest margin of safety for the ocular structures.
- Actions:
  - Used in collagen cross-linking of the cornea
  - Photosensitizer with UV rays
  - Limits the penetration of UV radiation.

What is this device used for?

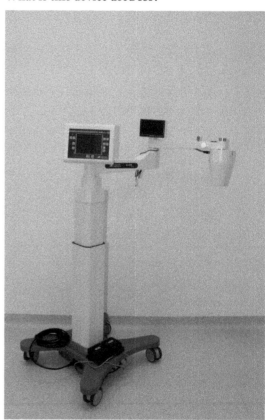

- This is a cross-linking device used for collagen cross-linking.

What are the indications?

- Corneal ectasias
  - Progressive keratoconus
  - Pellucid marginal corneal degeneration
- Post-LASIK ectasia
- Infectious keratitis
- Bullous keratopathy

What are the contraindications?

- Corneas thinner than 400 μm due to possible endothelial cell damage.
- Incisional refractive surgery (radial keratotomy or astigmatic keratotomy) as the stromal alteration can cause incisions to rupture.
- Central corneal scarring.
- Pregnant or nursing patients as these populations have not been sufficiently investigated.
- Relative contra indications are risk factors that might lead to delayed healing responses and complications after treatment.
  - Rheumatism
  - Keloid formation
  - Dry eyes

What is the mechanism of action?

- Riboflavin acts as photosensitizer.
- It is applied to cornea and activated by UVA (370 nm).
- UVA excitation of riboflavin in triplet state leads to formation of reactive oxygen species, which interact with collagen fibrils to form covalent bonds which bridge amino groups and increase the biomechanical stability.
- It induces keratocyte apoptosis.
- Anterior stroma has more effect than posterior stroma.

What are the preoperative investigations?

- Refraction
- Slit-lamp examination
- Keratometry
- Corneal topography
- Specular microscopy

What is the procedure?

- Topical anesthesia is applied.
- Utmost sterile precautions are followed.
- Painting and draping commence.
- Instrument is calibrated.
- Original Seiler cross-linking (Dresden protocol):
  - Complete epithelium scraping manually by blunt spatula (7 mm).
  - Riboflavin 0.1% in 20% Dextran T500 in NS (pH = 7, hyperosmolar), 1 drop every 3 minutes for 30 minutes.

- Check saturation of cornea with riboflavin, i.e., slit-lamp examination with blue light—look for green fluorescence in AC.
- Check calibration irradiance.
- Intraoperative pachymetry is performed should be >400 mm.
- Patient is instructed to look at the center of the light.
- UV-A irradiation at the rate of 3 mW/cm^2 or 5.4 J/cm^2 for 30 minutes.
- Riboflavin drops every 5 minutes.
- BSS to prevent desiccation during procedure.
- BCL applied at the end of the case

What are the modifications in surgical technique?

- Epithelium removal:
  - Removal of epithelium by excimer laser PTK
  - Partial removal of epithelium
  - Transepithelial or Epi-On technique
  - Advantages:
    - Significantly less postoperative discomfort
    - Less risk of serious infections
    - Much faster healing
  - Disadvantages:
    - Penetration of riboflavin still questionable
    - UV damage to the endothelium
- Factors used to increase riboflavin penetration:
  - Benzalkonium chloride (BAK)
  - Tetracaine
  - Ethylenediaminetetraacetic acid (EDTA)

What are the modifications in riboflavin application?

- Can use a well for constant exposure to riboflavin
- Hypotonic riboflavin
  - Used to swell thin corneas
  - 0.1% riboflavin in 0.9% saline instead of dextran

What are the modifications in irradiation?

- Accelerated C3R
  - Total energy should be 5.4 J/sec

- Ranges from 3 mW for 30 minutes to 30 mW for 3 minutes

What can cross-linking be combined with?

- With PRK as a procedure for refractive correction and cross-linking called topo-guided PRK (T-PRK)
- With INTACS
  - Additive effect
  - Hence greater refractive correction
- With MMC 0.02%

What are the side effects?

- With epithelium off technique:
  - Pain
  - Delayed epithelium healing
- Corneal haze
- Endothelial damage (if thickness <400 mm)
- Corneal scarring
- Infective keratitis
- Persistent corneal edema
- Corneal melt
- Bilateral ring-shaped corneal opacities
- Reactivation of viral keratitis
- Discomfort, glare, colored halos, diplopia, accelerated cataract formation, IOP overestimation

Define and describe keratoconus?

- It is defined as a non-inflammatory paracentral/central corneal stromal thinning leading to apical protrusion of cornea and irregular astigmatism.
- It has a bimodal curve of penetration:
  - First peak—late teens, early twenties
  - Second peak—late thirties and early forties

What are the signs of keratoconus?

- Frequent change of glasses
- Myopic astigmatism which increases progressively to irregular astigmatism
- Retinoscopy: Scissor reflex
- Fundoscopy: Oil droplet
- Keratometry: Irregular mires
- Slit lamp: Vogt's striae (disappear on pressure over eyes)

- Fleisher's ring: Epithelial iron deposits at the base of cone seen on blue filter
- Rizzuti's sign: Conical reflection of nasal cornea with slit lamp light from the temporal side
- Descemet's rupture due to hydrops
- Corneal scarring

What is the Rabinowitz–McDonnel criteria for diagnosis of keratoconus?

- Central K-value: >47.20 D
- Inferior-superior asymmetry (I-S value): >1.2
- Modified:
  - Skewed radial axis: >21°
  - Difference in central power: >1 D between two eyes

What are the causes and associations of keratoconus?

- Cause:
  - Idiopathic (4:1000)
  - Autosomal dominant (10%)
- Associations:
  - Systemic
  - Chromosomal abnormalities like Down's or Turner's syndrome
  - Connective tissue disorders (Marfan's syndrome or Paget's disease)
  - Cutaneous—atopy
  - Ocular
  - Conjunctiva ocular abnormalities—Leber's congenital amaurosis, aniridia, retinitis pigmentosa
  - Vernal keratoconjunctivitis (VKC)

What are the other causes of prominent corneal nerves? (Table 4.9)

Table 4.9 Prominent Corneal Nerves

Ocular	Systemic
Keratoconus	Leprosy
Fuchs endothelial dystrophy	Neurofibromatosis
Congenital glaucoma	MEN type II B
	Refsum disease
	Icthyosis
	Idiopathic

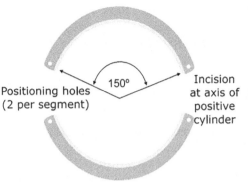 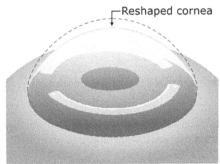

Figure 4.43 Intracorneal ring segments (ICRS)

What are the treatment options for keratoconus?

- Spectacles
- Contact lenses (rigid, piggyback, Rose K)
- Corneal collagen cross-linking
- Intracorneal ring segments (ICRs)
- Lamellar keratoplasty/DALK/penetrating keratoplasty
- Phakic IOLs (Toric PIOLs can correct the cylinder as well)
- Treatment of associations and complications, e.g., VKC, hydrops

4.16 INTRACORNEAL RING SEGMENTS (ICRS)

Identify the device.

- These are intracorneal ring segments (ICRS).
- INTACS is a type of ring segment manufactured by Addition Technology, Inc., Fremont, California, USA.
  - PMMA ring segments used intrastromally for keratoconus and keratectasia
  - Arc length: 150°
  - Hexagonal cross-section
  - Outer diameter: 8.1 mm
  - Inner diameter: 6.8 mm
  - Small hole at each end for ease of insertion and removal
  - The refractive effect is modulated by the INTACS thickness (0.25–0.45 mm, with 0.05 mm increments); current designs have

a predicted myopic range of correction from −1.00 to −4.10 D

Identify the ring.

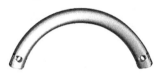

Figure 4.44 Ferrara intrastromal corneal ring

- Ferrara intrastromal corneal ring (Ferrara Ophthalmics, Belo Horizonte, Brazil)
- Computer-lathed PMMA and camphorquinone (CQ) acrylic segments
- Available in two diameters (6.0 mm for myopia up to 7.00 D, 5.0 mm for higher degrees of myopia)
- Thickness: 150–350 µm
- Internal and external diameters are 4.4 mm and 5.4 mm for the 5.0-mm optical zone and 5.4 mm and 6.4 mm for the 6.0 mm optical zone, respectively.
- Triangular cross-section
- Arc = 160°

Identify the instrument.

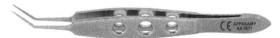

Figure 4.45 ICRS forceps

- Designed with a notched tip
- Conforms to the contour of the ring segment

- Uses:
  - Easy removal of the ring from carrier
  - Secure grip on segment
  - Ambidextrous

What are the other various rings commonly used?

- INTACS (Addition Technologies)
- Ferrara Rings (AJL Ophthalmic)
- KeraRing (Mediphacos)
- Myoring (Dioptex)

What is the difference between INTACS and Ferrara rings? (Table 4.10)

Table 4.10 Differences between INTACS and Ferrara Rings

	INTACS Rings	Ferrara Rings
Arc	150°	160°
OZ	5.0 mm	6.8 mm
Cross-section	Hexagonal	Triangular

What is the mechanism of action of ICRS?

- The cornea is imagined as a compressed arc of fibers.
- A spacer element inserted between them pushes them apart.
- The arc flattens to accommodate the element while maintaining positive asphericity of the cornea.
- The degree of corneal flattening observed after ICRS implantation is determined by two factors: the thickness of the implanted segment and the diameter of the cornea at the implantation site. Specifically, the flattening effect is directly proportional to the thickness of the ICRS segment and inversely proportional to the diameter of the cornea. In other words, if the implanted segment is thicker and the corneal diameter is smaller, the corneal flattening effect will be greater.

Who is a good candidate for ICRS implantation?

- 18 years and above
- Contact lens intolerance

- Corneal pachymetry >400 mm in the site of the corneal tunnel (depending on the thickness of ICRS to be implanted)
- Absence of central corneal scarring
- No pregnancy

What are the indications?

- Keratoconus and other keratectatic disorders
- Post-LASIK ectasia
- Refractive corrections

What are the contraindications?

- Absolute:
  - Uncontrolled immune deficiency
  - Pregnant/nursing (due to unstable refraction)
  - Post-RK (due to fear of intrusion/extrusion)
- Relative:
  - Pachymetry at incision site <400 μm
  - Progressive keratoconus
  - Pupil diameter >7.0 mm in dim light (due to increased glare)
  - Central/paracentral opacity/hydrops
  - History of HSV/HZO

What are the advantages and disadvantages?

- Advantages:
  - Safe and effective
  - Can be removed or exchanged, therefore reversible
  - Central clear zone not directly treated
- Disadvantages:
  - Specialized equipment required to create lamellar channels
  - Mechanically alters corneal curvature, not a solution to prevent progression of ectasia

Describe the procedure.

- Mechanical technique
- Femtosecond-laser-assisted method:
  - Infrared laser beam creates intrastromal cavitations.
  - Eventually a dissection plane at the desired depth is created.
  - A tunnel is created at about 80% of the corneal pachymetry in that area.

- Using special forceps, the segments are inserted into each channel.
- Advantages:
  - High level of precision
  - Minimal direct manipulation when creating the tunnels

What are the complications of ICRS?

- Keratitis
  - Infectious: Pain, borders fuzzy, treatment with antibiotics, explantation
  - Sterile: No pain, self-limiting, onset 1–2 weeks later, epithelium in the channel, treatment with NSAIDs, borders distinct
- ICRS placement: Shallow, deep, perforation, migration, extrusion, wrong placement, increase in corneal flatness in opposite quadrant
- Neovascularization at incision site
- Photophobia due to sterile keratitis
- Glare and halos: If pupil is >7 mm
- Rare: Channel deposits, channel haze, epithelial plugs in incision site

Glaucoma

5.1 TOPICS

- Instruments in trabeculectomy
- FAQs on trabeculectomy
- Instruments used in iridectomy
- FAQs on iridectomy
- Instruments used in congenital glaucoma surgeries
- Glaucoma drainage devices (GDDs)
- Other glaucoma surgeries and microinvasive glaucoma surgery (MIGS) devices

5.2 TRABECULECTOMY INSTRUMENTS

Note: The instruments which have been described in chapter 2 shall not be repeated in the current chapter. Only instruments pertaining to the surgery at hand shall be described.

What are the instruments used in trabeculectomy?

- Speculum
- Superior Rectus holding forceps
- Castroviejo calipers
- Forceps
  - Toothed
  - Non-toothed
  - Tying
- Tenotomy scissors
- No. 11 Blade
- Crescent blade
- Kelly's Descemet's punch
- Iridectomy scissors
- Vannas scissors
- Weck-cel sponges

- Cautery: Wet-field cautery
- Suture: 8-0 Vicryl, 10-0 Nylon, 4-0 Silk

Identify and describe the uses of the Khaw speculum in glaucoma surgery.

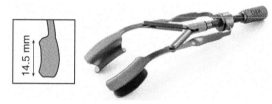

14.5 mm

- This is a Khaw speculum.
- Uses:
  - To lift the lids away
  - To avoid pressure on the globe
  - Central indent and side notch for maximum exposure and minimum pressure
  - For good exposure
  - Use a good speculum that produces minimal pressure and maximum exposure.
  - Corneal traction suture is better than a superior rectus suture as it avoids complications, such as superior rectus haematoma, conjunctival buttonhole, and postoperative ptosis.

Identify and mention the uses of the Khaw T-clamp conjunctival holding forceps.

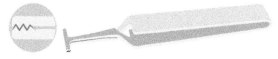

- Single-handed action
- Tip width is 4.0 mm
- Overall length is 7.45 cm

DOI: 10.1201/9781003455646-5

- Uses:
  - Holds conjunctiva securely and atraumatically.
  - Holds and protects the conjunctival edge during anti-metabolite application.
  - Useful particularly in fornix based conjunctival incisions.

Identify the Lims forceps and state its uses in glaucoma surgeries.

- Uses:
  - To hold tenons in limbus-based flap
  - Can be used as a fixing and tying forceps

Describe the Westcott tenotomy scissors and state its uses in glaucoma surgeries.

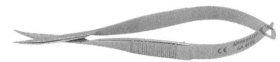

- 21 mm blade, gently curved
- Sharp-pointed tips
- Uses:
  - In trabeculectomy: To open the conjunctiva and tenons prior to making scleral flap.
  - Other uses:
    - SICS (small-incision cataract surgery)
    - Squint surgery
    - Scleral buckle surgery
    - Vitrectomy

Identify and state the uses of the side port blade in glaucoma surgery.

- Angle: 15°
- Thickness: 0.1 mm
- Uses:
  - Demarcation of the scleral flap margins before raising flap
  - The side port entry made in glaucoma surgeries is oblique to avoid inadvertent lens injury during hydrating. Sometimes the fluid used to titrate can cause cataract if it hits the anterior lens surface.

- Make the AC entry before using trabeculectomy punch
- For removal of the deep scleral block

What are the indications of performing a paracentesis?

- Diagnostic:
  - For aqueous tap for microbiological workup
  - To rule out malignancy
- Therapeutic:
  - CRAO
  - Hyphema drainage
  - Post anti-VEGF in NVG
- Intraoperative:
  - Cataract surgery
  - Scleral buckling surgery
  - Trabeculectomy surgery
  - Penetrating keratoplasty/DALK/DSEK surgery
  - Iridectomy

How important is it to perform a paracentesis in trabeculectomy?

- Controlled paracentesis prevents sudden hypotony and prevents rapid IOP fluctuation which can lead to complications such as choroidal detachment, suprachoroidal hemorrhage
- Helps avoid sudden iris prolapse while removing deep scleral flap/sclerostomy
- Forming the bleb at the end of surgery
- Easily allows anterior chamber reformation at the end of surgery
- Useful for checking the aqueous flow from the scleral flap and titrating the releasable scleral flap sutures
- Washes away a mild hyphema at the end of surgery

What are the ways to make the sclerostomy during trabeculectomy?

- Kelly's Descemet membrane punch
- Side port knife with Vannas scissors
- It should be 1–1.5 mm × 0.5 mm in size and the edges should be non-shelving.

Identify and state the uses of the Kelly's Descemet membrane punch.

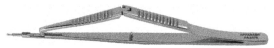

- Squeeze-action serrated handle
- Cuts clean 0.5 mm/0.75 mm/1 mm round hole
- 1 mm diameter tip
- Uses:
  - To punch out the deep scleral flap and trabecular meshwork, just anterior to the blue zone
  - Makes non-shelved, regular, clean margins of the deep flap with no tissue tags
  - Can also be used in combined phaco-trabeculectomy procedures

Identify and state the uses of the Vannas scissors in glaucoma surgeries.

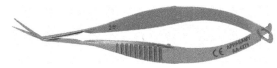

- This is a pair of Vannas scissors.
- Uses:
  - To make the sclerostomy in trabeculectomy, alternative to Kelly's punch
  - Can be used instead of iridectomy scissors
  - To cut fine sutures
  - Can be used to finely separate conjunctiva from tenons capsule

5.3 FAQs ON TRABECULECTOMY

What are the various glaucoma surgeries you know of?

- Glaucoma surgeries based on the penetration of sclera.
- Full thickness: Anterior sclerectomy
- Partial thickness
  - Penetrating surgery: Trabeculectomy
  - Non-penetrating surgery: Deep sclerectomy

What are advantages and disadvantages of full-thickness filtration surgery vs. trabeculectomy?

- Full-thickness procedures: Entire thickness of the wall from the corneoscleral surface to anterior chamber is removed.

- Scheie syndrome
- Anterior sclerectomy
- Posterior sclerectomy
- Iridencleisis
- Trephining
- Advantages: Provides lower pressure for longer times
- Disadvantages (This surgery is historical and no longer performed)
  - Thin-walled bleb: There is an increased incidence of endophthalmitis.
  - Excess hypotony can result in choroidal effusion, maculopathy, optic nerve edema, rapid progressive of cataract, refractive instability.
- Partial-thickness procedure: Partial thickness of the sclera, overlying the opening between the anterior chamber and subconjunctival space is removed, such as in trabeculectomy.
  - Advantages:
    - Decreased incidence of endophthalmitis
    - Decreased incidence of postoperative flat anterior chamber
    - With the advent of releasable sutures and anti-metabolites, the pressure lowering effects of trabeculectomy has results comparable to the full-thickness trabeculectomy procedure.
  - Disadvantage: Technically more challenging to perform

What are the pros and cons of partial-thickness penetrating surgeries and non-penetrating surgeries?

- Partial-thickness penetrating surgery: Trabeculectomy
  - Advantages:
    - Time tested procedure
    - Good lowering of intraocular pressure especially with use of anti-fibrotic agents
    - Versatile and therefore useful in all types of glaucoma
  - Disadvantage: Intraocular surgery, hence risk of endophthalmitis is present
- Partial-thickness non-penetrating surgeries
  - Deep sclerectomy
  - Viscocanalostomy
  - Advantages:

- Avoids sudden decompression of the globe.
- Decreases chances of suprachoroidal bleed and choroidal detachment.
- Decreased chances of sudden or prolonged hypotony (hypotony maculopathy, leaky blebs, blebitis, bleb dysthesia).
- Lower risk of endophthalmitis.
- Flat-AC-related complications are absent
- Iridectomy is avoidable and therefore avoids iris handling.
- Intraocular handling is negligible.
- Decreased inflammation/hyphema/malignant glaucoma.
- No need for atropine (good post-op vision).
- Can be combined with cataract surgery.
- Contact lens wear is possible.
- Can be done with local infiltration.
- Disadvantages:
  - More difficult and longer surgical time is required.
  - Pressure lowering effect is less.
  - Effect is not long-lasting.
  - May become penetrating during surgery if AC is entered accidentally.

What are the indications of trabeculectomy?

- Open-angle glaucoma
  - Progressive optic disc damage and visual field changes despite maximal medical management. Uncontrolled IOP with maximal medical therapy is an indication.
  - Cost, compliance, and complications of medical treatment.
  - An advanced glaucoma intervention study (AGIS) found that fluctuations in IOP are minimized due to surgery, which is a risk factor in progression of glaucoma.
  - Young patients with advanced glaucoma, where medical management alone is unlikely to be effective in achieving a low target IOP.
  - Lack of compliance/intolerance to AGMs (anti-glaucoma medications) or side effects
- Angle-closure glaucoma: Angle-closure glaucoma with uncontrolled IOP on maximal medical therapy

- Others
  - Developmental glaucoma
  - Traumatic glaucoma
  - Post-inflammatory glaucoma

What are the relative contraindications of trabeculectomy?

- Excessive conjunctival scarring in chemical burns, SJS, and repeated retinal surgeries
- In split fixation on HVF 10–2, trabeculectomy is performed after explaining to the patient the possibility of the wipe-off phenomenon.

What are the preferred sites for trabeculectomy?

- Superior, superonasal, and superotemporal quadrants for trabeculectomy are preferred
- They are also preferred as the upper lid provides better coverage of the bleb.
- Inferior blebs have higher rates of endophthalmitis.
- Nasal blebs are uncomfortable and have higher rates of dellen and endophthalmitis.

What are the pros and cons of limbus-based vs. fornix-based conjunctival flaps?

- Fornix-based conjunctival flaps
  - Advantages:
    - Good exposure of the surgical site.
    - Less chance of an overhanging bleb.
    - Posterior flow of aqueous is not circumscribed.
    - Can be combined with cataract, as tenon is not damaged.
    - Less chances of a conjunctival buttonhole.
    - Bleb is more diffuse, low lying, posterior as the conjunctiva is adherent at limbus.
    - Releasable suture techniques can be used with fornix-based incisions.
    - Easier to identify surgical landmarks (like scleral spur).
    - Closure by:
- Wise method: Continuous suture taken
- Khaw's method: Multiple 10-0 Vicryl mattress sutures from conjunctiva to the peripheral area
  - Disadvantages:
    - Technically difficult
    - More chance of leak compared to limbal-based procedure

- – Caution must be excised when doing argon laser suture lysis or subconjunctival injection of 5-FU in the early postoperative period.
- Limbal-based approach
  - Advantages:
    - – Tight closure possible.
    - – Technically easy, easier to excise tenons capsule.
    - – Early postoperative digital massage and injections of 5-FU are safer.
    - – Preferred in children and mentally challenged patients as they tend to rub the eye (fornix-based flaps may lead to bleb leak).
  - Disadvantages:
    - – Exposure of surgical site difficult resulting in more conjunctival manipulation.
    - – Overhanging bleb on limbus.
    - – Re-operations are difficult.
    - – Posterior flow of aqueous can get circumscribed due to scarring of the conjunctiva.
    - – Closure of limbus based must be in two layers.
    - – Tenons and conjunctiva.
    - – Small needles with small needle track to be used to prevent buttonholes.
  - Precautions: Use serrated non-toothed forceps for handling the conjunctiva and fine-tooth forceps for the tenons capsule.

Describe the scleral flap in trabeculectomy?

- Size and shape of the scleral flap can be variable.
- Thickness of the scleral flap is usually 1/2 to 2/3rd of the thickness of the sclera.
- Usual size of the scleral flaps is 3 × 3 mm.
- Bleeding from the perforating branch of the anterior ciliary vessel that perforates the sclera, to enter the ciliary body, 2–4 mm from the limbus at 12 o'clock, may result in bleeding.

What are the key points for scleral flap suturing?

- Scleral flap closure is usually done using interrupted, non-absorbable 10-0 nylon sutures.
- Long pass of the suture allows easy laser suture lysis later.

- Modifications include releasable sutures and suture lysis.

What are the key points for conjunctival suturing?

- Conjunctival closure is a very important step in trabeculectomy. Ensure watertight closure.
- Depending on whether it is limbal-based or fornix-based, closure should be water-tight.
  - Limbus-based: Continuous sutures.
  - Fornix-based: Khaw's sutures or Weiss sutures are taken.

When do we do tenonectomy in trabeculectomy?

- Tenon removal is optional, and some may remove it as it is a source of fibroblasts that can cause bleb scarring.
- May be removed only when tenons is exuberant and suture lysis is contemplated.
- Not done if anti-metabolites are used.

What are the complications of trabeculectomy?

- Intraoperative:
  - Conjunctival buttonholes
  - Scleral flap buttonhole
  - Vitreous loss
  - Damage to lens in phakic eyes
  - Intraoperative bleeding (hyphema) to rule out sickle cell trait/disease
- Early postoperative
  - Shallow AC with low IOP
    - – Choroidal hemorrhage or detachment
    - – Wound leak
    - – Over filtration
  - Shallow AC with high IOP
    - – Suprachoroidal hemorrhage
    - – Malignant glaucoma
    - – Pupillary bock
  - Visual loss due to wipe off phenomenon
- Delayed (months to years later)
  - Hypotony with maculopathy
  - Hypotony because of cyclodialysis
  - Late bleb leak
  - Bleb-related ocular infections/ endophthalmitis
  - Cataract
  - Cyst of tenons capsule
  - Malignant glaucoma
  - Sympathetic ophthalmia

How do you classify shallow AC post trabeculectomy?

- Spaeth et al. classified shallow AC post trabeculectomy as follows:
  - Grade 1: AC is peripherally flat with peripheral iris and cornea touching but with preservation of AC in front of pupillary space.
  - Grade 2: Shallow AC, but there is greater apposition between the mid-iris and cornea, but some space is retained between the lens and cornea in pupillary plane.
  - Grade 3: Complete contact of the iris and posterior surface of the cornea in the pupillary space

How do you manage shallow AC post trabeculectomy?

Shallow AC with low IOP

1. Wound leak
2. Excessive filtration
3. Cyclodialysis cleft

1. Wound leak
   a. Low IOP
   b. Shallow/absent bleb
   c. Seidel's test positive
   d. Management
   e. Medical:
      i. Conservative management
      ii. Often reforms spontaneously, needs AC reformation if centrally flat with iridocorneal touch
      iii. Topical steroids by suppression of cyclitis
      iv. Cycloplegics (atropine) relax the ciliary muscles cause posterior movement of lens and deepen the AC
      v. Pressure patch
      vi. Therapeutic bandage contact lens
      vii. Simmons scleral shell tamponade
   f. Surgical:
      i. Tissue adhesive cyanoacrylate glue with bandage contact lens or fibrin glue
      ii. Suturing the bleb or bleb revision, including conjunctival advancement or conjunctival or scleral patch grafts

2. Excessive filtration
   a. Low IOP
   b. High well-formed bleb
   c. Seidel's test negative in scleral flap leak and positive in bleb leak
   d. Management
   e. Compression sutures
   f. Atropine
   g. Steroids
   h. Firm patching
      i. Pressure patch
      ii. Large diameter bandage contact lens (BCL)
      iii. Simmons scleral shell tamponade
   i. Reform the AC with air or SF_6 and drain and choroidal detachment that may be present. Scleral and conjunctival flap is re-sutured.

3. Cyclodialysis cleft
   a. Separation of longitudinal ciliary muscle fibers from scleral spur
   b. Shallow AC
   c Definite diagnosis on gonioscopy
   d Management:
      i. Topical atropine 1% up to 6 weeks
      ii. Most resolve spontaneously
      iii. Repair of cyclodialysis cleft
      iv. Laser procedures: Argon laser photocoagulation, modified endophotocoagulation probe, transcleral YAG laser
      v. Surgical: Cyclopexy, ciliochoroidal diathermy, anterior scleral buckling with cryotherapy or diathermy

Shallow AC with normal or raised IOP

1. Pupillary block
2. Suprachoroidal hemorrhage
3. Malignant glaucoma

1. Pupillary block
   a. Non patent PI
   b. High IOP
   c. Flat bleb
   d. Seidel's test negative
   e. Management:
      i. YAG laser at iridectomy site
      ii. Can perform a new laser iridotomy
2. Suprachoroidal hemorrhage
   a. Diagnosis: Shallow AC intraoperatively
   b. Sudden shallowing of AC
   c. Eye becomes hard

    d. Loss of red reflex
    e. Prolapse of the intraocular contents out of the wound
- Management:
    a. Close the wound as quickly as possible.
    b. Sedate the patient.
    c. Posterior sclerotomy and vitreous aspiration.
    d. Defer the surgery for a later date.
- Prevention:
    a. Preoperative mannitol.
    b. Avoid peribulbar/retro-bulbar block; prefer general anesthesia.
    c. Avoid sudden shallowing of the AC; may use an AC maintainer.
    d. Preoperative sclerectomy and sclerotomy to drain any intraoperative effusion, especially in the eyes of nanophthalmos, Sturge–Weber, and choroidal hemangioma.

3. Malignant glaucoma (Aqueous misdirection)
    a. High IOP
    b. Absent bleb
    c. Seidel's test negative
    d. Management:
      i. Atropine: 50% of patients with malignant glaucoma respond to medical treatment alone. Dose of atropine 1% is three times daily, used to relax the ciliary muscles.
      ii. Topical phenylephrine 10% 4 times a day and topical α1 adrenergic agonist stimulate the iris dilator muscles.
      iii. Hyperosmotics, either glycerol 50% orally or mannitol (2 g/kg body weight), decrease the vitreous volume.
      iv. Topical or systemic aqueous suppressants decrease aqueous pooling posteriorly.
      v. Peripheral iridotomy should be performed to exclude pupillary block or to ensure the patency of an existing iridotomy.
      vi. Nd:YAG laser hyaloidotomy may be used to rupture the posterior capsule and anterior hyaloid membrane.
      vii. Pars plana vitrectomy.
      viii. Anterior segment approach: Irido-zonular-hyaloido-vitrectomy, or IZH, has the lowest relapse rate.

Which patients are at the highest risk of developing an expulsive hemorrhage?

- Nanophthalmos
- Sturge–Weber syndrome
- Uncontrolled glaucoma
- Buphthalmos
- Previously vitrectomized eye
- Hypertensives; patients with arteriosclerosis and bleeding disorders

What are the signs of a failing bleb?

- Elevated IOP
- Reduced height of the bleb
- Encapsulated bleb
- Vascularized bleb
- Lack of microcysts

What are the causes of failure of trabeculectomy?

- Preoperative:
    - Medication induced inflammation: Pilocarpine, topical medications (BAK preservative)
    - Increased fibrosis in uveitic glaucomas
    - Re-surgeries
    - ICE syndrome as the membrane can block the ostium
    - Neovascular glaucoma (NVG)
    - Angle recession/traumatic glaucoma
    - High-risk patients
    - Pediatric glaucoma as the thick tenons capsule in children
- Intraoperative:
    - Conjunctival buttonhole
    - Scleral flap buttonhole
    - Excessive bleeding in subconjunctival space
    - Hyphema
    - Vitreous loss
    - Lens subluxation
    - Over tight suturing
    - Use of MMC causing cystic blebs
- Postoperative:
    - Conjunctival closure is inadequate.
    - Shallow AC.
    - Plugging of sclerostomy by vitreous/iris/inflammatory products/blood clots.

- Management:
  - Compression:
    - Digital compression or with a sterile cotton bud at the edge of the scleral flap.
    - This is done to force aqueous fluid to flow through the surgical fistula.
  - Suture lysis:
    - 2 weeks post-surgery
    - Releasable sutures can be removed
    - Argon laser suture lysis using Hoskins suture lysis lens
  - Needling:
    - For encapsulated blebs on slit lamp
    - Can be done using a bent needle
  - Subconjunctival 5-FU injections:
    - Done in first 3 weeks
    - Dose: 5 mg (0.1 ml of 50 mg/ml solution) injected 10 mm away from the bleb; can be done twice a day for a week and then once a day for a week

How do you improve bleb formation?

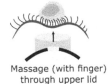 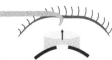

| Massage (with finger) through upper lid | Direct massage with blunt instrument (e.g., squint hook) through anesthetized conjunctive |

- Atraumatic conjunctival and tenons dissection
- Use of anti-metabolites intraoperatively and postoperatively
- Flap suture management: Either use releasable sutures or suturelysis. This can be done postoperatively. Suturelysis maybe considered depending on the bleb in the first postoperative week. However, if mitomycin C (MMC) is used, it must be considered after 1 month of surgery
- Massage:
  - Digital
  - Carlo–Traverso maneuver: After anesthetizing the cornea with a topical anesthetic, the center of the cornea is indented with a sterile swab stick for a few seconds. This pushes aqueous fluid in the subscleral space.
- Needling

- Adjustable suture forceps: Special fine smooth tips for trans-conjunctival suture adjustment without tearing conjunctiva.

How do you diagnose and manage bleb infection and bleb-related endophthalmitis?

- Risk factors: Long-term antibiotic use, thin blebs due to the use of 5FU and MMC, bleb leak, chronic anterior or posterior blepharitis
- Organisms: *H. influenza*, *Streptococcus*, and *Staphylococcus* are the more common organisms.
- Blebitis
  - Infection of the bleb without vitreous involvement
  - White bleb
  - Absent uveitis
  - Management
    - Conjunctival swab must be taken for culture and sensitivity
  - Topical and oral antibiotics
- Endophthalmitis
  - White milky bleb with severe anterior uveitis and vitritis
  - Management: Like that of post cataract endophthalmitis management.

How do you increase success rates in trabeculectomy?

- Intraoperative:
  - Good hemostasis, as hematogenous products stimulate fibroblasts.
  - Site selection should be correct.
  - Paracentesis to check intraoperative flow from scleral flap.
  - Fornix-based flaps.
  - Scleral flap with wide rectangular made 1 mm from limbus to ensure posterior flow.
  - Wide area of MMC application.
  - Intraoperative titration of fluid flow.
  - Placement of releasable or adjustable sutures to prevent postoperative hypotony.
  - Conjunctival closure should be watertight (vascular better than spatulated needle) to prevent wound leak.
- Postoperative:
  - Decrease inflammation (steroids, cycloplegics).
  - Avoid excess hypotony or rise in IOP.
  - Use antimetabolites.

What is the role of cycloplegics after trabeculectomy?

- They paralyze the ciliary muscle and therefore tighten the zonules, which cause deepening of the anterior chamber.
- Causes relief of ciliary spasm and dilated the pupil.
- Helps maintain blood aqueous barrier.
- Prevents the formation of posterior synechiae.

What are signs of a good filtering bleb?

- Diffuse posterior low-lying bleb with micro-cysts, vascularity should be similar to adjacent conjunctiva.
- Numerous microcysts in the epithelium.

How do you grade bleb morphology?

- Indiana classification: Scales for four parameters
  - Height (H0-H3)
  - Extent (E0-E3)
  - Vascularity (V0-V4)
  - Bleb leakage/Seidel's test (S0-S2)
- Moorfield's classification
  - Diffusion area
    - Central (1–5)
    - Maximal (1–5)
  - Bleb height (1–4)
  - Subconjunctival blood (0–1)

What are the indications for use of anti-metabolites in glaucoma surgeries?

Indications of MMC use in trabeculectomy are also the causes of increased risk of failure of trabeculectomy, and the answers are the same for both:
- Young patient
- Black race
- Chronic medications
- Previously failed trabeculectomy
- Pseudophakic patient
- Aphakic patient
- Inflammatory glaucoma
- Neovascular glaucoma
- ICE syndrome

How to use anti-metabolites?

- Dose of MMC: 0.2–0.5 mg/ml for 1–5 minutes
- Dose of 5-FU

- Subconjunctival: 0.1 ml of 50 mg/ml injected 1800 away from filtration site
- Intraoperative: 50 mg/ml placed for 5 minutes under the dissected flap of tenons capsule make sure edges of conjunctiva are not exposed to 5-FU

What are the precautions for use of anti-metabolites?

- Dissect conjunctiva and tenons well.
- Can be used subconjunctivally and subsclerally.
- Use Khaw's forceps to protect the conjunctiva as MMC should not encounter conjunctival edge and cornea.
- Thoroughly wash subconjunctival or subscleral space after the use of MMC.
- Keep instruments used to handle the anti-metabolites separately and pass them off to nurse without putting them back on surgical trolley to not contaminate the other instruments.
- Avoid massage especially in fornix-based flap in the postoperative period.

What are the complications of anti-metabolites in glaucoma surgery?

- Hypotony
- Choroidal detachment
- Hypotonic maculopathy
- Bleb leak
- Bleb infection
- Punctal occlusion with 5-FU
- Conjunctival wound leaks
- Sterile corneal ulcers

Who discovered Trabeculectomy?

- Sugar, in 1961, discovered this surgery

5.4 IRIDECTOMY INSTRUMENTS

Identify the curved iridectomy forceps (toothed) and state its alternatives?

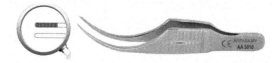

- Alternative instruments for iridectomy:
  - Plain iridectomy forceps (atraumatic)
  - Kelman–McPherson forceps

Identify and describe the uses of DeWecker iris scissors.

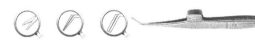

- 12 mm blades
- Uses:
  - Used to make the iridectomy
  - Manual anterior vitrectomy in absence of vitrectomy cutter

5.5 FAQs ON IRIDECTOMY

What are the indications of iridectomy?

- As an adjunct in other eye surgeries
  - Standard trabeculectomy
  - Complicated cataract
  - Penetrating keratoplasty
  - Silicone oil: Ando's iridectomy (inferior)
  - ACIOLs
- Where laser iridotomy is not possible
  - In very shallow AC
  - Hazy corneas
  - Children though some children may cooperate for a laser iridotomy.
  - Hyphema
- Excision of iris tissue:
  - For biopsy in iris cysts/tumors
  - Traumatic iris prolapse
  - Foreign body on iris
- Optical iridectomy

What are the types of iridectomy?

- Peripheral buttonhole iridectomy (PBHI)
- Keyhole iridectomy (KHI)
- Broad iridectomy (BI)

What are the contraindications of iridectomy?

- Rubeosis of iris

Why doesn't normal iris tissue bleed after iridectomy?

- Double-walled iris vasculature, which retracts after being cut

- Iris musculature compresses the vessels
- Axonal reflex causes constriction of vessels

How does iridectomy help in trabeculectomy?

- Keeps iris tissue from prolapsing in the sclerostomy site
- Prevents pupillary block in postoperative period

What are the indications for laser peripheral iridotomy (LPI)?

- Angle-closure glaucoma
- Acute primary angle-closure glaucoma
- Fellow eye of primary angle-closure glaucoma
- Primary angle closure (PAC)
- Primary angle-closure suspect (PACS)
  - One-eyed patients
  - Patients with a family history of angle-closure glaucoma
  - Those who require frequent dilation: Diabetic retinopathy (DR), age-related macular degeneration (ARMD)
  - Patients who cannot come for follow-up/ who do not understand the nature of their disease

5.6 INSTRUMENTS USED IN CONGENITAL GLAUCOMA SURGERIES

Identify and describe the Harms trabeculotomy probe.

- 9 mm long pointed tips
- Curved shaft with 3 mm spread

Identify and describe the McPherson trabeculotomy probe.

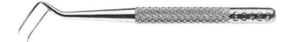

- 8 mm long pointed tips, curved shaft with 3 mm spread
- Angulated

What are their uses?

- To perform trabeculotomy in primary congenital glaucoma.
- One arm enters the Schlemm's canal, and the other arm works as a guide.

How can one identify the Schlemm's canal during trabeculotomy?

- Under 15× magnification of the microscope and under the superficial scleral flap, a radial scratch incision is made across the blue zone just in front of external scleral spur.
  - One can directly visualize the Schlemm's canal in wall of scratch incision just in front of the scleral spur (scleral spur identification—where the crisscross scleral fibers become circumferential)
  - *Or* an aqueous rivulet will be seen oozing through the Schlemm's canal.
  - *Or* there will be presence of blood in the Schlemm's canal.
  - One can also thread the Schlemm's canal with 5-0 prolene suture to confirm its presence.

What are the advantages of trabeculotomy (over goniotomy)?

- Most surgeons are familiar with approach and surgical landmarks.
- Can be converted into trabeculectomy.
- Can be added to trabeculectomy.
- No multiple lens system (as used in goniotomy)
- No dependence on special knives and lenses (as required in goniotomy).

Describe Barkan's knife

- Triangular blade tip with cutting edges on both sides (so no need to turn knife inside AC) .
- Simultaneous AC maintenance must be done with AC maintainer to prevent collapse of the anterior chamber.

Figure 5.13 Barkan's goniotomy knife

- Used for goniotomy in primary congenital glaucoma.
- Requires:
  - Clear cornea
  - Good operating microscope
  - Good goniotomy lenses like Barkan, Swan–Jacob, or Worst

What are the disadvantages of goniotomy?

- Multiple lens system is required to view the angle.
- Tilting of microscope is required to view the angle.
- Requires an experienced surgeon.

5.7 GLAUCOMA DRAINAGE DEVICES (GDDs)

Identify and describe the glaucoma drainage devices (GDDs)?

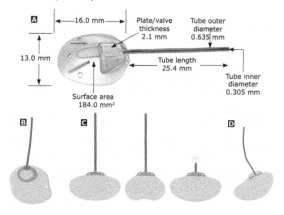

- Helps in filtration from anterior chamber to equatorial subconjunctival space
- Consists of tube and plate and a valve
- Made either of silicon or polypropylene
- Size varies from 135 mm^2 to 500 mm^2

What are the GDDs you know of?

- No resistance (non-valved)
  - Molteno
  - Baerveldt
  - Schocket
  - Indian made non-valved device or AADI (Aurolab Aqueous Drainage Device)
- Flow restricted (valved)
  - Ahmed glaucoma valve
  - Krupin slit valve
- Variable resistance

- Molteno dual ridge
- Baerveldt bio seal

Where can the tube be placed?

- Anterior chamber (bevel is up)
- Sulcus
- Pars plana (bevel is down)

What are the indications of GDDs?

- Failed trabeculectomy with anti-fibrotics
- Neovascular glaucoma
- Conjunctiva inadequate
- Excess scarring in
  - Trauma
  - Post-RD surgery
- Glaucoma in which trabeculectomy has a high failure rate such as
  - Uveitic glaucoma
  - Aphakic glaucoma
  - Post-PK glaucoma
  - ICE syndrome
  - Sturge–Weber syndrome

What are the contraindications of GDDs?

- Excessive scleral thinning
- Malignant glaucoma
- Poor patient compliance for self-care

What are the complications of GDDs?

- Early postoperative complications:
  - Wound leak
  - Suprachoroidal hemorrhage
  - Tube corneal touch
  - Tube block with fibrin, blood clot, vitreous, iris
  - Valve dysfunction
  - Iritis
  - Hypertensive phase
- Late postoperative complications:
  - Failure
  - Tube erosion
  - Tube migration
  - Endophthalmitis
  - Corneal decompensation
  - Dellen formation
  - Motility disturbances and diplopia
  - Bleb encapsulation is the most significant late complication resulting in failure.

5.8 OTHER GLAUCOMA SURGERIES AND MICROINVASIVE GLAUCOMA SURGERY (MIGS) DEVICES

What are the indications and contraindications of non-penetrating glaucoma surgeries (NPGS)?

- Indications:
  - POAG
  - Pigmentary glaucoma
  - High myopia
  - Pseudoexfoliation
  - Sturge–Weber syndrome
  - Aniridia
  - Uveitic glaucoma
- Contraindications:
  - Neovascular glaucoma (NVG)
  - Narrow angle
  - Congenital glaucoma

What are the types of NPGS?

- Deep sclerectomy: After peritomy, superficial scleral flap of 5 × 5, 1/3rd scleral thickness is made, and a deep scleral flap of 4 × 4 of 95% thickness is made and excised. The inner wall of Schlemm's canal is then removed, and a collagen implant is placed, and then the superficial flap is sutured, and the conjunctiva is closed. This creates a Descemet window, which allows seepage of aqueous fluid from the anterior chamber into the subconjunctival space. The long-term success may be enhanced by using a collagen implant.
- Viscocanalostomy: High-molecular-weight viscoelastic is injected into Schlemm's canal. A trabeculo-descemet's window is created.
- Ab-externo trabeculectomy: Deep sclerectomy removes the inner wall or roof of Schlemm's canal and juxtacanalicular trabecular mesh-work. Thin superficial scleral flap is then sutured to cover it.
- Sinusotomy: Lamellar band of sclera and outer wall of Schlemm's canal removed from 10–2 o'clock keeping inner wall intact with overlying conjunctiva closed.

What is the Ologen implant?

- Ologen collagen matrix is a Type I atelocollagen with porous structure and pore diameter between 10–300 µm comprising > 90% atelocollagen and <10% glycosaminoglycans.
- It is designed to promote and modulate the postoperative tissue regeneration.
- Its porous structure allows fibroblasts to grow within the matrix to avoid scarring.
- Ologen implant only functions as a wound modulator in trabeculectomy surgery but does not have any antifibrotic properties to counter the scarring response.
- Indication: Used as an adjunct in trabeculectomy, when MMC cannot be used in view of scleral thinning or in high myopes.

What is Healaflow?

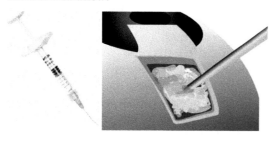

Figure 5.16 Healaflow

- Consists of 22.5 mg/ml of cross-linked sodium hyaluronate viscoelastic gel
- Injected under the scleral flap and conjunctiva
- Acts as drainage implant
- Limits postoperative fibrosis and improves rates of surgical success
- Precautions while using Healaflow: Must not be injected intracamerally as it can lead to an intraocular pressure spike
- Uses:
  - Can be used in all types of glaucoma surgeries
  - Trabeculectomy
  - Deep sclerectomy
  - Viscocanalostomy
  - Shunts/stents/tubes
  - Unlike EX-PRESS device, it can also be used in angle-closure glaucoma

EX-PRESS device?

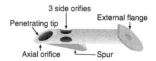

Figure 5.17 EX-Press glaucoma filtration device

- It is a small stainless-steel device that diverts aqueous humor through the implant from the anterior chamber to intrascleral space.
- Parts:
  - A cannula for draining aqueous humor from anterior chamber to intrascleral space
  - Plate to prevent excessive penetration
  - Spur to prevent extrusion from eye
  - Reserve orifices near distal end as alternative conduit in case of occlusion of primary opening
- The surgical procedure is the same as trabeculectomy except that this device is placed instead of the ostium created.
- Procedure: Scleral flap is made of 5 × 5 mm and the device is injected just anterior to the scleral spur.
- MRI of head is permitted in patients with the EX-PRESS device.
- Advantages:
  - It enables controlled flow through the ostium, hence preventing hypotony.
  - Multiple shunts can be implanted in one eye if greater pressure-lowering effect is needed.

What are the complications of EX-PRESS shunts?

- Iris touch
- Exposure
- Malfunction
- Malposition
- Cornea touch
- Obstruction

What is Trabectome?

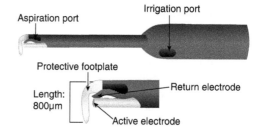

Figure 5.18 Trabectome

- Trabectome, manufactured by NeoMedix Corp., USA, is FDA approved.
- Consists of a handpiece with a 19G infusion sleeve, an aspiration port, and an ablation tip, which is triangular and facilitates penetration of the Schlemm's canal.
- Works by ablating and removing a 600–1200 strip of trabecular mesh work and inner wall of Schlemm's canal (ab interno trabeculectomy).
- Uses focused electro-surgical impulses delivered through a microcautery.
- Continuous irrigation and aspiration during the procedure removes debris and regulates temperature.

What are the various suprachoroidal devices used in glaucoma surgeries?

- Ab externo devices:
  - Gold Micro-Shunt (GMS, SOLX Corp, Waltham, MA)
  - STARflo (iStar Medical, Isnes, Belgium)
  - Aquashunt (OPKO Health, Miami, FL)
  - Advantage: Allows for more extensive tissue dissection and greater IOP lowering compared to an ab interno approach.
  - Disadvantage: Requires both conjunctival and scleral manipulation, making additional glaucoma filtering surgeries difficult in the future due to scarring.
- Ab interno devices:
  - Cypass Micro-Stent (Transcend Medical Inc, Menlo Park, CA)
  - iStent Suprachoroidal Bypass System (iStent Supra, Glaukos Corporation, Laguna Hills, CA)
  - Advantage: Simple insertion of devices that avoid conjunctival manipulation, sparing the conjunctiva for future bleb surgeries

What is Gold Misco-shunt?

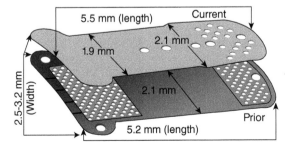

Figure 5.19 Gold micro-shunt

- The GMS+ is a revised model (3.2 mm × 5.5 mm).
- Composed of two rectangular fused leaflets with a rounded proximal end, and a distal end with fins to anchor the device in the suprachoroidal space.
- Fins are located at the proximal end of the device in the anterior chamber.
- It is made of medical-grade 24 karat gold as gold as a foreign body is well tolerated in the eye.
- Facilitates aqueous flow between the AC and the supraciliary/suprachoroidal space without the creation of a bleb.

What is Starflo?

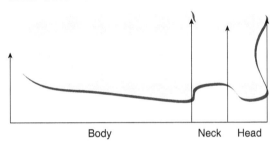

Figure 5.20 Starflo

- It is made of a flexible, micro-porous medical grade silicone called STAR Biomaterial, which is designed to optimize tissue integration and reduce fibrosis.
- Parts: Head, neck, and body.
- Received CE marking approval in Europe in 2012.

Describe the uses of the CYPASS micro stent.

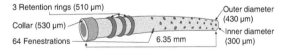

- 6.35 mm long polyimide tube
- Has fenestrations to facilitate outflow along the entire length of the device
- Implanted into the supraciliary space through a clear corneal incision
- Was FDA approved in 2016, but Alcon has issued a voluntary global recall, effective 2018, after research detected a dramatic rise in endothelial cell loss among patients during cataract surgery, compared with those who underwent cataract surgery alone

What is the Glaukos iStent?

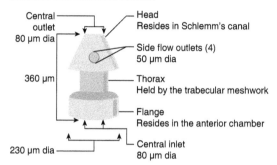

- iStent Supra (Model G3) is the newest IOP lowering stent from Glaukos.
- Received CE Mark approval in Europe.
- Lightweight heparin-coated L-shaped titanium device.
- Placed within Schlemm's canal.
- Has thrombolytic activity and prevents stenosis.
- Shaped like a half pipe and the part of the device within the canal is 1 mm in length with three barbed ridges that prevent loosening once placed.
- Inserted with the help of an applicator under gonioscopic guidance where the pointed tip engages the trabecular mesh work.

What are options for intractable glaucoma/painful blind eye?

- Diathermy
- Cyclodestructive procedures
- Diode laser cyclophotocoagulation
- Endo cyclophotocoagulation
- Retrobulbar alcohol and enucleation is now obsolete.

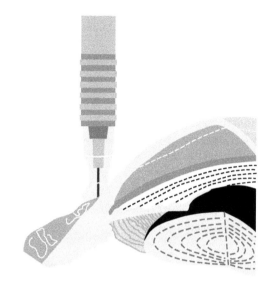

Figure 5.23 Cyclophotocoagulation

What are the indications of cyclophotocoagulation?

- To reduce IOP in an eye with poor visual potential.
- Temporary procedure in an eye to bring down the IOP before definitive procedure if it is deferred in view of systemic or ocular conditions.
- Inadequate conjunctiva due to multiple surgeries.

6

Retina

6.1 TOPICS

- Speculums
- Scleral depressors
- Scleral buckling surgery
- Instruments for cryotherapy
- Instruments for pneumoretinopexy
- Vitrectomy instruments
- Diathermy instruments
- Vitreous substitutes
- Intraocular magnets and foreign bodies

6.2 SPECULUMS

Identify and describe the Maumenee–Park eye speculum?

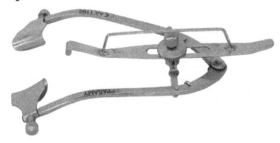

Figure 6.1A Maumenee–Park eye speculum

- Two types:
  - With solid blades which cover the eyelashes
  - With fenestrated blades
- Has a canthus hook and blade locking screw with three blades: For the upper lid, the lower lid, and the lateral canthus
- Uses:
  - Extraocular surgeries
  - Retinal detachment surgery

Describe the uses of the self-retaining universal eye speculum in retinal surgeries?

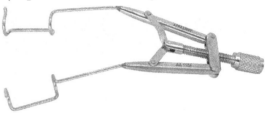

Figure 6.1B Self-retaining universal eye speculum

- A speculum with a larger exposed area gives an advantage in scleral buckle surgery as it provides better exposure and ease to pass the sutures.
- Can be used to perform fundus examination using portable fundus cameras and mobile devices.
- Can be used in children or patients with difficulty in keeping the lid open during ocular imaging procedures, like OCT and biometry.
- Peripheral retinal breaks can be lasered using laser indirect ophthalmoscopy with the help of a speculum to keep the lids open.
- Intravitreal injections like anti-VEGF and antibiotics in endophthalmitis.

6.3 SCLERAL DEPRESSORS

Identify and describe the scleral depressors.

- Schepens scleral depressor
- Thimble into which the finger is inserted for greater control
- The tip is designed to atraumatically depress the tissue for inspection
- Gass scleral indenter

DOI: 10.1201/9781003455646-6

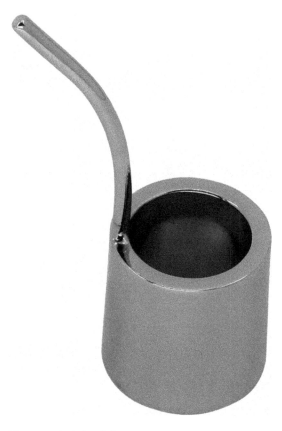

Figure 6.2 Scleral depressors

- Modified scleral indenter
  - Used to position over the hole while examining the retina during indirect ophthalmoscopy
  - Indentation gives a ring mark on the sclera, the center of which is then marked with a blue ink
  - Indent the spot with forceps and use indirect ophthalmoscopy to check the accuracy of the hole localization
  - Once the location of the hole is confirmed, scleral buckle can be used to indent the hole
- Schocket double-ended scleral depressor
  - Made from stainless steel
  - Has a slightly angled shaft
  - 16 mm in length from bend to tip

What are the indications and contraindications of scleral indentation?

- Indications:
  - Dynamic evaluation of retinal periphery

- Retinal break vs. retinal hemorrhage vs. retinal dialysis
- Flat vs. raised retinal lesions
- In ROP to examine the peripheral fundus
- Indentation is helpful while lasering the periphery viz. anterior edge of the break or lattice
- Contraindications:
  - Active inflammation such as uveitis/scleritis
  - Recent intraocular operation (for the fear of opening the wound)
  - Scleral thinning
  - Equatorial staphyloma

Identify and describe the Gass scleral indenter.

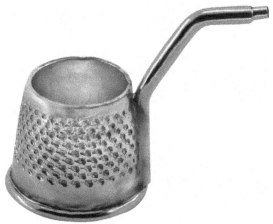

Figure 6.3 Gass scleral indenter

- It is a type of modified scleral indenter.
- It is used to position over the break while examining the retina during indirect ophthalmoscopy.
- Indentation gives a ring mark on the sclera, whose center is then marked with blue ink.
- Re-indenting the spot with forceps and indirect ophthalmoscopy checks the accuracy of the hole.
- Once the location of the hole is confirmed, the scleral buckling can be used to indent the hole.

What is a retinal break?

- Full-thickness defect in the neurosensory retina.
- Tears: Caused by dynamic vitreoretinal traction. U-shaped (horseshoe, flap) tears consist of

a flap, the apex of which is pulled anteriorly by the vitreous base being attached to the retina.

- Hole: Caused by chronic atrophy of sensory retina may be oval or round.
- Operculated hole: Piece of retina is torn away from the rest of the retina and floats anterior to the hole by the vitreous gel.
- Dialysis: Circumferential tear along the ora serrata with vitreous attached at the posterior margin.
- Giant retinal tear: A tear involving 90° or more of the globe circumference. Vitreous gel is attached to the anterior margin of the break.

What are the indications for prophylactic treatment of retina breaks and holes? What are the AAO guidelines for the same?

- These are general recommendations and are not absolute in nature. Each patient's case must be assessed individually and management charted accordingly.
- Indications for treatment of retinal breaks (Table 6.1)

What are the management options for sealing retinal breaks?

- In an attached retina
  - Laser by indirect ophthalmoscopy
  - Laser by slit-lamp delivery
  - Cryotherapy
  - Endolaser
- In a detached retina: Scleral buckling along with cryo, vitrectomy + laser/cryo, and pneumatic retinopexy + laser/cryo

What are the indications for prophylactic treatment to prevent retinal detachment (RD)?

- Any horseshoe shaped tear (symptomatic)
- Operculated symptomatic tear
- Subclinical RD (presence of SRF > 1 DD from retinal break but not more than 2 DD posterior to equator)
- Lattice (fellow eye)
- Asymptomatic HST and round hole in following:
  - Patient undergoing YAG capsulotomy
  - Patient undergoing LASIK
  - Associated with Marfan's syndrome with family history with involvement of fellow eye
  - High myopia
  - Where follow-up is unreliable or unavailable

What are the modes of prophylactic treatment?

- Laser: Argon green
  - Advantages:
    - Less cataractogenic
    - Less xanthophillic damage
  - Technique
    - 500 μm spot size
    - Intensity is grayish white
    - Done in 2–3 rows

Table 6.1 Indications for Treatment of Retinal Breaks

Type of Lesion	Treatment
Acute symptomatic horseshoe tears	Treat promptly
Acute symptomatic operculated tears	Treatment may not be necessary
Traumatic retinal breaks	Usually treated
Asymptomatic horseshoe tears	Usually can be followed up without treatment
Asymptomatic operculated tears	Treatment is rarely recommended
Asymptomatic atrophic round holes	Treatment is rarely recommended
Asymptomatic lattice degeneration with holes	Usually does not require treatment
Asymptomatic lattice degeneration without holes	Not treated unless PVD causes a horseshoe tear
Asymptomatic dialysis	No consensus on treatment and insufficient evidence to guide management
Eyes with atrophic holes, lattice degeneration, or asymptomatic horseshoe tears where the fellow eye has had an RD	No consensus on treatment and insufficient evidence to guide management

– confluent burns
– Adjust the power per intensity
• Indirect laser delivery system
• Slit lamp with Eisner's scleral indenter
• Cryocoagulation: Can be done through hazy media

Identify and describe the Gass retinal detachment hook.

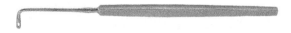

Figure 6.4 Gass retinal detachment hook

• Fenestrated therefore easy to tag the recti after threading the suture through the hook
• 1.5 mm oval hole
• Used in scleral buckle surgery

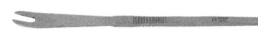

Figure 6.5 Forked orbital retractor

Identify and describe the Schepen's forked orbital retractor.

• 14 mm × 56 mm blade having 4.5 mm wide notch in the blade
• Overall length is 14.8 cm
• Forked retractor for better scleral exposure
• Used in scleral buckle surgery

Figure 6.6 Scleral marker

Identify and describe the scleral marker.

• 3 mm, 3.5 mm, and 4 mm standard size
• For directly marking the sclerotomy sites accurately

Identify and describe the uses of the cross-action (Castroviejo) plug forceps.

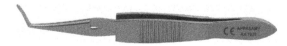

Figure 6.7 Cross-action (Castroviejo) plug forceps

• Metal plugs for 20G port closure and plastic plugs for 23G closure
• For temporary closure of sclerotomies for exchange of instruments before closure
• Uses:
  • To maintain the air-filled globe during vitrectomy
  • Vitreoretinal drug delivery with biodegradable scleral plugs (Foscarnet and Ganciclovir)
  • To seal the sclerotomies while performing temporary exchange of instruments during surgery

6.4 SCLERAL BUCKLING SURGERY

Identify and describe the forceps.

Figure 6.8 Bishop–Harmon forceps (A)

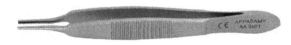

Figure 6.9 Alabama (B)

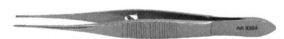

Figure 6.10 Elschnig (C)

• Bishop–Harmon: To fix soft tissue like sclera, conjunctiva
• Alabama: Grooved on one side and rounded on other side for suture tying, used to suture thicker materials
• Elschnig: To fix the lid while passing traction sutures
• Smooth forceps: To handle implant/band

Identify this blade.

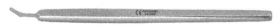

Figure 6.11 Scleral knife/crescent blade (hockey knife)

• Blade width: 1 mm
• Blade thickness: 0.38 mm

- Straight bi-bevel
- Used for lamellar scleral dissection prior to placement of implant
- Can be used for lamellar corneal dissection and dermoid dissection

Identify and describe the Watzke sleeve introducer/spreader forceps.

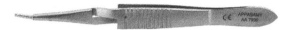

Figure 6.12 Watzke sleeve introducer

- Used to introduce the Watzke sleeve
- Used to stretch a silicone sleeve so that the two ends of the silicone band can be passed through during scleral buckling

Identify and describe the Watzke sleeve.

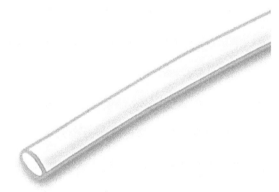

Figure 6.13 Watzke sleeve

- Made of silicone rubber
- Elastic and easy to use

What are the other methods of band fixation?

- Clove hitch suture (4-0/5-0 non-absorbable)
- Tantalum clips

What is an explant?

- Buckle element is sutured directly to the sclera.

Identify and describe the 240 band.

- This is a type of solid silicone explant in the pattern of encircling band; also known as encircling element or belt buckle.

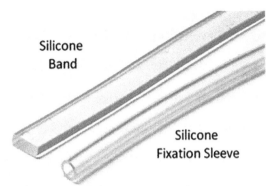

Figure 6.14A 240 band

- Solid silicone is practically non-compressible, hence preferred for this purpose.
- 2.5 mm width and 0.6 mm thickness with length being 125 mm.
- Used for 360° encirclage; usually combined with tire type of silicone explant like 277, 279, 286, etc. to enable better hold and appropriate tightness.
- Some gauge the obtained indentation height by using the circumference difference and horizontally stretching the ends of the bands an appropriate length obtained (e.g., for a 2 mm height indent, using the circumference formula of 2 × pie × radius, the difference between two global circumferences, we get an approximate length of 12 mm (assuming average axial length within normal range). Hence, when the 240 band is used for encirclage, mark each end when just apposed to the globe, keeping it as flat as possible. After crossing, stretch ends horizontally apart by about 12 mm (check horizontal distance between marked points on the band) to obtain 2 mm indent height and fixate using either Watzke sleeve or clove stitch or tantalum clips).
- It can also be used as encircling element—support explant, especially in vitrectomy combined with buckling for supporting vitreous base, passed beneath recti.
- For 360° encircling elements: Single mattress sutures are usually sufficient in each quadrant. Suture bites are just far apart to allow free movement of band. If high indent is required, two broad mattress sutures can be placed in each quadrant.

- Other encircling elements commonly used are 40 (2 mm width and 0.75 thickness), 41 (3.5 mm width and 0.75 mm thickness), and 42 (4 mm width and 1.25 mm thickness), all three having same length of 125 mm, but 41 and 42 are usually preferred when used without tire.

Identify and describe this buckle 279.

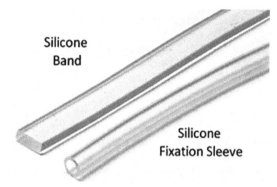

Silicone Band

Silicone Fixation Sleeve

Figure 6.14B Buckle 279

- Also known as scleral buckle or scleral tire. These are usually available as a ring of solid silicone with a groove for band with fixed size.
- 279 tire has one edge slightly thicker, with groove measuring 2.5 mm and horizontal width 9 mm with curvature of 11 mm. Its curve is concave toward globe. Thicker edge is placed posteriorly for better indentation.
- Used as either explant (using non-absorbable sutures) or implant (using scleral tunnel dissection) with band of size 2.5 mm width—commonly 240.
- Can be oriented either circumferential (generally preferred) or radial (sponges preferred).
- Circumferential buckles in the manner of 360° provide support in the region of the vitreous base where traction is usually more severe. They are theorized to support broad areas of pathology. Can lead to shortening of eye wall and radial retinal folds (may worsen radial traction) and can lead to fish-mouthing.
- Radial buckles support localized areas but prevent fish-mouthing and can be used for more posterior breaks.
- Circumferential segmental buckle covers a limited sector with the tire element, while the

band surrounds the globe 360°; some, however, prefer to use the tire alone. For the tire part, suture limbs are placed parallel to limbus. The tire chosen should cover the entire extent of the break appropriately.
- Other common tire elements used: 277 equally concave indent (groove: 2.5 mm; horizontal width: 7 mm with curvature 9 mm); 286 equally convex indent (2.6 mm groove, horizontal width 6 mm with curvature 6.6 mm); 280 asymmetric concave indent (2.5 mm groove, horizontal width 10 mm with curvature 12 mm).

Identify and describe silicone sponge.

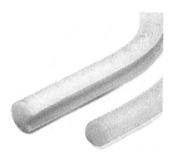

Figure 6.15 Silicone sponge

- Commonly available as cylinders in various diameters (4, 5, 7.5 mm)
- They can be oriented circumferentially or radially. But geometrically, radial orientation is preferred for retinal tears.
- Silicone sponges, due to their composition, are deformable and compressible.
- On initial suturing, it hence causes compression leading to IOP rise. As IOP drops back to normal, the sponge expands leading to apposition of the RPE to the NSD (Neuro-sensory detachment) leading to closure of break.
- As they enable greater indent height, which is a function of the separation of needle bite and diameter of explant, they are preferred for non-drainage (minimally invasive detachment surgery) buckling technique.
- Sponges, especially of circular cross-sectional profile, produce much higher central indent. Hence, accurate localization of break especially in the transverse meridian is critical with a circular cross-sectional profile. Sponges also

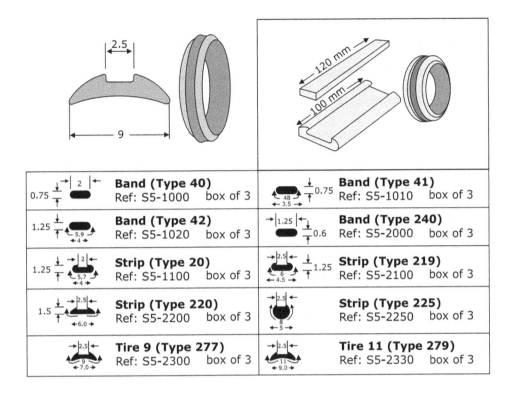

0.75 / 2	**Band (Type 40)** Ref: S5-1000 box of 3		48 / 3.5 / 0.75	**Band (Type 41)** Ref: S5-1010 box of 3
1.25 / 5.9 / 4	**Band (Type 42)** Ref: S5-1020 box of 3		1.25 / 0.6	**Band (Type 240)** Ref: S5-2000 box of 3
1.25 / 2 / 5.7 / 4	**Strip (Type 20)** Ref: S5-1100 box of 3		2.5 / 6 / 4.5 / 1.25	**Strip (Type 219)** Ref: S5-2100 box of 3
1.5 / 2.5 / 6.0	**Strip (Type 220)** Ref: S5-2200 box of 3		2.5 / 8 / 5	**Strip (Type 225)** Ref: S5-2250 box of 3
2.5 / 9 / 7.0	**Tire 9 (Type 277)** Ref: S5-2300 box of 3		2.5 / 11 / 9.0	**Tire 11 (Type 279)** Ref: S5-2330 box of 3

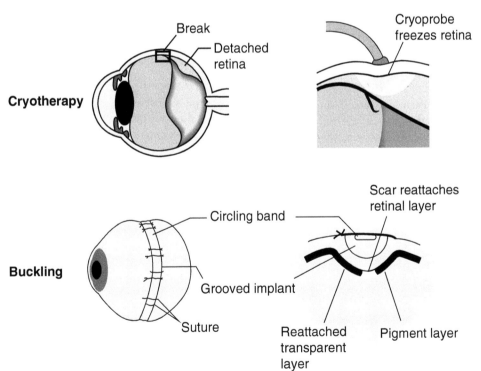

Figure 6.16 Circumferential buckling

provide greater posterior indent as compared to solid tire. They, however, can lead to greater astigmatism.

- Other shapes of sponges available are partial-thickness cylinders, grooved sponges, and oblong variants.
- Older sponges had communicating air cells, leading to increased infection risk, but newer ones have closed air cells, limiting infection.
- Newer materials like polyhydroxy-ethyl (hydrogel), a synthetic sponge, have micro-pores that absorb and release antibiotics slowly over a period, decreasing infections.
- However, granulomas and late displacements are still a problem, as is rare possibility of infection.
- Milder degrees of infection can be managed topically, and sponge removed after 3–4 weeks to allow for chorioretinal adhesions.

What are the management options of retinal detachment?

- Scleral buckling and its modifications
- Pneumoretinopexy
- Vitrectomy and its modifications

What are the principles of retinal detachment surgery?

- Identification of all retinal breaks and areas of vitreous and periretinal traction.
- Induction of aseptic chorioretinal inflammation around the breaks to seal them.
- Release of any vitreous and periretinal traction.
- Drainage of subretinal fluid.
- Ensuring chorioretinal apposition for at least a couple of weeks by either or both of the following:
  - External tamponade—silicone buckle, sponge, tire, encircling band
  - Internal tamponade—air, gases such as sulfur hexafluoride (SF_6)
  - Perfluoropropane (C_3F_8) or liquids such as silicone oil

What are the relative contraindications to scleral buckling?

- Thin sclera
- Prior glaucoma surgery
- Prior squint surgery
- GRT

- Posterior breaks
- PVR grade C or more

What are the steps of scleral buckle surgery?

- Classic technique:
  - Localization of the break: Done with IO and scleral depression
  - Chorioretinal adhesions: Done with cryotherapy the endpoint is choroidal and retinal whitening
  - Indentation of the break: Buckle and encircling band is used; buckle supports the break and encircling band supports the vitreous base
  - SRF drainage: Not indicated in all cases
  - Gas injection
- D-ACE technique: Described for those with high SRF levels, as apposition of RPE to neuro-sensory retina is difficult. However, visualization through gas is difficult therefore it did not gain popularity.
  - Drainage
  - Air
  - Cryotherapy
  - Explant

How does one localize a break?

- Indirect ophthalmoscopy with scleral indentation is a must
- Use the principles of Lincoff's rules
- Posterior extent of the most posterior break marked on sclera
- The base of the break also marked on sclera
- In rare situations, drain the SRF to locate the break
- Advantage of marking:
  - Allows to evaluate and sizing of explant
  - Allows antero-posterior positioning of the encircling band

What is three-point localization?

- It is a type of marking after localization of break, performed intraoperatively.
- Usually described for large horseshoe tears, where three points are marked.
- The posterior most extent of the break.
- And one side on each end of the lateral extent of the horns of the break.
- Marking is done after indirect ophthalmoscopy with a Gass like indenter, where pressure

is used to mark a circle around the localized break. After drying the bed, a methylene blue marker pencil is used or light cautery. After marking with dye, the bed should be dried again to prevent spreading.

How does one create chorioretinal adhesions?

- Cryocoagulation
- Diathermy
- Photocoagulation
- Cyanoacrylate glue

What is Lincoff's rules?

Lincoff's rules is used for locating primary break (**Table 6.2**).

Later Dr. Kressig added some general principals to determine possible location of break in cases of re-detachments (**Table 6.3**).

What is a retinal implant? What are the advantages & disadvantages?

- Silicone material when placed intrasclerally (2/3rd thickness of scleral bed)
- Advantages:
  - Support to the drainage site of the scleral flap
  - Good buckle height
- Disadvantages:
  - Increased time for scleral dissection
  - Fear of scleral perforation
  - Re-surgery more difficult

Table 6.2 Lincoff's Rules

Lincoff's Rules	Configuration of RD	Possible Location of the Break
1	Superior temporal or nasal detachments	The primary break that determines the shape of the detachment lies within 11/2 clock hours beneath the higher border of the detachment in 98%.
2	Superior detachments that cross the midline at 12 o'clock and advance down both sides of the disk eventually become a total detachment	In this type of detachment, the primary break will lie in a triangle the apex of which is at 12 o'clock and its sides are 11/2 clock hours to either side of 12 o'clock in 93%.
3	Inferior detachments	The higher border of the detachment indicates the side of the disk on which the inferior break is to be found in 95%.
4	Inferior bullae in rhegmatogenous detachments	Originating from a superior break

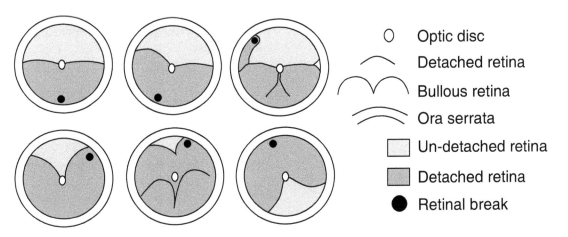

Figure 6.17 Lincoff's rules configuration of RD possible location of the break

Table 6.3 Kressig–Lincoff Rules for Re-Detachment

Kressig–Lincoff Rules for Re-detachment	Configuration of RD	Possible Location of the Break
1	When the superior border of a temporal or nasal superior detachment drops below the buckle	It implies an undetected break within 11/2 clock hours below the new superior border.
2	When the pattern of a detachment (superior, lateral, or inferior) converts from one pattern to another	It indicates an undetected break consistent with the new pattern (localize per classical rules).
3	When the borders of a detachment remain unchanged after a buckling operation and the buckle is in the correct position	This implies an undetected break above the buckle.
4	When a total detachment remains unchanged after being encircled and drained	It implies an undetected break anterior to the existing encirclage near 12 o'clock.

- Buckle intrusion in vitreous cavity
- Endophthalmitis risk if uveal tissue is exposed

What are the types of buckles used?

- Permanent:
  - Solid silicone
  - Sponge
  - Hydrogel
- Absorbable:
  - Gelatin
  - Synthetic suture
  - Donor tissue
- Radial explant:
  - Large U tears
  - Posterior tears
- Circumferential explant:
  - Multiple breaks in more than two quadrants
  - Anterior breaks
  - Further away from ora serrata
  - Wide breaks, GRT
- Encircling circumferential explant:
  - Break in more than three quadrants
  - Lattice degeneration in more than two quadrants
  - Along with vitrectomy

What is the role of an encircling element?

- It keeps the explant in place.
- If used in isolation, it creates narrow buckling effect and supports area of vitreoretinal traction.
- It provides buckling effect at vitreous base especially in vitrectomized eye.
- The amount of buckling is sufficient to keep RPE against the break and to prevent VRT.

What are the parameters to consider during buckle fixation?

Table 6.4 Configuration of the Buckle

Circumferential Buckle	Radial Buckle
Supports area parallel to vitreous traction	Focal support to the tear
Can be done 360°	Posterior breaks especially in large HST
Multiple breaks in different quadrants and in different AP locations can be done	Advantages: Decreased chances of fish-mouthing
Can be used in Retinal dialysis/GRT	Disadvantage: Accurate localization is essential
Large breaks	Can lead to higher astigmatism
Shortening of eye wall leads to radial retinal folds and may cause fish-mouthing	

- The width of the buckle should be twice of the tear (**Table 6.4**).
- The tear should be at the posterior aspect of the ridge.
- The height of the buckle depends on the distance between the anterior and posterior suture bites on the sclera.
  - If the width of the suture bites is 2 mm more than the width of the explant, it gives a low buckle height.
  - If the width of the suture bites is 3–4 mm more than the width of the explant, it will produce a high buckle height.
  - The diameter of the buckle.
  - The tightness/placement of the suture.
  - The asymmetric shape with thicker posterior edge will produce more buckling effect.
- Effect depends on:
  - Type of material
  - Location and tension of scleral sutures
  - Circumferential tightening of scleral band

What are the materials used for scleral buckling?

- Non-absorbable:
  - Solid silicone:
    - Not affected by temperature
    - Can be autoclaved
    - Water insoluble
    - Low toxicity
    - Elastic
  - Silicone rubber sponge:
    - Can be used for radial indentation
    - Can cause infection, however
  - Polyhydroxyethylacrylate (synthetic sponge):
    - Hydrogel acrylic co-polymer packed in saline
    - Not used as hydration levels are inconsistent
    - Advantage: No dead space like silicone rubber, so technically lesser chance of infection
  - Other non-absorbable materials:
    - Polyethylene: Disadvantage is that it can get eroded and infected
    - Polyviol can cause irritation and infection
    - Teflon mesh is difficult to remove
    - Large gauge non-absorbable suture
- Absorbable:
  - Fascia lata: Fear of HIV and other transmissible diseases
  - Gelatin: Unpredictable hydration and absorbs in 24 months so buckling effect is lost
- Temporary buckle techniques:
  - Lincoff's balloon
  - Modifications of above technique

What are the indications of SRF drainage?

- To aid localization of breaks (D-ACE)
- Avoid non drainage in those with high-risk toward rise of IOP (open angle glaucoma, rupture of recently treated anterior segment wound, ipsilateral poor ocular perfusion, thin sclera)
- Long-standing retinal detachment (RD)
- Significant PVR
- Bullous retinal detachment
- Inferior detachment
- Patient having preoperative glaucoma
- Need for intravitreal gas injections
- Unhealthy RPE (elderly patients)
- All re-operations
- Large breaks located posterior to equator

What does the site for SRF drainage depend on?

- Depends on configuration of RD
- Associated vitreoretinal traction (VRT)
- Select the site:
  - Preferred below the buckle bed
  - Beneath the area of vitreoretinal traction (VRT)
  - Away from retinal break (One does not want vitreous to pass through the break into subretinal space)
  - Dependent area of maximum fluid
  - Preferably slightly anterior to equator
  - Preferred meridian just above the plane of horizontal recti muscles
  - Posterior drainage considered in re-surgeries of large retinal breaks

What are the methods of SRF drainage?

- Prang:
  - Digital pressure applied to central retinal artery occlusion occurs and choroidal vasculature gets blanched
  - Full-thickness perforation made with 27G hypodermic needle
  - SRF drained and air injected
- Cut down
  - Radial sclerotomy made at the area of deepest SRF
  - Prolapse a choroidal knuckle and examine it with a +20 D lens to ensure there are no large choroidal vessels
  - Apply light cautery to the knuckle
  - Perforate with 25G hypodermic needle

What are the complications of SRF drainage?

- Choroidal hemorrhage
- Ocular hypotony
- Retinal incarceration
- Vitreous prolapse
- Endophthalmitis
- Damage to long posterior ciliary arteries and nerves

What are the complications of scleral buckling procedure?

- Intraoperative:
  - CRAO
  - Vitreous hemorrhage
  - Vitreous prolapse from SRF site or a mistaken full-thickness suture in thin sclera
  - Raised IOP
  - Corneal abrasions
  - Globe perforations
  - Muscle tear/hematoma/lost muscle especially in staphylomatous eyes
  - Iatrogenic break
- Early postoperative:
  - Raised IOP (especially if non-drainage)
  - Choroidal detachment
  - Endophthalmitis
  - Orbital cellulitis
  - Failure to reattach
- Late postoperative:
  - Endophthalmitis
  - Extrusion/exposure of implant

- Ptosis
- Maculopathy
- Cataract
- PVR changes
- EOM imbalance
- Refractive change

Mention indications for non-drainage buckling procedure and probable mechanism.

- Non-drainage buckling is usually effective if summit of buckle lies within 3 mm of retinal break.
- Though the exact mechanism is not explained, even if the break is not perfectly apposed to the underlying buckle, non-drainage works probably due to changes in vitreous forces after buckle.
- Cryotherapy does not induce fluid resorption, as non-drainage performed without cryo, also works in a similar manner—absorption of fluid despite gap between detached neural retina and RPE.
- Breaks without vitreous detachment (atrophic holes, retinal dialysis), non-drainage is specially effective.
- It is even effective in certain detachments with multiple breaks (if same latitude) and even with proliferative vitreoretinopathy (PVR) grade C1–C2 (though chances of success lesser comparatively).

When would you choose intraocular tamponade during scleral buckling?

- Intraocular tamponade can be in the form of fluid/gas.
- Indications of intravitreal fluid:
  - After the retina is settled and the break is on the buckle, to counter the ocular hypotony and to flatten the circumferential retinal fold
- Indications of gas at the end of the surgery:
  - To prevent fish-mouthing
  - To counter ocular hypotony
  - As an internal tamponade

What is fish-mouthing?

- Radial fold behind the explant communicating with open break on ridge

- Etiology: Circumferential buckle with excessive radial folds due to increased buckle height
- Clinical importance: Prevents settling of retina
- Treatment:
  - Reduce the buckle height (loosen the scleral suture/band)
  - Inject saline
  - Inject gas
  - In suspected cases, like large horseshoe tears, use a radial buckle
  - Photocoagulation posterior to the radial tear

What is D-ACE surgical sequence for treating retinal detachments?

- D-ACE stands for drainage of subretinal fluid, intravitreal injection of air, transscleral cryopexy, and episcleral explant
- Indicated in:
  - Small-/medium-sized breaks in superior quadrant without PVR
  - In patients with thin sclera, where placement of a bulky scleral buckle is difficult
  - Select cases of GRT
  - Tear under superior rectus muscle

Describe Lincoff's orbital balloon.

- It is a non-drainage procedure advocated in a single break.

- The aim is to create temporary scleral buckling effect.
- Procedure:
  - Cryo-application is done and deflated balloon is kept is area of localization after making 2 mm conjunctival incision near ora serrata.
  - Partial inflation is done.
  - Localization is verified and the balloon is fully inflated with 1.25 cc of saline.
  - Monitor for the development of CRAO.
  - The tube of balloon is patched to forehead.
  - One week later, the balloon is decompressed to ½ it's volume and after another week complete deflation is done.
- Advantages:
  - Safe, effective especially in single HST without PVR
  - Especially beneficial for HST below superior rectus muscle as the muscle imbalance due to the explant is minimized
- Disadvantages:
  - Decreased IOP
  - Shift in location of balloon
  - Corneal abrasion due to silicone catheter
  - Infections

Who invented scleral buckling?

- Ernst Custodis is credited to inventing scleral buckling.

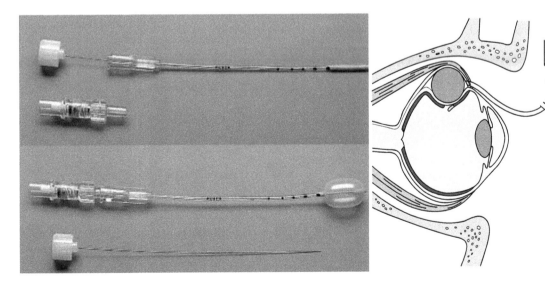

Figure 6.18 Lincoff's orbital balloon

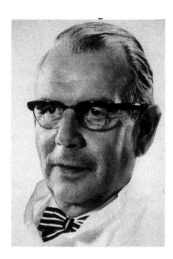

Figure 6.19 Ernst Custodis

6.5 INSTRUMENTS USED FOR CRYOTHERAPY

Identify and describe the cryo probe and mention the principle of cryotherapy.

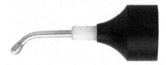

Figure 6.20 Cryo probe

- It causes freezing of the intracellular and extracellular water to ice, and this leads to tissue death. The ultimate scar seals the break.
- The principle is called the Joule–Thomson principle: Gas under pressure released through a narrow aperture causes a temperature change.
- Compressed N_2O gas at 400–625 psi is used.
- Nitrous oxide and carbon dioxide are effective refrigerants.
- Boiling point of N_2O: −88.5°C.
- Boiling point of CO_2: −56.6°C
- Therefore, nitrous oxide can produce a greater amount of cooling than carbon dioxide.
- Probe size 2.5 mm is used in scleral buckling surgery or for external cryotherapy for retinal breaks.

When is cryotherapy preferred over retinal laser therapy?

- Hazy media
- Very peripheral tears not seen on LIO

What is the technique of cryotherapy?

- Each break is given cryotherapy till there is blanching of the retina and cryotherapy over bare choroid is always avoided to prevent RPE fallout, which can be a precursor for PVR.
- Avoid re-freezing.
- Use tip and not the shaft till effect is seen on the RPE layer.
- Do not pull the probe until it is completely defrosted.

What are the advantages and disadvantages of cryotherapy?

- Advantages:
  - No sclera/muscle damage
  - Can be applied to full-thickness sclera and conjunctiva
- Disadvantages:
  - Ocular:
    - Excess cryo reaction can lead to retinal necrosis.
    - Cystoid macular edema.
    - Choroidal effusion/exudative RD.
    - Phthisis bulbi.
    - Pigment dispersion in the vitreous/subretinal space leads to an increase in the incidence of PVR.
    - In gas-filled eyes, the effect of cryo is prolonged and intense and causes retinal necrosis.
  - Systemic:
    - N_2O is teratogenic in animals. There is decrease in vitamin B_{12}, which affects methionine synthetase, and DNA production is hampered.
    - Exhaust from the cryo unit should be collected. Otherwise, there is a theoretical risk of occupational hazard.

What is the role of photocoagulation in retinal surgery?

- The retina needs to be in contact with RPE around the break, so it can be done only after settling the retina unlike the previously mentioned techniques.
- It can be external drainage/internal delivery systems.

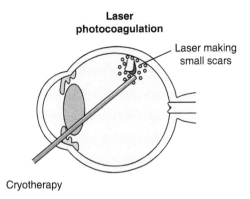

Laser photocoagulation — Laser making small scars

Cryotherapy

Cryotherapy — Feezing tissue together

Figure 6.21 Cryotherapy technique

- Advantages:
  - Posterior breaks can be treated well.
  - There is less RPE fallout in photocoagulation compared to cryotherapy and therefore decreased incidence of PVR.
- Disadvantage: There maybe suprachoroidal and subretinal fluid collection if there is incomplete penetration.

What are the parameters to be kept in mind with regards bottle height?

- Standard bottle height is 40 cm (18 in), which should be the height of the drip chamber from the eye level.
- Increase the bottle height:
  - If there is intraocular bleeding to arrest it temporarily till you can use diathermy/eraser.
- Disadvantages: CRA occlusion, ON perfusion decreased, Corneal edema
- Decrease the bottle height:
  - If there is corneal edema
  - Disadvantages: DM folds, miosis of the pupil, bleeding

6.6 PNEUMORETINOPEXY

What is pneumoretinopexy and what is its mechanism of action?

- It is a procedure in which gas is injected in vitreous cavity for closure of retinal breaks (George Hilton).
- Surface tension and buoyancy push the retina toward the underlying RPE, and hence, vitreous fluid cannot enter the subretinal space.

- The healthy RPE absorbs the remaining fluid and helps in reattachment of retina
- The break is closed by cryotherapy or laser photocoagulation

What are the indications and contraindications of pneumoretinopexy?

- Indications:
  - A single break no larger than 1 clock hour in the superior 8 clock hours of the fundus or a group of small breaks within 1 clock hour
  - Superior retinal tear
  - Clear media
  - PVR grade A or B
  - Small horseshoe tear preferably <1 clock hour
  - Ability to follow up patient for at least 6 months with diligent patient cooperation
  - Prior to RD history of good vision in the eye
  - Shorter diameter of detached area must be at least 6 disc diameters
- Contraindications:
  - PVR grade C and above
  - Beyond 1 clock hour
  - Break in inferior 4 clock hours
  - Known case of glaucoma
  - Patients who cannot maintain position due to illness/mental incompetence
  - Need for immediate air travel
  - Large HST >2 clock hours
  - Anterior chamber lenses (ACIOLs)
  - PCIOL with PC rent
  - Recent intraocular surgery
  - Cloudy media
  - Glaucoma

What are the prerequisites for pneumoretinopexy?

- Clear media
- Patient able to maintain position
- Superior single break
- No PVR
- No glaucoma

What is the technique of pneumoretinopexy?

- IOP should be low.
- Localize breaks.
- Antibiotic/betadine solution is instilled.
- Chorioretinal adhesion in the form of cryopexy or photocoagulation.
- Gas injection—SF_6 or C_3F_8.
- Can be done as a one-step or two-step procedure.
- One-step procedure: Cryopexy first followed by gas injection
  - Convenient
  - It is especially helpful if media opacity prevents laser
  - Pigment atrophy preventing adequate laser burns
- Two-step procedure: Gas injection followed by laser photocoagulation 1–2 days later
  - In larger extensive breaks
  - Tears overlying a scleral buckle or posterior tears

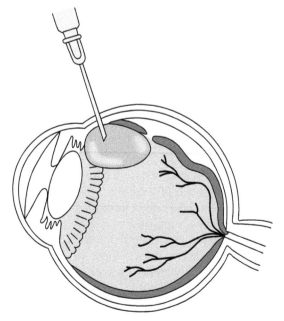

Figure 6.22 Pneumoretinopexy technique

- Transconjunctival cryotherapy
  - Localizes and seals the break
  - Also causes hypotony
  - Avoid in steam roller technique
- Pneumoretinopexy:
  - Standard
  - Steam roller
- Head position:
  - Therapeutic position should be maintained for 18 hours a day for 5 days
  - After 5 days sleep on the side to avoid contact with lens surface

What is steamroller technique?

- Is advocated when superior RD is threatening macula.
- In this technique, the gas is injected, and the patient is in a prone position.
- Over a period of 20–30 minutes, the patient is prone to straight head positions so that fluid is slowly absorbed.
- This is to prevent immediate involvement of macula unlike standard procedure.
- Either C_3F_8 (0.3 ml) or SF_6 (0.6 ml) is injected through 30G needle through upper most pars plana.
- Single large gas bubble should be injected.
- Check for CRAO: If there are no pulsations, then do a paracentesis or a vitreous tap
- Injection site should be away from site of retinal break or pars plana detachment 0.3 cc of SF_6 covers 90 degrees of arc of retinal surface.

What are the complications of pneumoretinopexy?

- Intra-op complications:
  - Elevated IOP
  - Vitreous hemorrhage
  - Vitreous incarceration
  - Subconjunctival gas
  - Extension of detachment
  - Multiple gas bubbles
  - Subretinal gas
  - Enlargement of tears
- Post-op complications:
  - New retinal breaks
  - Infective endophthalmitis
  - Cataract
  - Intravitreal proliferation
  - Lower initial anatomic success rate

Table 6.5 Volumes of Gas Injected for Pneumoretinopexy

	Air	SF$_6$	C$_3$F$_8$
Amount required (these are 100%, i.e., concentrations without dilution)	0.9 ml	0.6 ml	0.3 ml
Expansion of gas	Same	2 times	4 times
Duration for which gas lasts	5 days	10 days	1.5 months
Time taken for maximum expansion	Immediate	1.5 days	3 days

What are the advantages and disadvantages of pneumoretinopexy?

- Advantages over scleral buckling:
  - Reduced ocular trauma
  - Reduced hospitalization
  - Reduced complications, like muscle imbalance, refractive errors, and retinal incarceration
- Disadvantages:
  - Need for clear media, superior 1/2 breaks, and proper case selection
  - Lower success rate
  - Induce PVR
  - New retinal break formation
  - In case of failure, scleral buckling is required

What are the volumes of the gases to be injected?

6.7 VITRECTOMY INSTRUMENTS

Identify and describe the infusion sleeve tips?

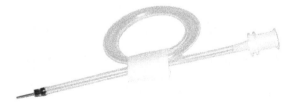

Figure 6.23 Infusion sleeve

- It is first in and last out in retinal surgeries.
- Infusion sleeve tip visibility is a must throughout placement of the cannula.
- Site of insertion of the infusion sleeve from the limbus:
  - Aphakic: 3 mm
  - Phakic: 4 mm
  - Infants: 2 mm
- Do not confuse it with AC maintainer.

- Infusion sleeve tip sizes:
  - 2.4, 4, and 6 mm (20 G)
  - 4 and 6 mm (23 G)
- Flange is for placement and fixation of suture such that sleeve sits snugly on sclera (**Table 6.5**).
- Uses:
  - During vitrectomy surgery, to maintain vitreous volume with irrigating fluids to prevent globe collapse
  - Infusion sleeve tip inspection for complete penetration through the ocular coats is a must before starting infusion

How do you differentiate between an infusion sleeve tip and an AC maintainer?

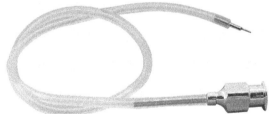

Figure 6.24 AC maintainer

- AC maintainer does not have a flange while the infusion sleeve tip (20G) usually has a flange.
- AC maintainer usually has threads for screwing mechanism, while infusion sleeve is smooth.

What are the uses of the various lengths of infusion tips?

- 4 mm infusion sleeve tip:
  - In phakic vitrectomy
  - It is the commonest infusion sleeve tip used
- 6 mm infusion sleeve tip:
  - In significant anterior PVR

- When RD is associated with CD
- Disadvantages:
  - Lens touch may occur.
  - Peripheral breaks may occur.
- 2.4 mm:
  - In pediatric cases
  - In ROP (The provided tip is not subretinal, or else the risk of suprachoroidal infusion exists. This is especially important in premature eyes.)

What is placement distance from the limbus for the infusion cannulas?

- In phakic patients: 4 mm (to avoid lens touch)
- In pseudophakic patients: 3 to 3.5 mm (preferred over 4 mm to avoid risk of anomalous ora levels and hence avoid retinal breaks in periphery during insertion)
- In pediatric patients: 3 to 3.5 mm (depending on age of patient, as growth compensation needed while inserting to avoid retinal breaks)

What are the different sizes in mm for the various gauge range?

These are inner diameters of the trocar system or the insertion blade:
- 20G: 0.89 mm
- 23G: 0.64 mm
- 25G: 0.51 mm
- 27G: 0.40 mm

Describe the 23G valve cannula.

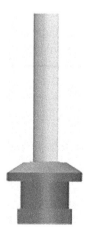

Figure 6.25 Valve cannula and trocar systems

- 23G valve entry ports (0.64 mm)
- Advantages:
  - Decreased wound leakage, less chances of incarceration at port site
  - Faster postoperative recovery
- Disadvantages:
  - Not as sturdy, especially for moving eyeball for peripheral vitrectomy
  - May need suturing of ports, especially if hypotony is expected

Identify and describe the vitreous cutter.

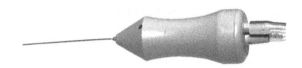

Figure 6.26 Vitreous cutter

- Basic mechanism of vitreous cutters is the utilization of suction with simultaneous inclusion of a shearing force to cut vitreous while inducing minimal traction.
- Broadly classified as electrodynamic (fixed duty cycle, heavy, leads to fatigue and can exacerbate tremors) and pneumatic (can alter duty cycle, lighter, ergonomically better, and cheaper)
- By mechanism of action:
  - Rotatory
  - Oscillating (Peyman type, less shearing than rotatory)
  - Guillotine: Two tubes, outer fixed with port of aspiration and inner tube slides vertically across the port of the outer tube, cutting the vitreous as it is aspirated into the port
  - Classical (single actuation) pneumatic cutters were based on spring return mechanism—diaphragm inside the probe was pushed by air pulse (port closed position) which simultaneously compressed a spring that forced the diaphragm to open port position. This limited the control over the duty cycle (DC). DC is the percentage of time the port is open during each cut cycle. As cut-rate increases, DC decreases; hence, the classical cutters had the issue of limited aspiration flow with increasing cut rates.

- Newer dual pneumatic probes have two separate air lines that control the port position of the vitrectomy tube. Hence, the DC can be controlled independent of the cut rate, leading to customized modes being possible.
- Lower DC limits port-based flow and provides better fluidic stability with less pulsatile vitreoretinal traction (called "shave" mode).
- Slit-based and hole-based modifications of the 23G guillotine cutters by creating a 0.1 mm hole or slit in the inner tube leads to least amount of acceleration and minimal dependence on blade motion in the slit type. This helped achieve the "constant flow" motion desirable in vitrectomy.
- The twin duty cycle (TDC) cutter technology uses a double port—two-dimensional cutter featuring a large rectangular aperture in the piston or inner tube with two sharp cutting edges. Aperture allows continuous and even flow due to two open cutting ports while the two sharp edges in the cutting port allows vitreous cut during both forward and backward movement, thus effectively doubling the cut rate. This reduces vitreous traction, decreases surgical time, and increases safety.
- A modification of the dual pneumatic actuator with a limited angles rotary cutting scheme has been described (InnoVit).
- A combination of the mentioned modifications has also been in the dual actuated diaphragm cutters (Advanced UltraVit by Alcon). It eliminates spring, eliminates friction from piston seals, and enables variable duty cycle. It has axial cutting design and larger port opening with bevel tip. This places the tip closer to the retina

and coupled with higher cut rates of 10,000 CPM reduces traction and backflow through the port. This is useful for dissection of broad diabetic membrane (plaque like) where the higher cut rates help in segmentation of the edges and the bevel tip acts like a shovel to create a tissue plane between the plaque and retina. The plaque edge is then cut while feeding into the port (shovel and cut). The combination of this with the above dual cutting technology has also been described (HyperVit), which is theorized to give CPM of about 20,000.

- Most recent cutters are disposable having reduced weight, described as being self-sharpening tips to ensure smooth cut during the procedure. This however leads to shearing of the material at edges; hence efficiency reduces if used again.

What are the types of vitrectomy cutters per mode of power supply?

What are the uses of the vitrectomy probe?

- Vitrectomy (**Table 6.6**)
- Lensectomy
- Membranectomy
- Primary posterior and anterior capsulotomy in pediatric patients as well as adults
- Surgical iridectomy
- Pupilloplasty
- Induction of PVD
- Retinotomy

What are the indications of performing a retinotomy?

- Drainage of subretinal fluid
- Relieve traction
- Subretinal IOFB or cyst removal

Table 6.6 Differences in Cutter Types

Pneumatically Driven	Electrically Driven
Axial guillotine	Rotary and solenoid
Inner tube moves in a longitudinal axis	Inner tube spins inside the outer tube
Less traction on the vitreous	More traction on the vitreous
Disposable	Reusable
DC is adjustable	DC is not adjustable
(DC is the duty cycle, i.e., the amount of time the port remains open in each cut)	

- Subretinal blood removal
- Subretinal band removal

What are the advantages and disadvantages of small gauge vitrectomy (23, 25, 27G)?

- Advantages:
  - Cutting port is closer to the tip; therefore, there is better control of fine tissue manipulation near the retinal surface.
  - Modifiable duty cycle: It is the percentage of time the port remains open during cutting.
    - Reduced DC: Safer shaving of vitreous base
    - Increased DC: Good efficiency for core vitrectomy
  - Ultra-high-speed cutting (5000 cps)
  - Decreased vitreous surge
  - Cutting close to mobile retina safer
- Disadvantages:
  - Hyper-flexibility of instruments
  - Low light levels
  - Decreased flow rate
  - Less efficient for angled instruments like scissors and pick forceps

What are the surgeries not feasible through small incision vitrectomy?

- Crystalline lens removal
- IOFB removal
- Pediatric surgeries where it is better to suture, even if small gauge instruments are used

What are the advantages and disadvantages of 23G/25G vitrectomy?

- Advantages:
  - Decreased postoperative inflammation and CME
  - Less conjunctival scarring (those who had multiple ocular surgeries or glaucoma patients)
  - Flexibility of port use
  - Increased patient comfort
  - Decreased corneal astigmatism
- Disadvantages:
  - Incision related:
    - Risk of postoperative hypotony
    - Wound leakage
    - Endophthalmitis
  - Instrument related:
    - Hyper-flexibility of instruments
    - Low light levels
    - Higher resistance to aspiration
    - Decreased flow rate
    - Less efficient for angled instruments like scissors and picks
    - Fragmatome and dual function instruments like IOFB removal forceps are mostly 20G
- Miscellaneous:
  - Costly instrumentation
  - Pave syndrome: Presumed air by vitrectomy embolization, where an unsecured cannula slips under choroid during FAE causing venous air embolization which can be fatal

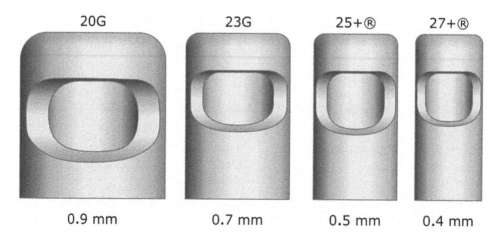

20G	23G	25+®	27+®
0.9 mm	0.7 mm	0.5 mm	0.4 mm

Figure 6.27 Small gauge vitrectomy

Figure 6.28 Intravitreal scissors

Identify and describe the scissors. State its uses.

- Vertical or curved scissors
- Uses:
  - To cut the fibrous vascular fronds, bands
  - During segmentation or delamination of ERM

What is the classical Charles flute needle and mention the modifications that you know of?

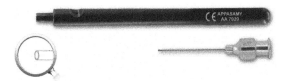

Figure 6.29 Flute needle

- The classical Charles flute needle is a blunt ended (20G diameter when used with the ocutome system) connected by a Luer lock to a handle.
- Within the handle, the male Luer terminal connects to an exit port in a depression on the side of the handle.
- When needle is introduced in a closed micro-surgical environment of posterior segment via pars plana sclerotomy, closure of the exit channel by the surgeon's thumb prevents flow of fluid or gas.
- Removal of finger/thumb allows egress of fluid/gas along the needle and through the handle outward as along as the infusion line maintains the IOP above the atmospheric pressure. This is passive aspiration.
- Modification by McLeod and Leaver involved moving the exit port on a mount on the handle adjacent to the Luer terminal. They have also slightly increased the size of the exit port.
- The needle tip can be modified with a silicone tip or brush.
- Further modifications in the way of decrease diameter gauge and disposable cannulas have become common.
- The handle attachment has been modified with the silicone reservoir to enable backflush.

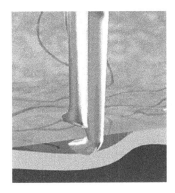

Figure 6.30 Segmentation

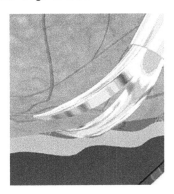

Figure 6.31 Delamination

What are the types of membrane dissection techniques? (Table 6.7)

Table 6.7 Membrane Dissection Methods

Segmentation	Delamination
Blades perpendicular to retina	Blades parallel to retina
In PVR to decrease tangential traction	In PDR for removal of ERM
In PDR with atrophic retina	
Segmentation (Figure 6.30)	Delamination (Figure 6.31)
Re-proliferation can occur	Re-proliferation less commonly occurs
Innermost limiting layer damage	Less damage to innermost limiting layer
Late rhegmatogenous RD can occur	Entire membrane can be removed

Identify and describe the silicone-tip needle. Mention its uses.

Figure 6.32 Silicone-tip needle

- Silicone-tip needle comes with a needle with a soft silicone tip for atraumatic removal of intraocular fluids.
- Silicone-brush needle (straight/curved) comes with 20G needle with a soft silicone tip that is split to create a brush like quality.
- Uses: Used along with a flute handle
  - For non-traumatic brushing of the retinal surface with simultaneous aspiration
  - For repositioning of retinal folds or breaks

Identify and describe the uses of the flute handle.

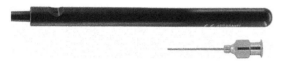

Figure 6.33 Flute handle—backflush handle

- Silicone backflush reservoir on the conventional flute needle
- Use: Passive aspiration of fluid
- Advantage: Safe backflushing of the incarcerated tissue during passive aspiration of intraocular fluids

Identify and describe the microvitreo retinal (MVR) blade and mention its uses in retinal surgeries.

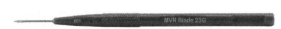

Figure 6.34 MVR blade

- Has a lancet tip that makes a symmetrical incision around the initial entry point
- 1.4 mm blade width to make 0.89 mm incision for 20G tools

- Shaft is 20G to make a round opening from the linear incision
- 23G stiletto blade produces 0.72 mm sclerotomy opening for 23G vitrector
- Prevents ciliary epithelium from being pushing forward
- Older name: Myringotomy blade; earlier use in ENT surgeries as well
- Uses:
  - Sclerotomy incision
  - Incision in capsule before lensectomy/membranectomy
  - Incision into the capsule of IOFB
  - ROP stage 5 surgery
  - To cut into the central part of the ERM

Identify and describe the mayo infusion cannula?

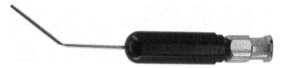

Figure 6.35 Mayo infusion cannula

- 20G infusion with 30 bent blunt cannula.
- It is useful for anterior infusion for performing lensectomy using vitrectomy techniques.
- It can be used for infusion directly into the posterior segment using pars plana approach in the case the 4 mm/6 mm cannulae cannot be viewed due to lens/ROP/large SRF/choroidal detachment/etc.
- Used for bimanual approach with vitrectomy probe in:
  - Lensectomy
  - Membranectomy
  - In ROP when the pars plana can't be seen
  - Vitreocorneal touch
  - Aphakic pupillary block
  - Hyphema
  - PHPV
  - In routine vitrectomy until tip of regular infusion sleeve is seen correctly
- Can be used:
  - Translimbal (cataract/hyphema)
  - Through ciliary body (ROP/PHPV)
  - Through pars plana (membranectomy/retro IOL membrane)

- Advantages:
  - Maintains globe
  - Can be interchanged with cutter
  - Access to periphery is easy

Identify and describe the membrane pick.

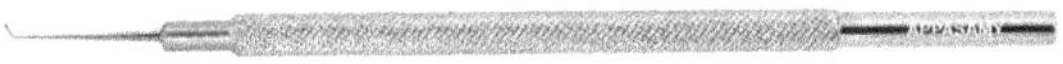

Figure 6.36 Membrane pick

- Non-illuminated and illuminated.
- Short blunt round-ended membrane picks are the safest way of initiating peeling if an edge is present.
- Longer tips are available but can cause damage to the retina.
- Use: Dissecting and peeling epiretinal membrane.

Identify and describe the membrane scratcher.

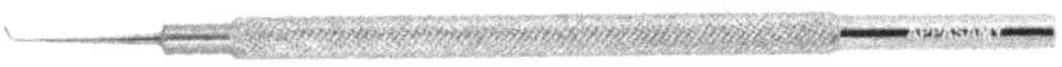

Figure 6.37 Membrane scratcher

- Blunt triangular tip
- Has a tip diameter of 3 mm with 90 mm length made of nickel and chrome on a stainless steel handle
- Has 4 small teeth which are 0.15 mm wide
- 4 mm long angled at 45°
- Uses:
  - To raise the edge of epiretinal/preretinal membrane
  - Explore the membrane between the retinal folds

Identify and describe the membrane peeler.

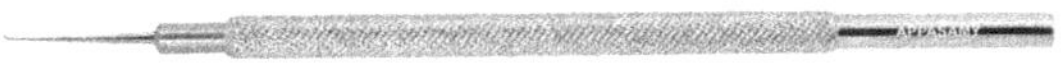

Figure 6.38 Membrane peeler

- Blunt triangular tips correspond to membrane peeler
- It has tip diameter of 3 mm with 90 mm length made of nickel and chrome on a stainless steel handle
- To separate weakly adherent preretinal membrane
- Atraumatic exploration of membrane between deep retinal folds.

Identify and describe the microspatulas.

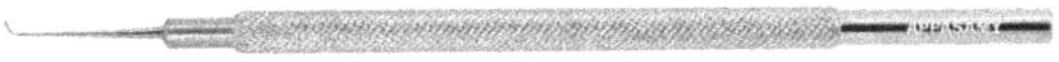

Figure 6.39 Membrane spatula

- With tip angulation.
- 30°, 45°, 60°, 80°.
- Bottom is diamond-dusted.
- Being an abrasive surface, when rubbed on preretinal membrane, it is easy to separate edge of membrane which can be later held by end-ripping forceps.

Identify and describe the membrane spatulas.

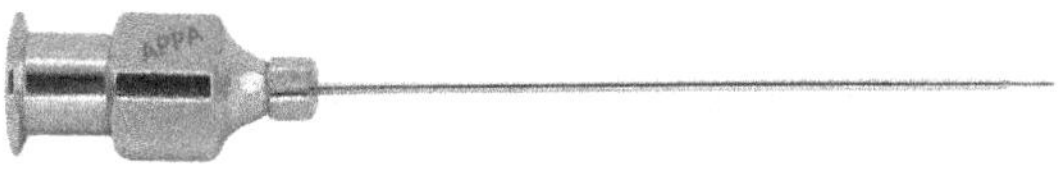

Figure 6.40 Diamond-dusted membrane scraper

- Hooked
- Bent at 45°, 5 mm from rounded tip
  - Use: To separate fibrovascular membrane adhesions between retinal folds
  - Curved: Tip curved at 45° angle, hence easy to pick up preretinal membranes in a narrow funnel RD
  - With knife: Edges are sharp

Identify and describe the diamond-dusted membrane scraper.

- Silicone-tipped for non-traumatic contact with retina
- Coated with chemically inert diamond dust, leads to traction while scraping
- Lifts the epiretinal membrane or internal limiting membrane

What are the types of forceps and their uses?

Identify and describe the ILM forceps.

- To remove ILM (do not confuse with NFL) (**Table 6.8**)
- To lift the edge of epiretinal/preretinal membrane
- To hold and peel the delicate membrane on the surface of retina
- Modification of end grasping forceps with a fine serrated platform at the tip to ensure gripping of fine membranes like the ILM

Table 6.8 Intravitreal Forceps

Forceps	Uses
Pick forceps: Tip curved, hollow, 20 G, 25 mm long	Lifts the edge of the preretinal membrane Holds and peels the membrane
End-gripping forceps: Tip blunt with a small platform	To hold delicate membranes on surface of retina (especially for ILM peeling)
End-gripping forceps with tapered Tip	Membrane between narrow retinal folds can be held
Forceps with serrated jaw (Crocodile forceps)	To hold: Dense thick membranes Lens capsule Small foreign body

Figure 6.41 ILM forceps

Describe the foreign body forceps.

Figure 6.42 Foreign body forceps

- Basket type—three prongs (retractile)
- To hold the foreign body after it is freed from vitreous
- Types:
  - Claw
  - Diamond-coated
  - Memory snare IOFB extractor
  - Micro alligator forceps

Identify and describe the subretinal forceps (duck beak forceps)?

Figure 6.43 Subretinal forceps

- Use: To remove/pull the subretinal bands through a retinotomy

Identify and describe the end grasping forceps.

Figure 6.44 End grasping forceps

- Serrated or flat tips that open when the handle is pressed (can also close on pressing handle—depending on the type preferred)
- Useful to peel ILM, ERM
- Available in both disposable and reusable handles

Identify and describe these intraocular scissors.

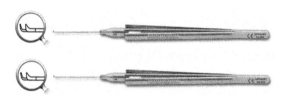

Figure 6.45 Intraocular scissors

- Vertical or curved or horizontal scissors (horizontal scissors are angled at 135 with straight blades)
- Used to cut the fibrous vascular fronds, bands
- Uses:
  - Segmentation: Membranes are cut in between the epicenter for which vertical scissors are commonly used
  - Delamination: Shearing of the membrane from epicenter for which curved and horizontal scissors are used
  - Segmentation and delamination are possible with the cutter therefore separate scissors are not required (especially with small 25/27G)

What are the types of subretinal membranes?

- Annular
- Dendritic
- Placoid

Identify and describe the endo illuminator instrument.

- Co-axial fiber optic illumination
- More divergent angle (74%), therefore better illumination, which reduces glare
- Inflexible
- Minimum intensity light, therefore less photo toxicity
- Use: Visualize retinal structures during surgery and check that the infusion cannula is correctly placed at the beginning of surgery
- Complications: Phototoxicity, lens touch, and retinal tears

What are the sources of illumination?

- Halogen: Most common; used in 20G; not used with 23G or 25G as illumination is reduced by 50%
- Metal halide lamps: Have a low life span
- Xenon: Requires cooling; costly and space occupying (commonly used in Constellation Vision System, Alcon; Stellaris, Bausch and Lomb; and Bright Star, DORC vitrectomy machines)
- Mercury vapors: Green yellow in color, lesser retinal toxicity than xenon light
- LED (light-emitting diodes): Latest and brightest with least heat (safest) and have a long life

What are the types of endo illuminators?

- Focal: Handheld light pipes
- Wide-angled: Chandelier illuminator
- Illuminated instruments: Illuminated picks, scissors

Identify and describe the chandelier system of light source.

- Illumination system
- Available in 20G, 23G, 25G, and 27G
- Use: Fixed wide-angle for bimanual surgery
- Advantages:
  - Preferred in tractional and combined retinal detachment surgeries where bimanual dissection of membranes is required

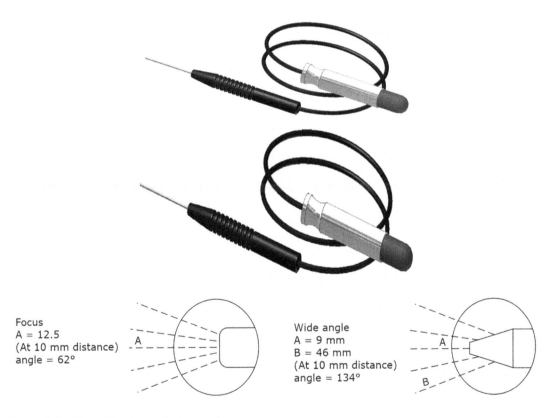

```
Focus
A = 12.5
(At 10 mm distance)
angle = 62°
```

```
Wide angle
A = 9 mm
B = 46 mm
(At 10 mm distance)
angle = 134°
```

Figure 6.46 Endo illuminator instrument

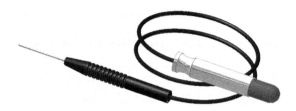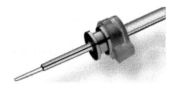

Figure 6.47 Chandelier system of light source

- Extensive PVR
- Constant illumination from a fixed distance therefore area illuminated is larger
- Preferred in long duration surgeries
- Disadvantages:
  - Illumination possible only at one area
  - Shadow of the instrument may obstruct the view (dual 29G chandelier has smaller trocar and dual light which eliminates this shadow)
  - Extra port is needed

6.8 DIATHERMY INSTRUMENTS

Identify and describe the diathermy instrument.

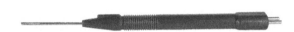

Figure 6.48 Diathermy instrument

- Diathermy along with illumination
- Disadvantages: Tissue shrinkage, break, NF damage
  - Limit diathermy to 1 mm away from the disc while cauterizing neovascular fronds to avoid disc damage

What is the principle of diathermy?

- Radio frequency current is produced by crystal controlled; solid state amplifiers powered by Ni/Cd (nickel/cadmium) batteries

What are the types of diathermy?

- Penetrating
- Non-penetrating

What are its uses?

- Penetrating sclera
  - For perforation and SRF drainage
  - Tumor destruction

- Non-penetrating surface diathermy
  - When implant was used, diathermy was performed at the bed of the implant to create chorio-retinal adhesions at the site of the break in implant, it was used to create a bend in the area of break to create chorioretinal adhesions (however, it produced scleral thinning and therefore was discontinued for the same).
  - Localization of break.
  - Various color-coded electrode diodes are available depending on their use.
  - Diathermy with trans-illumination—for accurate localization.

What is an endolaser? What are its uses?

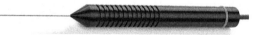

Figure 6.49 Endolaser

- It is available in 20G, 23G, 25G, and 27G sizes.
- Probe design can be straight or curved.
- Uses:
  - To stop active bleeding in diabetic vitrectomy
  - Intraoperative photocoagulation of retinal tears and retinotomies
  - Photocoagulation intraoperatively in proliferative retinopathies such as PDR in Diabetic retinopathy, vascular occlusions vasculitis and other conditions

Identify and describe the cautery.

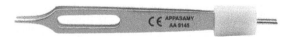

Figure 6.50 Bipolar forceps

- Bipolar available in 20G, 23G, and 25G
- Used for achieving hemostasis or controlled drainage retinotomy

What are the indications of Primary vitrectomy for RD?

- Posterior break
- Macular hole
- Giant retinal tear
- Large, multiple tears in various locations
- PVR grade C and above
- Combined RD
- Vitreous hemorrhage
- Presence of anterior PVR
- Media opacities, choroidal detachment, viral retinitis
- Dislocated IOL, lens fragments
- Retinoschisis, coloboma

What are the principles of retinal detachment surgery?

- Identification of all retinal breaks and areas of vitreous and periretinal traction
- Induction of aseptic chorioretinal inflammation around the breaks to seal them
- Release of any vitreous and periretinal traction
- Drainage of subretinal fluid
- Ensuring chorioretinal apposition for at least a couple of weeks by either or both of the following
  - External tamponade: Silicone buckle, sponge (half- or full-thickness), tire, encircling band;
  - Internal tamponade: Air, gases such as sulfur hexafluoride (SF_6), perfluoropropane (C_3F_8), or tamponading liquids such as silicone oil

What are the principles of vitreous surgery?

- Aims of vitreous surgery
  - To remove any vitreous abnormalities; e.g., hemorrhage, traction bands
  - To restore retinal anatomy by removal of epiretinal membrane or drainage of subretinal
  - To treat abnormal retinal vessels or breaks by endophotocoagulation or cryotherapy
  - To provide tamponade to maintain chorioretinal apposition, internally by silicone oil and gases or externally by encirclage or plomb (buckle)
  - To obtain tissue for biopsy:
    - Endophthalmitis

- Tackling giant retinal breaks (GRT), proliferative vitreoretinopathy (PVR)
- General trans–pars plana vitrectomy algorithm
  - Lens removal
  - Removal of anterior hyaloid face unless proliferative diabetic retinopathy and clear lens
  - Truncation of cone (frontal plane of posterior vitreous detachment [PVD])
  - Vacuum cleaning sub-posterior vitreous detachment and preretinal hemorrhage
  - Peeling, segmentation and delamination of epiretinal membrane (ERM)
  - Subretinal surgery
  - Internal drainage of subretinal fluid during retinal break
  - Complete internal drainage of subretinal fluid
  - Inducing retinal adhesions around breaks after apposition achieved endophotocoagulation/cryo/diathermy

Identify the machine. What are the general steps of pars plana vitrectomy?

Steps of pars plana bitrectomy (general):

- Drape and insert a lid speculum.
- Incise the sclerotomy.
- Secure the infusion cannula and check its penetration into the vitreous cavity.
- Construct the other two sclerotomies.
- Insert the endo-illumination and focus the viewing system.
- Insert vitrectomy cutter and excise the vitreous after inducing PVD.
- Take as much vitreous as possible, with settings of highest cut rate and lowest vacuum

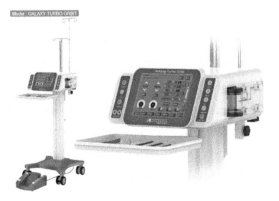

Figure 6.51 Vitrectomy machine

during steps close to the retina—like vitreous base shaving, macular manipulation, etc.
- Perform the requisite steps for the particular indication of vitrectomy—clear hemorrhage, close retinal break, remove ERM, etc.
- Search the retina for iatrogenic or pre-existing breaks with endo-illumination and indentation
- Tamponade as required.
- Close the sclerotomies.
- Subconjunctival injection of antibiotic + steroid as needed.
- Eye pad and patient counsel.

Explain gas internal tamponade?

- Principal: Fick's diffusion equation: Two gases on either side of a semipermeable membrane will pass across the semipermeable membrane until their concentrations are equal on both sides.
- N_2 from air, lungs, and blood passes into eye to enlarge the SF_6 or C_3F_8 bubble. Hence, pure gases are expansile and must be diluted before injection into eye. The high surface tension of these gases does not allow the bubble to enter retinal breaks and prevent fluid from entering the break as high buoyancy (maximum at apex of angle of bubble).
- Additional surgical steps for gas internal tamponade
  - Attach the air pump tubing to the three-way tap on the infusion line; confirm cannula in place then switch on the air pump at 30–40 mmHg.
  - With a flat retina, place the tip of a flute cannula close to the optic nerve head to drain the vitreous cavity fluid, while patient position is supine and head facing straight
  - Close one sclerotomy.
  - Prepare the long-acting gas (mixed to the desired concentration with filtered air) by inserting into a 50 ml syringe (make sure any tubing for drawing up gas is flushed through with the gas before drawing up gas into the syringe)
  - Draw up the gas; for 30% gas, you need 15 ml of gas followed by 35 ml of air to give a total of 50 ml (you may need more in a high myope; preferable to use two syringes). To check how much gas was inserted by holding up the syringe to the light and observe for a condensation line

where the syringe stopper was drawn up to with the long-acting gas. Mistakes can occur with gas mixtures with resultant under fill if less long-acting gas or severe IOP rise with too much. Hence, it is important to observe the processes during gas mixing to ensure the correct dosages are used. Some prefer to use a 100 ml syringe to avoid conversion of ml to percentage, i.e., 30 ml = 30%
  - Attach the syringe to the three-way tap, and flush out the air by inserting 35 ml but keep 15 ml balance in syringe in case of hypotony during closure of the surgical wounds.
  - At the end of the operation, the air in the vitreous cavity must be flushed with a volume of gas.
  - Close the second sclerotomy.
  - With 23G, remove both upper trocars and insert a 26G needle through the pars plana to allow exhaust of the gases, attach the 50 ml syringe onto the three-way tap and flush through the gas to 15 ml.

Explain silicone oil internal tamponade.

- The high surface tension of silicone oil (albeit lower than gases) prevent fluid from entering the break as high buoyancy (maximum at apex of angle of bubble).
- Its immiscible usually used for long lasting tamponade (PVR, trauma, etc.)
- But can emulsify.
- Needs removal.
- Additional surgical steps for silicone oil:
- Method 1 (Adv: The retina can be manipulated during the oil insertion.)
  - Attach a silicone-oil-filled syringe linked to the silicone oil pump set to 50 psi to the three-way tap.
  - Reduce the pressure to 30 psi with 23G to avoid separation of tubing from the infusion trocar.
  - Insert a flute needle and drain intraocular fluids in order of first SRF, then vitreous cavity fluids and then heavy liquids while actively inserting the oil
  - Drain fluid off the disc.
  - Prefer end point of IOP at approximately 10 mmHg.

- Method 2 (Adv: Inserting the oil onto the macula first, allowing egress of SRF through anterior retinal breaks, may reduce the risk of subretinal oil)
  - Fill the eye with air completely.
  - Insert the oil through a sclerotomy allowing the air to egress from another sclerotomy, which should be kept open till active insertion is taking place.
  - Prefer end point of IOP at approximately 10 mmHg.

What are the steps of silicone oil removal?

- Whenever silicone oil has been inserted, the aim must be to remove the oil at the appropriate time, to maximize vision and reduce the chance of complications.
- Additional steps 20G method 1:
  - Prepare for the vitrectomy as before. Enlarge one superior sclerotomy (or in aphakic patients, create a 2 mm clear corneal wound).
  - Hold the sclerotomy open while the infusion is on.
  - Allow the silicone oil to extrude (block the microscope light from entering through the pupil).
  - Sew up the sclerotomy (instruments can be inserted through the sewn up sclerotomy).
  - Perform an internal search.
- Additional steps 20G method 2 (preferred):
  - Prepare for the vitrectomy as before. Use a 10-mm-long 18G cannula attached to an oil injector pump set on extract.
  - Actively extrude the oil (block the microscope light from entering through the pupil).
  - Perform an internal search.
- Additional steps 23G:
  - Prepare for the vitrectomy as before. Use a 4-mm-long 23G cannula attached to an oil injector pump set on extract inserted through one of the trocars (if not available, create a 20G sclerotomy as mentioned).
  - Actively extrude the oil (block the microscope light from entering through the pupil).
  - Perform an internal search.

What are the uses of PFCL heavy liquid?

- Principle: Heavy liquids are vitreous substitutes used as intraoperative tools.
- These agents may cause emulsification, vascular changes, and structural alterations of the retina and are therefore usually removed at the end of surgery.
- They are biologically inert, with a specific gravity higher than water, immiscibility with water or blood and with a high gas-binding capacity
- Additional surgical steps:
  - Use a heavy liquid-filled syringe and a two-way cannula with the tip close to the fovea.
  - Expand the bubble of heavy liquid with the distal orifice within the bubble and the proximal orifice in the vitreous cavity fluid.
  - Keep the heavy liquid away from breaks if these are on tension (e.g., in PVR) because the liquid easily separates into different bubbles and enters the subretinal space.
  - For removal, use a flute needle in the bubble, and try to remove in one smooth action to avoid losing the bubble when it is small.

What is the surgical technique of performing vitrectomy in a case of retinal detachment?

- Place encircling band near ora to support the vitreous base but may not be necessary if good vitreous base removal has been done.
- Access vitreous via three sclerotomies.
- Remove posterior vitreous.
- Induce PVD.
- Complete vitrectomy up to the equator, with indentation and base shaving.
- Inject 1–2 cc of PFCL to stabilize posterior retina (occasionally).
- Complete peripheral vitrectomy.
- Peel membranes if present.
- Remove flap of retinal tear.
- Settle retina with PFCL or air:
  - Settling with air—posterior retinotomy
  - Settling with PFCL—peripheral retinotomy
- Retinopexy with laser or cryopexy
- Tamponade with gas or silicone oil
  - SF_6: Non-expansile concentration $\approx$ 18%
  - C_3F_8: Non-expansile concentration $\approx$ 14%
  - Silicone oil: 1000 or 5000 centistokes

What are the complications of vitrectomy?

- Intraoperative:
  - Iatrogenic retinal breaks
  - Cataract by lens touch
  - Incarceration of retina at sclerotomy site
  - Choroidal hemorrhage
  - Subretinal infusion of fluid
- Postoperative:
  - Cataract
  - Glaucoma
  - Fibrin formation
  - IOL subluxation

- Macular pucker
- CME
- Choroidal detachment/hemorrhage
- Endophthalmitis

What is the Modified Retina Society Classification of grading of PVR? (Table 6.9)

How do you differentiate rhegmatogenous retinal detachment from retinoschisis? (Table 6.10)

How do you differentiate retinal detachment from a choroidal detachment? (Table 6.11)

Table 6.9 PVR Classification—Modified Retina Society

Grade	Characteristics
A	Vitreous haze, vitreous pigment clumps
B	Wrinkling of inner retinal surface, rolled edge of retinal break, retinal stiffness, vessels are tortuous
C	Full thickness folds in
C1	One quadrant
C2	Two quadrants
C3	Three quadrants
D	Fixed retinal folds in four quadrants
D1	Wide funnel RD
D2	Narrow funnel-shaped RD (anterior end of the funnel visible by IO with 20D lens)
D3	Closed funnel (optic nerve not visible)

Table 6.10 RD Differentiation from Retinoschisis

	RRD	Retinoschisis
Symptoms	Photopsia and floaters present	Photopsia and floaters absent
Location	Can occur anywhere	Commonly infero/superotemporal
Refractive error	Often myopic	Often hyperopic
Laterality	Usually unilateral	Usually bilateral
Detachment	Convex with undulated appearance and mobility	Convex, smooth, immobile
Surface	Corrugated	Smooth
Mobility	More	Less
Tobacco dusting	Present	Absent
Demarcation lines/ Subretinal cyst	Present	Absent
Laser	Does not create burn due to SRF	Creates burns
Choroidal vessels	Not seen	Easily seen
Sclerosed vessels	Not seen	Maybe present with beaten metal appearance
Scotoma	Relative scotoma	Absolute scotoma

Table 6.11 Differentiation RD vs. CD

	RD	CD
Symptoms	Flashes and floaters maybe present	Absent as there is no traction
Appearance	Convex, undulated, mobile	Brown, convex, smooth, relatively immobile
Ora seen	Ora seen with depression	Ora seen without depression
Field defect	Present	Absent
Posterior pole and macula	May or may not be involved	Posterior extension limited due to adhesions between suprachoroidal lamellae and sclera where vortex veins perforate
Hypotony	Low	Very low IOP
AC	Normal	Shallow

Who performed the first vitrectomy?

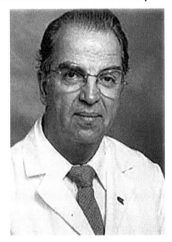

- Robert Machemer performed the first vitrectomy using a 17G cutter (1970).

Who is the father of retinal detachment surgery?

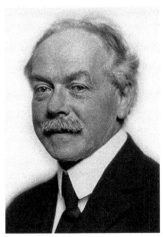

- Jules Gonin treated the first retinal break by ignipuncture (1923)

6.9 VITREOUS SUBSTITUTES

What are the various vitreous substitutes used?

- Intraocular gases:
  - Air
  - SF_6
  - C_3F_8
- Special fluids:
  - Silicone oil
  - Perfluorocarbon liquids (PFCL)

Identify the silicone oil solution.

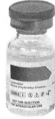

SILICONE OIL 1000 CST

Figure 6.54 Silicone oil solution

- Silicone oil of 1000 cSt (cSt = centistokes indicates density).
- Also available in 5000 and higher densities.
- Silicone oil is used as intraocular tamponade.
- It is a clear, inert, hydrophobic polymer.
- The length of the polymer determines its viscosity.
- Range of viscosity is 1000–12,500 cSt.
- Refractive index is 1.4035.
- Density is 0.975, which is less than water, and therefore, it floats up.
  - Interfacial tension of silicone oil is high but less than gas water interface. (Therefore, air

is used first to flatten retina, and then air is replaced with silicone oil.)

- Immiscible with water or blood.

What are the commonly used oils?

- Polydimethyl siloxane (PDMS)
- Trifluoromethyl siloxane

Identify and describe silicone oil injector.

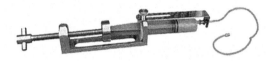

Figure 6.55 Silicone oil injector

- This is a steel silicone oil injector system used for manual insertion of silicone oil using a 20G port.
- It utilizes 10 ml syringe and steel cannulae, usually adjusted into the steel injector system.
- Can also be used for removal of silicone oil.
- Other options for SO insertion are the automated machine-driven system using special disposable cannulae (VFI, or viscous fluid injection cannula)
  - Available as metal or polyamide with Luer-lock system) and injector system with tubing (usually a high-pressure system), attached to the machine.
  - The latter are specific to the particular modern vitrectomy machine system, usually have a rubber stopper with a glass type syringe to ensure high vacuum and VFI attached at the other end.

What are the uses of silicone oil?

- Long-term retinal tamponade.
- RD with significant PVR or at high-risk of developing PVR (giant retinal tear)
- Patient who can't maintain position for gas such as children or patients with orthopedic problems
- Diabetic vitreous hemorrhage with membrane peeling (Since oil is immiscible, postoperative bleeding is compartmentalized and visibility is better. It also prevents recurrent bleed.)
- Other indications of silicone oil in diabetics:
  - Severe TRD
  - Combined RD

- Recurrent VH
- If break is present, it can cause tamponade, which leads to decreased angiogenesis and photocoagulation is possible
- In one-eyed and certain patients who need faster visual rehab (as it gives media clarity, in contrast to intraocular gas
- Patient needs air travel or goes to higher altitude
- Other indications such as those where the conventional scleral buckle will not work well are
  - Infectious retinitis: CMV, ARN, PORN
  - Multiple holes
  - Gliotic retina
  - Formed vitreous

When does one avoid silicone oil?

- Patient with silicone lenses
- If repeat surgery for silicone oil removal is not possible.

What are the complications of silicone oil?

- Intraoperative:
  - Overfill
  - Zonular rupture with silicone oil in AC
  - Sub retinal silicone oil migration
- Postoperative:
  - Refractive changes, post-op refraction is determined by shape of anterior surface of silicone oil; e.g., hyperopic shift in phakic patients
  - Cataract
  - Glaucoma
  - Silicone-oil-induced keratopathy
  - Sub retinal silicone oil
  - Subconjunctival silicone oil
  - Peri silicone oil fibrosis
  - Emulsification of silicone oil in AC (inverse pseudohypopyon)
  - Iritis/endophthalmitis/inflammatory membrane
- Be careful while performing cataract surgery in a silicone-oil-filled eye. Try to keep the PC intact as intact lens capsule prevents anterior migration of silicone oil

What are the advantages of silicone oil over gas?

- Longer-lasting tamponade
- Position maintenance required is less which is useful in children and patients with orthopedic problems

- Air travel is possible
- Multiple breaks in different meridians better suited for oil
- One-eyed patients have faster visual recovery

What are the indications of silicone oil removal?

- Emulsification of the silicone oil
- Secondary glaucoma
- Keratopathy
- Along with cataract extraction

Make a comparison of silicone oil and gas tamponade? (Table 6.12)

What are perfluorocarbon liquids (PFCLs) and what are their types?

- Perfluorocarbon liquids are used intraoperatively to manipulate the retina as they have a high density and high surface tension.
- Types:
    - Perfluoro-octane: C_8F_{18}
    - Perfluoro-decalin: $C_{10}F_{18}$
    - Perfluoro-phenanathrin: $C_{14}F_{24}$
- Properties:
    - Biologically inert.
    - Heavier than water.
    - Specific gravity 1.7622; therefore, it can flatten the retina forcefully.
    - Low viscosity, 2–3 centistokes; therefore, it can be injected easily.
    - Optically clear, immiscible with saline and silicone oil; therefore, it forms an immiscible interface with saline.
    - No change in the refractive power of the eye; hence, the same lens system can be used.
    - Does not absorb radiation between 488–810 nm; therefore, photocoagulation can be done through PFCL.

- C_8F_{18} has a low boiling point and high vapor pressure and hence vaporizes faster.

What are the indications of PFCL?

- PVR grade C3–D
- Giant retinal tear with RD
- Complicated diabetic retinal detachment
- Traumatic RD
- Subretinal hemorrhage
- Vitreous hemorrhage
- Dislocated lens fragment/IOL
- RD due to macular hole

What are the advantages and disadvantages of using PFCL?

- Advantages:
    - Stabilizes the posterior retina
    - Traction can be identified
    - Ease of membrane detection
    - Anterior PVR can be tackled
    - Avoids posterior drainage retinotomy
    - Controls intraoperative bleeding for endophotocoagulation to be possible
    - Unfolds GRT flap
- Disadvantages:
    - Metallic foreign body may sink through it.
    - Corneal endothelial damage occurs.

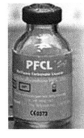

Figure 6.56 Perfluorocarbon liquid (PFCL)

Table 6.12 Silicone Oil vs. Gas Tamponade

	Silicone oil	Gas
Media clarity	+	-
Long-term tamponade	+	-
Repeat surgery for removal	Required	Not required
Positioning of the head (Children, mentally retarded, and orthopedic patients)	Not required	Required
Air travel	Possible	Not possible

- PFCL can seep into the subretinal space if injected without relieving the traction.
- Secondary cataract.
- Secondary glaucoma.
- PFCL must be removed completely and cannot be left in the eye postoperatively.

What are the indications of gases in intraocular use?

- Injectable gases are C_3F_8 and SF_6
- Indications of gases at the end of the surgery
  - To prevent fish mouthing
  - To counter ocular hypotony
  - Used as an internal tamponade

What are the refractive changes in the eye after various retinal surgeries?

- Scleral buckle surgery
  - Induced myopia after scleral buckling surgery.
  - Amount of increase in axial length depends on the height of the scleral buckle.
  - More in phakic than aphakic eyes.
  - Gradually diminishes over time.
  - High astigmatism is infrequent, possibly more in segmental buckles placed close to the cornea.
- Silicone-oil-induced changes
  - Depends on the status of the lens.
  - Silicone oil is in the eye for a limited period, therefore these changes are not permanent.
  - Phakic eyes:
    - Silicone oil forms a concave surface behind the lens, thereby acting as a minus lens inside the eye making the eye hyperopic.
    - Average hyperopia of 6D.
  - Aphakic eyes:
    - Silicone oil produces a convex surface, bulging through pupil thereby creating a myopic shift
    - Amount of myopia depends on the size of the pupillary aperture
    - Average myopia of 7.4D
  - Management
    - If prolonged intraocular oil is anticipated, contact lens wear is suitable to minimize aniseikonia.
    - IOL with plano-posterior surface can be used.

6.10 INTRAOCULAR MAGNETS AND FOREIGN BODIES

What is the intraocular magnet, and what are its uses?

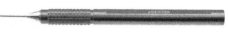

Figure 6.57 Intraocular magnet

- Steel/titanium shaft with magnetic tip and a cap to secure it to the shaft
- Use: For intraocular metallic foreign body removal
- Disadvantage: Cannot remove nonmetallic foreign bodies
- Complications:
  - Retinal tears
  - Vitreous incarceration

What are the types of magnets?

- Lancester's working criteria for magnet: To be effective, a giant magnet should pull a steel ball of 1 mm with a force of over 50 times its weight over a distance of 20 mm
- Giant magnet:
  - Bronson's electromagnet
  - Use: For trans-scleral route of removal of the IOFB after accurate localization
- Rare earth magnet (intraocular magnet):
  - Small and low in intensity
  - Use: If the foreign body is within 1 mm of its tip

What is maximum size of IOFB, which you can remove through PP?

- 5 mm
- If >5 mm: Vitreous base related complications can occur, and so do lensectomy, and use the translimbal route. Though some manipulate the foreign body such that 5 mm is along the axis, this needs experience and can still be dangerous.

What are the various ocular effects of IOFB?

- Mechanical: Associated traumatic findings
- Because of chemical nature: Siderosis, chalcosis, argyrosis, chrysiasis
- Associated infections

What are the clinical findings raising a suspicion of intraocular IOFB?

- Wound of entry—corneal/scleral (suprachoroidal hemorrhage)
- Iris hole
- Shallow AC
- Wound tract through lens
- Presence of hypotony
- Fixed semi-dilated pupil
- Heterochromia (long-standing iron foreign body)
- Presence of foreign body in AC/angle/vitreous/retina/subretinal space
- Double perforation when there is an exit wound posteriorly

What are the associated features that can complicate the management?

- Corneal tear
- Traumatic cataract
- Subluxated lens
- Vitreous hemorrhage
- Retinal detachment
- Endophthalmitis
- Sympathetic ophthalmia

What are the chronic changes with retained iron foreign body?

- Electrolyte dissociation of metal causes formation of ferrous ions which combine with intracellular proteins and can cause damage to the cells—the lytic effect.
- Retinal degeneration (secondary RPE-like picture).
- Corneal stain.
- Lens deposits can cause complicated cataracts.

How does one come to a diagnosis of siderosis?

- Clinical:
  - History of trauma
  - Wound of entry
  - Semi-dilated pupils
  - Heterochromic iris
  - RPE-like picture
  - IOFB seen
- Pathological:
  - Prussian blue reaction with Perl's micro chemical stain

What are the clinical signs of a copper IOFB?

- Chalcosis: Copper gets deposited extracellularly along the limiting membranes when copper is in the form of alloy
- Pure copper causes severe reaction similar to endophthalmitis
- Signs:
  - Kayser–Fleischer ring (KF ring)
  - Sunflower cataract
  - Greenish tinge to iris
  - Golden sheen of retina

How do you investigate a case of IOFB?

- Aim:
  - To diagnose
  - To localize
  - To find out magnetic or not
  - Chemical analysis rare
- Investigations:
  - Radiologic:
    - X-rays
- Before CT, X-ray was used to detect IOFBs where detection rates were 90% for metallic, 70% for glass, and 0–15% for other materials.
- Advantage: Can detect all metals except aluminum. Hence, if aluminum is suspected, take a bone-free picture, as aluminum density is equal to that of bone.
- Disadvantages:
  - Radiation exposure.
  - <0.5 mm size foreign bodies can be missed.
  - Localization is not possible.
- Views:
  - PA view
  - Water's view (nose chin in contact with the plate)
  - Lateral view (affected side toward the film)
- Importance of localization is to plan the site of incision if scleral route surgery is contemplated.
- Various radiological methods
- With the help of marker:
  - Where AP view is taken with lead markers to localize the IOFB
- Contact lens method with a Zeiss contact lens was popularized by Coomberg
  - Disadvantages:
    - Eyeball is presumed to have AL of 24 mm.

- – Lens cannot be put in a badly perforated eye.
  - – Improper lateral view can affect the calculations.
- By geometric construction (Sweet's method)
  - Two X-rays are taken with X-ray tube in known position.
  - Two metal indicators are kept at 10 mm from corneal vertex and films from two views are taken.
  - Disadvantages:
    - – Patient has to fixate well such that the corneal vertex does not alter in position.
    - – Eyeball AL is presumed to be 24 mm.
- Stereoscopic method:
  - Marker is put on the globe and two X-rays at two fixed angles at different positions are taken.
  - Foreign body position is calculated in relation to its placement with respect to the marker.
- Bone-free X-rays (Vogt's method):
  - Dental films are used to localize aluminum foreign body.
  - Anterior segment foreign body can be localized by this method.
- Other lenses:
  - Lorac contact lens: Has a central opening and it can be held in place by rubber suction tube
  - Limbal ring: Disadvantage: AL—24 mm presumption
    - – CT scan
- Cuts suggested are 0.5–1.5 mm
- A negative CT is must before an MRI
- Advantages:
  - Allows detection of <0.5 mm IOFB.
  - Multiple IOFB can be localized.
  - Extremely sensitive method.
  - No globe manipulation.
  - Little patient cooperation is required.
  - Can distinguish between metallic and non-metallic foreign bodies.
- Disadvantages:
  - Difficult to localize radiolucent foreign bodies.
  - Metallic foreign bodies can cause scattering artifact.
    - – MRI
- Advantage: Non-metallic: Wood or plastic can be visualized.

- Disadvantage: Contraindicated in magnetic foreign bodies as they can move on exposure to the magnetic field and cause damage to intraocular structures.
  - Ultrasonography
- Diagnosis on B-scan: Acoustic highly reflective shadow with ringing phenomenon with orbital shadowing
- Diagnosis on A-scan: 100% reflective spike
- Advantages:
  - No radiation exposure.
  - <0.5 mm bodies are detected.
  - Metallic and non-metallic foreign bodies can be detected.
  - Intraocular and extraocular foreign bodies can be detected.
  - Can detect endophthalmitis, PVD, RD, VH.
- Disadvantages:
  - Not advisable in open globe injuries
  - Two-dimensional
  - Electrophysiology:
    - – To assess the visual prognosis in old retained metallic foreign bodies
    - – The height of the B-wave is diminished and the oscillatory potentials on ascending part of B-wave have reduced amplitudes
    - – More characteristic phenomenon is that ERG shows changes first in B-wave, followed by a wave, indicating siderosis toxicity moves from vitreous to inner retina.
    - – Electrophysiological changes precede visual loss.

How do you manage a case of IOFB?

- Confirm the diagnosis.
- Localize the IOFB.
- Remove IOFB—usually via PPV with intravitreal antibiotics given for prophylaxis.
- Treatment of associated complications: RD, endophthalmitis, VH, subluxated lens, cataract, iridocyclitis.
- Treatment of effects of foreign body.
- Prevention of endophthalmitis.
- Prevention of sympathetic ophthalmitis.
- Enucleation within 2 weeks of injury of badly perforated eye (if severe uveal tissue loss however controversial).
- Treatment with systemic steroids.
- Siderosis:

- Removal of IOFB
- Galvanic deactivation
- Chelating agents
  - IV EDTA
  - Desferrioxamine
- Chalcosis:
  - Removal of IOFB
  - Chelating agents
    - BAL
    - Sodium Thiosulphate
    - Sodium Hyposulphate

What are the surgical principles of IOFB removal?

- Primary repair of the perforation.
- Endophthalmitis prophylaxis with empirical antibiotics covering bacteria and fungi.
- EVS studies not applicable to this scenario.
- Use of steroids is controversial as they might cause flaring up of the infection, but it can reduce the chances of sympathetic ophthalmia.
- Localize the foreign body and its removal by selecting correct approach.
- Manage complications like VH, RD, endophthalmitis.
- Manage sympathetic ophthalmitis

What would the route of surgery in IOFB removal depend on?

- Location of foreign body:
  - Anterior segment
  - Posterior segment
    - Intravitreal
    - Subretinal

- Magnetic/non-magnetic
- Clear/opaque media
- Associated complications such as RD/endophthalmitis
- Visualization
  - Well visualized: Trans-scleral route maybe used
  - Non well visualized: Vitrectomy to be done
- Size of FB: If size of FB <5 mm, it can be retrieved via pars plana ports else a translimbal approach can be used.

What are the various approaches to its removal?

- Through pars plana vitrectomy with removal of foreign body by:
  - Rare earth magnets
  - IOFB forceps
- Through the trans-scleral approach in extreme peripheral suprachoroidal or subretinal foreign body.
- Through limbal approach with removal of even the clear lens if the foreign body measures >5 mm.

Which foreign body has a better prognosis?

- Copper has better prognosis as iron in the long run causes siderosis bulbi, which causes intra-ocular cell death.
- But copper IOFB causes a more severe inflammatory response.
- In chronic cases if vision is already lost, removal of a copper IOFB itself can cause flaring of severe inflammation hence late removal is not advisable.

7

Lens

7.1 TOPICS

- Blades in cataract surgery
- FAQs on blades in cataract surgery
- Capsulorrhexis instruments
- FAQs on capsulorrhexis
- Phacoemulsification instruments
- FAQs on phacoemulsification
- Other instruments for manual cataract extraction
- Instruments for IOL handling
- Intraocular lenses (IOLs)
- Instruments used in small-pupil cataract surgery
- Instruments used in the management of subluxated cataracts
- Historical instruments
- Femto-laser-assisted cataract surgery (FLACS)

7.2 BLADES IN CATARACT SURGERY

Identify the instrument and describe the blade and mention its uses.

15° knife

- Thickness: 0.1 mm
- Straight, sharp pointed tip
- Width of incision made: 1.7 mm
- Uses:
  - Operative:
    - Phacoemulsification, Extracapsular cataract surgery (ECCE), and Small incision cataract surgery (SICS) surgery to make paracentesis and incisions for introducing the I-A handpiece

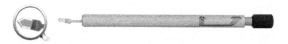

Figure 7.1 This is a 15° side port knife

- To cut sutures
  - To mark final alignment axis for toric IOLs
  - Glaucoma filtration surgeries
- Therapeutic:
  - Iridectomy
  - To drain hyphema
  - CRAO to make a paracentesis to lower the IOP

Identify the blade and describe the uses.

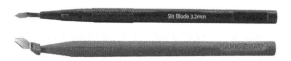

Figure 7.2 Keratome blade

- Triangular blade with cutting edges
- Available in 2.2 mm, 2.8 mm, or 5.2 mm size
- Angled at 45° to the handle
- Uses:
  - Used for making stab incision in phacoemulsification
  - Helps make a wound with minimal force and SIA (surgically induced astigmatism)
  - 2.2 mm, 2.4 mm, 2.8 mm blade: Phacoemulsification, DSEK
  - 3.2 mm blade: SICS, IOL explantation
  - 5.2 mm blade: SICS extension of wound

Identify the instrument and describe.

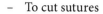

Figure 7.3 Diamond keratome

DOI: 10.1201/9781003455646-7

- 0.2 mm blade thickness
- Angled clear cornea keratome with sharp sides, tip angle at 45°
- Uses: For anterior chamber entrance, wound extension
- Advantage: Diamond keratome can be reused

Identify the instrument and describe the blade and its uses.

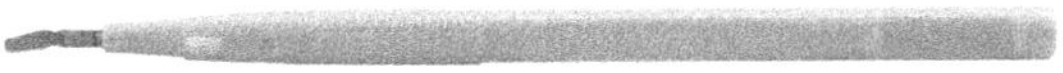

Figure 7.4 Crescent knife

- Blade with cutting and dissecting property
- 2 mm, 2.2 mm, 2.4 mm, 2.6 mm width
- Uses:
  - SICS
  - Scleral flaps in trabeculectomy
  - Pterygium surgery
  - Lamellar dissection in keratoplasty
  - Dermoid excision

Identify and describe the instrument and state the advantage of performing a limbal relaxing incision.

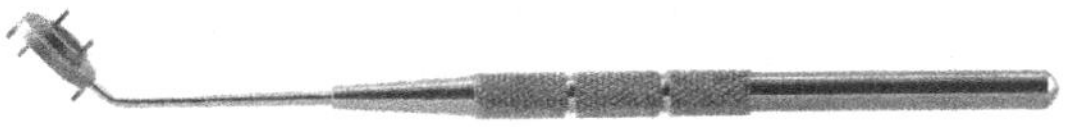

Figure 7.5 LRI marker

- Limbal relaxing incisions (LRIs) are refractive surgical procedure to correct astigmatism of 0.5 D–1.5 D
- Most used along with cataract surgery

7.3 FAQs ON BLADES IN CATARACT SURGERY

What is the astigmatic neutral funnel?

- Derived from two equations
  - Corneal surgically induced astigmatism is directly proportional to the cube of the length of the incision.
  - Corneal surgically induced astigmatism is inversely proportional to the distance of the incision from the center of the cornea.
  - The mouth of the funnel is 3.0–3.5 mm at the limbus, and it flares out posteriorly.
  - Making the incision within this funnel will result in least astigmatism.

What are the various types of tunnels made in small incision cataract surgery (SICS)?

- Straight (with or without backcuts)
- Smile
- Frown
- Chevron

Mention some complications of SICS tunnel making you may have encountered?

- Scleral buttonhole
- Superficial tunnel
- Blunt ragged blades
- High myopia due to scleral thinning
- Premature entry due to very deep wound
- Avulsion of the roof of the tunnel
- Multiple planes of tunnel
- Anterior chamber entry is not uniform

What are the types of corneal incisions made in phacoemulsification surgery?

- Clear corneal incision (CCI):
  - Triplanar
  - Biplanar
  - Uniplanar
- Limbal incision

Mention some complications of corneal incisions during phacoemulsification?

- Wound leak
- Wound burn
- Premature entry
- Long or short tunnels
- Torn tunnel

What are the indications and contraindications of LRIs?

- Indications: To correct 0.5 D–1.5.0 D of astigmatism
- Contraindications:
  - Keratoconus
  - Autoimmune disease
  - Peripheral corneal disease
  - Prior corneal surgeries, particularly incisional procedures (e.g. Radial Keratotomy)

What are the advantages and disadvantages of LRIs?

- Advantages:
  - Easy to perform
  - Quick postoperative stabilization
  - Best for low astigmatism

- Disadvantages:
  - Infection
  - Less predictability
  - Undercorrection
  - Overcorrection
  - Perforation of the cornea
  - Regression

How is the procedure performed?

- Select a nomogram and track results with said nomogram.
- Instill topical anesthetic agent.
- Mark 6 and 12 o'clock meridians on the cornea in upright position with a pen marker or with a needle.

- Usual depth range is 450–650 μm (depending on the peripheral corneal thickness which should be measured prior to avoid perforation).
- Arc-shaped incision is made in the clear cornea close to the limbus.
- Some may place the cataract incision within the LRI incision.
- Many surgeons use online surgical calculators based on preoperative keratometry and surgeons induced astigmatism (SIA).
- A commonly used nomogram developed by Dr. Louis Nichamin as mentioned below for reference.
- NAPA Nomogram: Nichamin Age & Pachymetry-Adjusted (**Tables 7.1** and **7.2**)
- Blade depth setting is at 90% of the thinnest pachymetry.

Table 7.1 With-the-Rule Astigmatism (Steep Axis 45–135°)

Pre-op Cylinder (D)	Paired Incisions in Degrees of Arc					
	20–30 years	31–40 years	41–50 years	51–60 years	61–70 years	71–80 years
0.75	40	35	35	30	30	
1	45	40	40	35	35	30
1.25	55	50	45	40	35	35
1.5	60	55	50	45	40	40
1.75	65	60	55	50	45	45
2	70	65	60	55	50	45
2.25	75	70	65	60	55	50
2.5	80	75	70	65	60	55
2.75	85	80	75	70	65	60
3	90	90	85	80	70	65

Table 7.2 Against-the-Rule Astigmatism (Steep Axis 0–44°/136–180°)

Pre-op Cylinder (D)	Paired Incisions in Degrees of Arc					
	20–30 years	31–40 years	41–50 years	51–60 years	61–70 years	71–80 years
0.75	45	40	40	35	35	30
1	50	45	45	40	40	35
1.25	55	55	50	45	40	35
1.5	60	60	55	50	45	40
1.75	65	65	60	55	50	45
2	70	70	65	60	55	50
2.25	75	75	70	65	60	55
2.5	80	80	75	70	65	60
2.75	85	85	80	75	70	65
3	90	90	85	80	75	70

What are the various other treatment options for astigmatism during cataract surgery?

- 0.5–1.5 D = LRI
- Up to 1.5 D = Opposite clear corneal incisions
- Up to 6.0 D = Toric IOLs
- > 6.0 D = Toric IOLs ± LRI or bioptics, custom toric IOLs

7.4 CAPSULORRHEXIS INSTRUMENTS

Identify the instrument and describe it. Mention the advantages of this instrument.

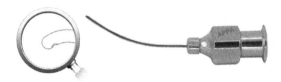

Figure 7.6 Khokhar capsule painting cannula

- 23G cannula has a curved terminal with a closed tip
- The posterior part of the polished curved part has three pores arranged in a linear fashion over 1.5 mm each
- Advantage: Minimal amount of dye is used at the appropriate plane and maintains a stable anterior chamber during staining

Identify the instrument and describe and mention the use.

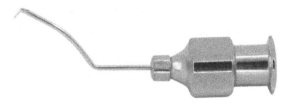

Figure 7.7 Kratz cystitome

- Sharp tipped with curve
- Hollow shaft: Shaft angled at 60°
- 2 ml syringe attached to the hub of the cystitome
- Use: For continuous curvilinear capsulorrhexis

Identify the instrument and describe.

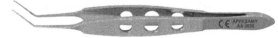

- Utrata capsulorrhexis forceps
- Angled forceps with sharp bent tip

- 45° angled (better visualization) curved shafts, tip to curve length 13.0 mm
- Use: To initiate, hold the flap and complete capsulorrhexis and hold the flap

Identify and describe the instrument.

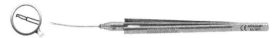

- Reverse capsulorrhexis forceps
- When you release the handle, it holds the tissue which is why it is also known as cross-action forceps.
- 21G forceps, can be introduced through a side-port incision.
- 45° tip is for better visualization.

What is the advantage over regular capsulorrhexis forceps?

- Reduced stress on interossei of the surgeon's hands while completing capsulorrhexis
- Can be done through the side port, resulting in less fluctuations of the anterior chamber
- Sharp tip of the forceps works as a cystitome

Identify and describe the instrument.

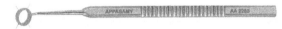

- Capsulorrhexis marker
- Designed to simplify the capsulorrhexis.
- It is used to make a mark on the cornea, which reflects on the capsule; this helps create an adequately sized capsulorrhexis.
- Sizes range depends on the size of the capsulorrhexis required.

7.5 FAQs ON CAPSULORRHEXIS

What are the techniques are used to make a continuous curvilinear capsulorrhexis (CCC)?

- Needle cystitome (preferably bent 26G needle)
- Utrata capsulorrhexis forceps, microrrhexis forceps
- Femtosecond-laser-assisted cataract surgery (FLACS)
- Zepto nano-pulse precision capsulotomy
- Fugo blade

What is the ideal size of capsulorrhexis?

- Approximately 5 to 5.5 mm
- Should cover the optic of the IOL by 0.5 mm circumferentially

What are the types of forces while making a capsulorrhexis?

- Ripping forces:
  - Many fibers are pulled at different angles and with differing force.
  - The breakpoint will not be simultaneous.
  - Tear is uncontrolled.
- Shearing forces:
  - One fiber is broken at a time.
  - Tear is more controlled.
  - Requires less force.

What are the advantages and disadvantages of a larger capsulorrhexis?

- Advantage: Better nuclear maneuverability in SICS surgery
- Disadvantages:
  - Decreased IOL instability
  - Less risk of PCO
  - Peapod effect, where the optic pushes forward from the bag

What are the advantages and disadvantages of a small capsulorrhexis?

- Advantages:
  - Greater IOL stability
- Disadvantages:
  - Increased risk of capsular phimosis
  - High risk of bag instability while dialing the lens out during SICS
  - More chances of PCO

What are the indications of a small or large capsulorrhexis?

- Small capsulorrhexis:
  - Subluxated cataracts
  - Intumescent cataracts
- Large capsulorrhexis:
  - In dense brown/black cataracts, very soft cataracts
  - Retinitis pigmentosa (due to increased chances of subsequent capsular bag phimosis)

What are the various dyes used to stain the anterior capsule?

- Trypan blue (0.5%)
- Indocyanine green (0.1%)
- Fluorescein sodium
- Techniques for staining:
  - Staining from above under an air bubble
  - Intracameral sub-capsular injection of the dye with or without blue light enhancement
  - Soft-shell stain technique described by Akahoshi
  - Dye solution can be mixed with viscoelastic agents
- Adverse effects:
  - Trypan blue should be avoided in pregnant women due to possible teratogenic effects (animal studies)
  - Hydrophilic acrylic lenses having a high-water content (>70%) may get permanently stained on contact with trypan blue.
  - Should be avoided in patients with sub-luxated lens as the dye passes through the area of sub-luxation to stain the posterior capsule compromising the surgical view.

7.6 PHACOEMULSIFICATION INSTRUMENTS

Identify and describe the following instrument.

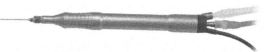

- Phacoemulsification handpiece
- Metal handpiece is used in the surgery of phacoemulsification.
- The body has two, four, or six piezoelectric crystals for ultrasonic power generation.
- The frequency varies between 35 and 40 kHz (35,000–40,000 strokes/second)
- It has three tubings: one for infusion, one for aspiration, and one an electric line for creation of ultrasound energy.

Identify and describe this part.

- Silicone chamber or test chamber
- Collapsible silicone chamber

- Filled with BSS
- Used during tuning of the phacoemulsification handpiece.
- If during surgery the tip is blocked with a nuclear piece, it can be remove using the phacoemulsification sleeve while applying energy in foot pedal 3.

Identify the following phacoemulsification instrument? What is it used for?

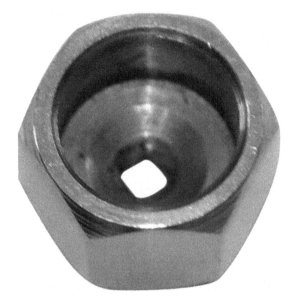

- Wrench
- Device used to remove and fix phacoemulsification tips to the handpiece
- Has a screw like mechanism
- Is usually specific to various handpieces and tips of different manufacturers
- Different designs are available for various company tips
- Use: To change or tighten the tip to the phacoemulsification handpiece

Identify the instrument and describe.

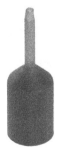

Silicone Sleeve mounted on Phacoemulsification Tip.

- Sleeve
- Material: Silicone
- Sizes: 19G, 20G, 21G, 23G
- Has two lateral holes at the side for irrigation
- Uses:
  - Insulation and protection of sclerocorneal tissue from thermal/mechanical damage
  - Prevents leak from corneal phacoemulsification wound
  - Keeps phacoemulsification energy localized at the tip
- Modifications
  - Double walled sleeve (e.g., Mackool system of Alcon)
  - Polyamide (Alcon) and Teflon (Surgic) coating between the tip and silicone sleeve decreases friction between tip and sleeve

What is sleeveless phacoemulsification?

- Phacoemulsification is performed with a tip without a sleeve thus reducing the incision size to sub 1 mm.

Describe the following instruments.

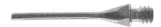

Figure 7.15 Phacoemulsification Tip

- Tip
- Made of titanium
- 20 mm in length
- Angulation of cutting end of the tip can vary from 0° to 60°
- Larger angle tips help in better excavation and better cutting
- Small-angle tips help produce quick occlusion and buildup of vacuum providing better hold
- Distal opening is for aspiration
- Lateral openings are for irrigation
- Uses:
  - Acoustic energy produced in the handpiece is transmitted to the tip which ultimately emulsifies the nucleus
- Types of tips:
  - Standard
  - Kelman
  - Mackool

- Aspiration bypass system (ABS)
- Cobra
- TurboSonics tip

What is the diameter of a tip?

- Tip diameter is variable.
- Internal diameter:
  - Standard: 0.9 mm (20G tip)
  - Micro tip: 0.5 to 0.7 mm
- Advantages:
  - Smaller wound of entry
  - Reduction of surge
  - Easier to occlude
- Disadvantages:
  - Less ability to aspirate and hold nuclear fragments
  - Requires more levels of vacuum

Identify and describe these tips.

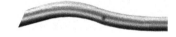

Figure 7.16 Intrepid balanced tip

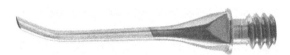

Figure 7.17 Kelman tip

- Manufactured by Alcon Laboratories for the Centurion Vision System Phacoemulsification machine
- Has enhanced sideways tip displacement at the tip end and greatly reduced tip action along the shaft
- Therefore, more efficient in reducing thermal damage at wound
- Lower CDE (cumulative dissipated energy) was observed with the balanced tip as compared to the Kelman tip
- Axis is bent at 22.5°, 3.5 mm from the tip
- Downward angulation ideal for hard cataracts in deep-set eyes
- Kelman flared tip: Bell-shaped tip the flare allows more power transmission; therefore, it provides better hold for hard cataracts.
- Advantages:
  - Less clogging
  - Better tissue holding
  - Easier occlusion

Identify the instrument.

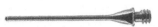

Figure 7.18 Fragmatome needle

- Used for removal of dropped nuclear fragments

How do you differentiate a fragmatome needle from a phacoemulsification tip?

- Fragmatome is longer (22.5 mm) than a tip

Mention some energy delivery systems you know of.

- Centurion (Alcon): OZiL ultrasound delivery, which utilizes both longitudinal and torsional energy delivery systems.
- Whitestar Signature (AMO): Has both Longitudinal and transversal or elliptical (Ellips) ultrasound delivery systems.

Identify and describe the instrument.

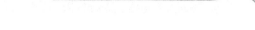

Figure 7.19 A: Sharp tip B: Blunt tip Chopper

- Round bodied with blunt or sharp tip
- Blunt tips are better for peripheral (horizontal) chopping whereas sharp which are better for direct (vertical) chopping
- Uses:
  - To divide the nucleus during phacoemulsification (horizontal or vertical)
  - Stabilizes the globe
  - Can rotate the nucleus
  - Feed nuclear pieces to the tip

Identify and describe the instrument.

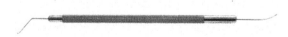

Figure 7.20 Friedman-Koch universal chopper spatula

- Uses of the chopper:
  - Double cutting surface enhances chopping
  - Rounded tip protects posterior capsule
  - Can be used by a left- or right-handed surgeon

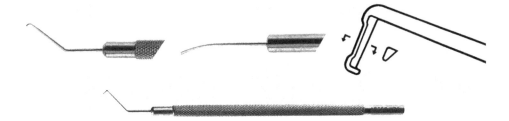

Figure 7.21 Olson chopper

- Uses of the spatula:
  - Manipulation of nucleus and epinuclear fragments
  - Notch of spatula can stretch iris and break posterior synechiae

Identify and describe the instrument.

- Blunt tip to protect posterior capsule
- Inner long cutting edge
- Front surface has two raised portions, which act as iris retractor
- Good for horizontal chop

Identify and describe the instrument.

Figure 7.22 Nagahara chopper

- Angled shaft, 45 degrees
- Flat interior cutting edge

Identify and describe the instrument.

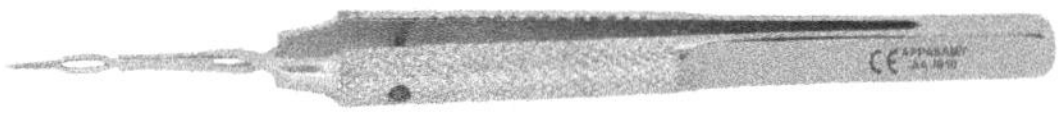

Figure 7.23 Akahoshi prechopper

- Prechopper: For directly inserting in core of nucleus for cracking the nucleus, thus avoiding the need of sculpting and therefore reduces phacoemulsification time
- A pin-and-rocker mechanism in the prechopper neck keeps tips together when the forceps are closed
- Inserted through a side-port incision or micro-phaco incision

Identify and describe the instrument.

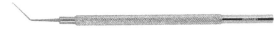

Figure 7.24 Sinskey hook

- Round body instrument with straight or angled shaft
- Has a 0.18–0.2 mm diameter blunt bent tip
- Tip to angle length is 10.0 mm
- Uses
  - To prolapse the nucleus from the bag into anterior chamber in SICS
  - As a chopper during phacoemulsification in soft/medium density nuclei
  - IOL dialing and centering
  - IOL explantation
  - Mark the visual axis before LASIK
  - Insertion of CTR/CTS

Identify and describe the instrument.

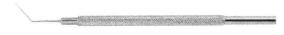

Figure 7.25 Reverse Sinskey hook

- Sinskey should not be confused with reverse Sinskey hook used for endothelial scoring in DSEK surgery

Identify and describe the instrument.

Figure 7.26 Osher Y-hook

- Blunt two pronged tips
- Use: To mechanically dilate the pupil by stretching it prior to phacoemulsification

What are the various instruments used in cortex removal?

- Irrigation and aspiration ports located on a single handpiece.
- Tip can be straight or angled, up to 90° for easier sub-incisional cortex removal.
- Tips may have roughened surfaces or are made from silicone to allow for posterior capsular polishing.
- Sleeve can be made of metal or silicone.
- Irrigation Aspiration (IA) handpiece is generally thinner than the phacoemulsification handpiece; therefore, a well-constructed main wound is crucial to minimize the efflux of fluid around a metal handpiece.

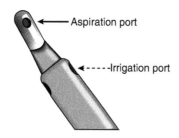

Figure 7.27 Unimanual/coaxial

- Aspiration port: 0.3 mm
- Irrigation port: 0.5 mm
- Irrigation maintains chamber integrity
- For pediatric cataracts and for patients with low scleral rigidity
- Uses
  - To remove cortex prior to IOL placement, easier subincisinoal cortex aspiration

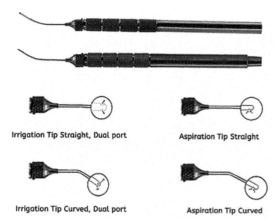

Figure 7.28 Bimanual irrigation and aspiration

- For removal of viscoelastic material after IOL placement
- Posterior capsular polishing

7.7 FAQs ON PHACOEMULSIFICATION

Describe the various parts of the phacoemulsification instrumentation.

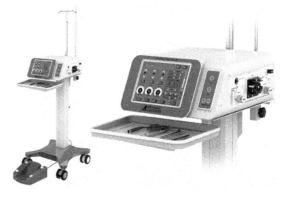

- Phacoemulsification machine
  - Machine with sensors that controls inflow and outflow of fluid
  - Delivers electrical energy to the handpiece
  - Foot pedal connected to the machine. Excursion of the foot pedal decides what happens at the phacoemulsification tip:
    - Step 1: Irrigation
    - Step 2: Irrigation + aspiration
    - Step 3: Irrigation + aspiration + phaco-emulsification energy delivery
- Phacoemulsification handpiece
  - Phaco instrumentation consists of ultrasonic handpiece having a transducer and a titanium tip.
  - Usually, tips have varying number of crystals (four–six).
  - The piezoelectric property of these crystals (quartz) is used to expand and contract when an electric current is delivered.
  - Frequency: 27–60 kHz, cannot be changed for a given machine.
  - Stroke length: It is the excursion of the tip in a longitudinal direction (1.5–3.75 milli inches), which is altered when one increases the phacoemulsification power.
  - Tip delivers ultrasound energy and aspirates (i.e., vacuum).

- Surrounding the tip is the sleeve, which allows for irrigation around the tip lowering the resulting temperature.
- Irrigation typically exits the sleeve from side ports.
- Tip angulation refers to the shaft of the tip.
- These may either be straight (0° tips) or angled.
- The bevel of the tip determines the slant at the tip opening (30°, 45°).

- Irrigation and aspiration systems:
  - Importance:
    - Maintaining intraocular pressure
    - Maintaining temperature and keeping the handpiece cool
    - Providing anterior chamber depth
    - Ideally, fluid lost from the eye due to aspiration and fluid leaks should equal the fluid entering the eye through irrigation.
  - Aspiration flow rate (AFR):
    - The rate of removal fluid from the eye
    - Measured when phacoemulsification tip is not occluded
    - Controls followability of pieces
  - Vacuum:
    - Helps in holding pieces at the tip to emulsify
    - Force of suction at the tip
    - Created by the pump
    - Only occurs when tip is occluded
    - Both AFR and vacuum are a function of the phacoemulsification system pump
- Aspiration:
  - Peristaltic system (flow based, ml/min):
    - A negative pressure, and therefore vacuum, is created by rotation of the rollers by the pump which pinches the silicon tubing by drawing fluid
    - The faster the rollers rotate, more is the fluid withdrawn, therefore producing a higher flow rate.
    - Aspiration flow rate and vacuum can be set independently in a peristaltic system unlike the venturi system.
    - Vacuum will be built up only after the tip is occluded.

- Venturi system (vacuum based, mmHg):
  - Compressed gas creates vacuum, inside a closed chamber.
  - The vacuum is transmitted to a handpiece.
  - The level of vacuum developed in the cassette depends on the amount and speed of the gas.
  - The amount of vacuum generated is controlled by the foot pedal (Not AFR).
  - Here the flow rate is a fixed fraction of the vacuum.
  - Advantage: Vacuum is directly transmitted to the tip therefore there is better followability.

Describe the modes of phacoemulsification?

- Conventional/longitudinal US mode:
  - The ultrasound power to emulsify the lens is derived from the longitudinal excursion of the phacoemulsification needle.
  - Phacoemulsification tip moves forward and backward at a high frequency in a jackhammer manner.
  - May sometimes induce repulsion of the pieces at the tip as it pushes the nucleus away with each stroke as it moves forward.
  - Thus, the efficiency of phacoemulsification is compromised.
- Torsional phacoemulsification:
  - Alcon surgical incorporated OZil torsional into the Infiniti Vision System in January 2016
  - Includes a handpiece that produces rotary oscillations of the phacoemulsification tip at a frequency of 32 kHz
  - Reduces the amount of energy required to emulsify the nucleus

What are the various mechanisms in which phacoemulsification occurs?

- Jackhammer energy
- Cavitation energy
- Acoustic energy
- Thermal energy

What are the various power settings?

- Fixed continuous mode:
  - Power is fixed according to hardness of nucleus and remains same throughout position 3 of foot pedal.

- Linear continuous mode:
  - Power is regulated from foot pedal. The greater the depression, the greater the amount of power delivered within position 3 of the foot pedal.
- Pulse mode:
  - In pulse mode each pulse of energy is followed by a gap of equal duration (on and off cycles), the frequency of the pulses is fixed, the energy delivered in each pulse depends on the amount the pedal is pressed in a linear fashion.
  - The power is delivered at preset intervals, the frequency of which is preset and decided by the surgeon.
  - The duration of on and off time can also be decided by the operator, which is called duty cycle (DC), thereby further reducing heat generation and increasing followability.
- Burst mode
  - Power delivery is in bursts.
  - Each burst has same power.
  - Interval between the bursts decreases as foot pedal is further depressed.
  - Where maximum power is delivered at intervals, which vary with the amount one depresses the foot pedal.

Phaco continuous

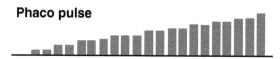

Phaco burst

Phaco pulse

- Modified pulse mode
  - E.g. Whitestar, Hyperpulse
  - Range of pulse rates (20–120 pulses/sec) and adjustable pulse duration (4–30 ms)
  - The rapid short pulses produce relatively more transient cavitation that increases ultrasound efficiency of emulsification—these facilities improved followability and thermal protection

What is surge?

- Collapse of the anterior chamber due to temporary persistence of high-pressure gradient between aspiration line and anterior chamber following release of occlusion.
- Results in uncontrollable amount of fluid aspirated into the tubing
- Factors controlling surge
  - Vacuum level: Higher surge with higher vacuum
  - Tip size: Smaller lumen restricts fluid during surge
  - Sleeve size: Larger sleeve allows more fluid during surge
  - Infusion pressure: Higher bottle pushes more fluid into the eye
  - Tubing compliance: Softer tubing causes more surge
  - Diameter of aspiration line: Less diameter, less surge

What are the mechanisms to control surge?

- Venting:
  - Main anti-collapse system
  - Machine has a sensor which detects occlusion break and releases fluid/air
  - Activated upon release of foot pedal
  - Immediate release of tissue aspirated accidentally
- Surgeon:
  - Decreasing the flow rate
  - Increasing the irrigation
  - Use of AC maintainer
  - Proper wound construction
- Less compliant tubing
- Aspiration bypass system (ABS) tip: When occlusion occurs fluid flows through the ABS hole
- Partial occlusion phacoemulsification: Micropulse phacoemulsification is used to avoid total occlusion thus preventing surge. The nuclear fragment is brought close to the tip with a 4-millisecond period of aspiration until the fragment partially occludes it. With the onset of the 4-millisecond burst of phacoemulsification energy, the fragment is emulsified before it can totally occlude the tip. Therefore, flow never falls to zero and vacuum never builds to maximum preventing surge.

- CASE technology: The Signature (J & J) phacoemulsification machine has the CASE (Continuous Anterior Segment Evaluation) technology. When the vacuum reaches a pre-determined threshold, the system reacts, within 26 milliseconds, by reducing the vacuum to a second, lower level that has been pre-set. This adjustment aims to enhance cataract stability in the eye's chamber during surgery and has demonstrated a reduction in post-occlusion surge.

What is reflux?

- Backward flow of fluid into the eye from the aspiration line
- Used to release material, which is caught in the aspiration port, e.g., posterior capsule or iris
- Mechanism:
  - Inverting direction of aspiration pump
  - Blocking aspiration line and opening second infusion line connected to it
- Disadvantage: Risk of contamination

What is chopping?

- Technique of nuclear management during phacoemulsification

What are the advantages of chopping?

- Can manage hard cataracts
- Decreased phacoemulsification time
- Decreased chances of corneal burns
- Decreased turbulence
- Increased efficiency of ultrasound

What are the various chopping techniques? (Table 7.3)

Table 7.3 Chopping Techniques

Horizontal Chop	Vertical Chop
Needs a large, dilated pupil so that equator of lens can be viewed	Can be done through a small pupil
Need to go underneath the capsulorrhexis	Not required to go underneath the capsulorrhexis
All grades of cataract can be chopped	Mainly used for chopping hard nuclei

7.8 OTHER INSTRUMENTS FOR MANUAL CATARACT EXTRACTION

Identify and describe the instrument.

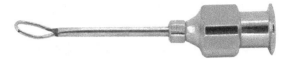

Figure 7.31 Irrigating vectis

- One forward and two reverse irrigating ports
- Used for nucleus delivery during ECCE/SICS

Non-irrigating vectis

- Nucleus delivery in dislocated lens or after PCR for removal of nucleus/nuclear fragments

Identify and describe the instrument.

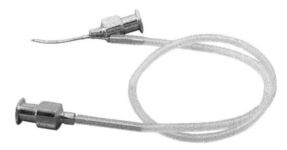

Figure 7.32 A–B Simcoe irrigation and aspiration cannula

- Two ports:
  - 23G front opening irrigation port
  - Has a 15 mm long 0.3 mm diameter aspiration port
- Aspiration through tubing hub attached to a 2 or 5 ml syringe and irrigation through Luer-lock hub
- Other models: Reverse Simcoe, U-shaped Simcoe (right- and left-sided)

Identify and describe the instrument.

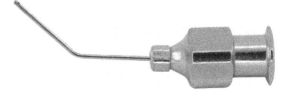

Figure 7.33 Single-port aspiration cannula

- Used for aspiration of cortex in SICS with AC maintainer by Blumenthal technique

Identify and describe the instrument.

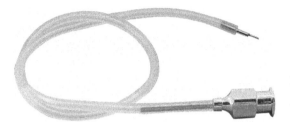

Figure 7.34 AC maintainer

- No flange
- Has serrations
- Do not confuse it with the infusion sleeves used in vitreoretinal surgery
- Uses:
  - To maintain the anterior chamber stability during SICS in Blumenthal technique
  - Suprachoroidal hemorrhage drainage
  - Used with single-port aspiration cannula

Identify and describe the instrument.

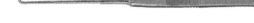

Figure 7.35 A Smith lens expressor

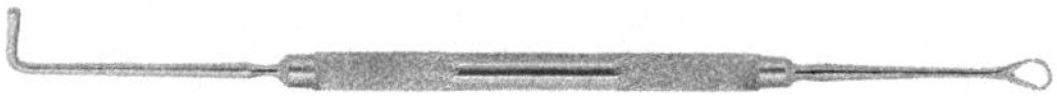

Figure 7.35 B Kirby lens expressor and spatula

- Use: To manually express the nucleus in ECCE

Identify and describe the instrument.

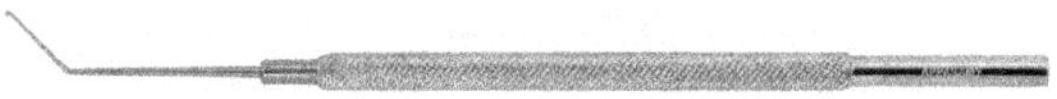

Figure 7.36 Mackool–Kuglen hook and IOL rotator

- Has a hemispherical ball at the tip which is 0.8 mm
- Rotator tip with an angled shaft
- Uses:
  - To dial and center IOLs especially which has no dialing hole

- IOL explantation
- Nucleus delivery into the AC in SICS surgery
- Better safety profile as less chances are there of damaging the PC in comparison to Sinskey hook
- Can also be used to retrieve sutures form the anterior chamber

Identify and describe the instrument.

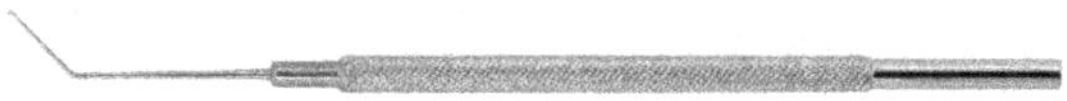

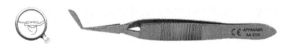

Figure 7.37 Lester lens manipulator

- Straight shaft with 0.2 mm hourglass shape tip
- Use: For IOL manipulation

Identify and describe the instrument.

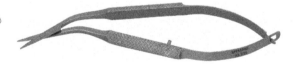

Figure 7.38 Faulkner lens inserting forceps

- Use: Holding and inserting soft IOLs through small incisions

Identify and describe the instrument.

Figure 7.39 Soft IOL cutter

- 6 mm long blades; for cutting soft IOLs
- Lower blade is fixed and goes under the IOL, and upper blade moves, so surgeon can see the movement

Identify and describe the following instrument.

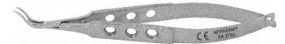

Figure 7.40 Akahoshi IOL scissors

- Use: To cut acrylic lenses

Identify and describe the instrument.

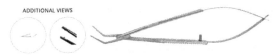

Figure 7.41 Implant removal forceps

- Angled, cross-action, thin shafts
- Tooth in top jaw with grooves in bottom jaw
- Designed to grasp the lens optic or lens segment to efficiently remove from the anterior chamber

Identify and describe the following injectors?

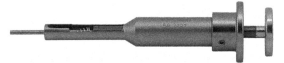

- Plunger or screw-style IOL injector
- Slot for insertion of cartridge which contains the IOL
- Metallic injectors are reusable but preloaded; disposable injectors are also available
- Used to inject loaded foldable intraocular lens

Identify and describe this.

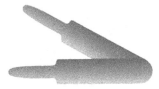

- **Lens glide**
- Double-ended
- Made of polypropylene
- Narrow end used during phacoemulsification
- Broader end used during manual cataract surgery
- Use: To guide the lens out of the AC or the guide the IOL into the bag during IOL placement.

7.9 INTRAOCULAR LENSES (IOLs)

What are the various materials used to make IOLs?

- Rigid: PMMA
  - Water content <1%
  - Refractive index = 1.49
  - Usually, single piece

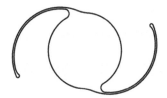

Figure 7.44 PMMA IOL

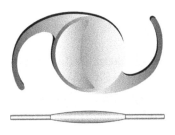

Figure 7.45 Hydrophilic acrylic posterior chamber foldable IOL

- Flexible materials
  - Silicones
  - Acrylic
  - Hydrophilic
  - Hydrophobic
  - Hydrogen
  - Collamers

Identify and describe these following IOLs.

- Rigid
- Inert
- Optic size: 6–6.5 mm
- Overall size: 12.5–13.5 mm
- Refractive index: 1.47–1.55
- Advantages
  - Cheap
  - Higher memory retention (retaining original capsular bag shape)
  - Can be placed in sulcus in case of posterior capsular dehiscence

Hydrophilic acrylic posterior chamber IOL

- Single- or three-piece IOLs
- May have C loops or plate haptics
- Higher incidence of PCO than silicone IOLs
- Good uveal and capsular biocompatibility
- Dipped in physiological saline

Hydrophobic acrylic posterior chamber IOL

- Could be single- or three-piece
- Hydrophobic acrylic is a copolymer of phenyl ethyl acrylate (PEA) and phenyl ethyl methacrylate (PEMA)
- Has higher memory and rigidity
- Better optics than hydrophilic, which remains more pliable in aqueous environment of eye

Mention some of the known modifications made to IOLs.

- Blue-blocking IOLs
  - Blue-light filtering IOLs attenuate wavelengths up to 500 nm
  - UV and visible wavelengths up to 600 nm are capable of photochemically damaging the retina
  - Human lens provides some protection against phototoxicity and removing the lens removes this protective barrier
  - Risk for ARMD and choroidal melanomas may potentially increase
  - Blue-light filtering IOLs attenuate wavelengths up to 500 nm
  - To mimic the protective yellow pigments of the crystalline lens chromophores are included within the IOL
  - Disadvantage: Blue-light-filtering lenses could theoretically decrease melatonin production, which may cause sleep disturbances
- Square edge IOLs: Mechanical barrier for cellular proliferation to prevent posterior capsular opacification (PCO)
- Aspheric IOLs:
  - IOL has a prolate surface, which induces negative spherical aberrations, which neutralize the positive spherical aberrations of the cornea
  - Done to increase contrast sensitivity under mesopic conditions

Identify and describe the following IOL and classify its various types.

- Refractive:
  - Refractive models reach multifocality by their different refractive power annular zones
  - Sometimes the near vision provided by them is inadequate
  - Pupil dependent
  - Sensitive to centration defects
- Diffractive:
  - Diffractive models are composed by diffractive microstructures in concentric zones that get closer to each other as they distance from the center
  - Sometimes the intermediate vision provided by them is inadequate
  - Not very pupil dependent
  - More tolerant to centering defects
- Combined

What is apodization?

- Principle: Based on the greater need for distance vision in conditions of dim illumination (when pupils are large)
- There is a gradual reduction in diffractive step heights from center to periphery and a subsequent distance-dominant lens for large pupil
- In addition, a greater focus of light to the distant focal point reduces the defocused near light with its subsequent visual phenomena of glare and halos

Mention some refractive technology multifocal intraocular lenses.

- Mplus (Oculentis) +3
- Mplus X (Oculentis)
- Rayner M-flex

Mention some diffractive technology multifocal intraocular lenses.

- Fine Vision (PhysIOL): Neutral asphericity; near add: +3.5/trifocal/+1.75
- ReStor (Alcon): −0.1—0.2 asphericity; near add: +4/+3/+2.5
- Seelens MF (Hanita): Neutral asphericity; near add: +3
- Tecnis MF (J & J): −0.27 asphericity; near add: +4/+3.25/+2.75

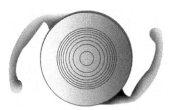

Figure 7.46 Multifocal IOL

Mention their advantages and disadvantages of multifocal IOLs.

- Advantages: Spectacle independence for distance, intermediate and near vision
- Disadvantages:
  - Patient dissatisfaction occurs sometimes due to posterior capsule opacification (PCO), residual ametropia, IOL decentration, dry eye, inadequate pupil size, and wavefront abnormalities
  - Decrease in contrast due to splitting of available light
  - Photic phenomenon—glare and halos sometimes occurs.
  - Dysphotopsias

What are extended depth focus IOLs? How are they different from multifocal IOLs?

- Tecnis Symfony IOL (J & J) is the first FDA-approved lens.
- AcrySof Vivity (Alcon): Non-diffractive extended depth of focus IOL with Alcon's proprietary non-diffractive X-WAVE technology.
- Known to enhance intermediate and near vision.
- Creates a single, contiguous, elongated focal point that enhances depth of focus

What are trifocal IOLs?

- Trifocal diffractive lenses address the intermediate vision limitations of multifocal IOLs.
- The FineVision® (FV) IOL (PhysIOL, Liège, Belgium): It is a hydrophilic acrylic IOL with a 6.15 mm optical diameter which has 26 diffractive rings across the entire optic; the lens provides 1.75 and 3.5 D add powers.
- AcrySof® Panoptix® IOL (Alcon, Fort Worth, TX, USA): It is a hydrophobic acrylic IOL with a 6.0 mm optical diameter. It has a central 4.5 mm region with 15 diffractive rings. It has an outer annulus that is purely refractive.

Identify and describe the following IOL.

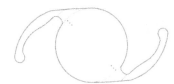

Figure 7.47 Toric IOL

- Toric IOLs are used to correct pre-existing corneal astigmatism
- Indications: Pre-existing corneal astigmatism in a range of 1 D–6 D
- Contraindications:
  - Subluxated cataracts
  - Irregular corneal astigmatism due to advanced ectatic corneal disorders
  - Patients having undergone VR surgery, glaucoma surgeries
  - PC rupture during surgery as it will not ensure stable bag IOL complex postoperatively.

Identify the following instrument.

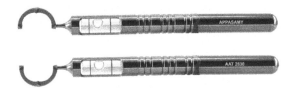

Figure 7.48 Preoperative toric IOL marker

- Preoperative markings for toric IOL placement.
- Bubble level aids in accurately marking the eye temporarily.
- Used temporarily to make 0°, 90°, and 180° reference marks on the cornea.
- Bubble is sensitive to 0.5° to confirm the horizontal axis.
- Bubble marker is sensitive to steam sterilization and can be cleaned using alcohol swabs.

Identify the following instrument.

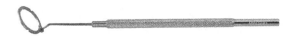

Figure 7.49 Yeoh thin toric gauge

- Markings are at every 5°.
- Four slots are at 0°, 90°, 180°, and 270°.
- Slots at 0° and 180° are for the inner ring.
- Slots at 90° and 270° are for the outer ring.
- Surgeon can insert a marking pen tip in the slot for marking.

Identify the following instrument.

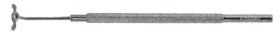

Figure 7.50 Appa axis marker

- Marking blades are curved to conform to the globe
- Used along with the gauge to mark the final alignment axis
- Marks at 3, 6, and 9 o'clock

How does one place a toric IOL?

- Reference marks to identify the horizontal and vertical meridian are made on the limbus.
- Reference marks account for cyclorotation (usually 2–4°); however, some patients may have up to 15° of cyclorotation from sitting to standing position.
- Marking the eye in sitting position ensures correct IOL orientation.
- Done with toric pre-markers designed for marking the reference axes preoperatively.
- Under the operating microscope two marks are made—axis of the incision and axis of IOL alignment.
- Limbus must be dry before making these marks as wet tissue causes the ink to spread to a span of around 10° making axis identification difficult.
- The IOL is rotated until it is 5° or 10° shy of the final desired axis of orientation.
- The viscoelastic is then removed from the eye.
- Once the viscoelastic is removed, the final orientation is achieved.
- The three dots on the IOL must be perfectly aligned with the marks on the limbus.

Identify the instrument.

- Toric lens manipulator

- Allows gentle positioning of the lens under the iris plane
- Tip maximizes surface contact with the IOL which allows for easy manipulation

What are the causes of residual astigmatism after placing a toric IOL?

- Preoperative measurement errors
- Incorrect marking of reference points on the cornea
- Incorrect placement of the IOL
- Failure to take into account the impact of surgically induced astigmatism
- Incorrect IOL power at the corneal plane
- Measurement variability
- Failure to account for posterior corneal astigmatism
- Incomplete viscoelastic removal leading to IOL rotation
- IOL rotation post-operatively

What are the options to treat it?

- Redialing the IOL post-surgery
- Excimer laser ablation with LASIK/PRK
- Incisional treatment with LRI
- Glasses or contact lenses

Do you know of any newer methods of toric alignment?

- Verion image-guided system
  - Manufactured by Alcon.
  - It is a modified keratometer which captures a high-resolution image that automatically detects scleral vessels, pupil, iris, and other features and shows where the steep axis is relative to a picture of the eye.
  - The data captured by this reference unit is displayed in the Verion digital marker, which is compatible with the LenSx laser and some microscopes.

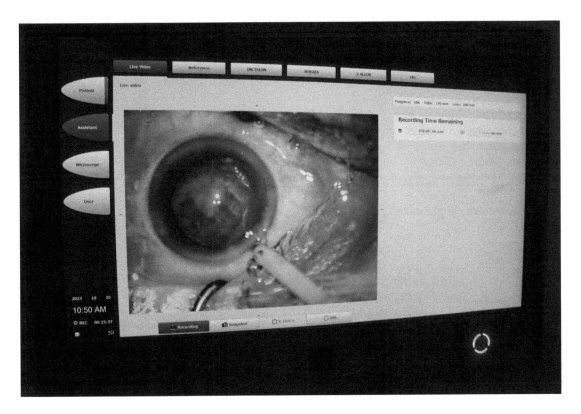

Figure 7.52 Callisto Eye

- Callisto Eye
  - Manufactured by Carl Zeiss Meditec
  - IOL Master captures an image of the eye while taking measurements
  - The information is transferred to the Callisto eye system
- Osher Toric Alignment System
  - Manufactured by Eye Photo Systems
  - During the initial pre-op examination, a detailed, high-resolution photograph of the dilated pupil is captured.
  - Iris fingerprinting is employed to improve the accuracy of toric implant alignment.
  - The Osher Toric Alignment System utilizes a Zeiss microscope's eyepiece to overlay templates of planned surgical incisions, limbal relaxing incisions, the capsulorrhexis, and the toric lens target axis onto the eye.

Identify and describe the following IOL.

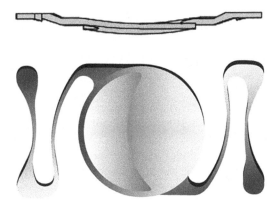

- Anterior chamber IOL
- PMMA material
- Optic diameter: 5.5 mm
- Haptic design: Kelman Multiflex
- Overall diameter: 12–13 mm

- Equiconvex
- Vault: Usually about 0.5 mm

What are the contraindications of ACIOL placement?

- Peripheral anterior synechiae
- Reduced endothelial cell count (Fuchs endo-thelial dystrophy)
- Shallow anterior chamber
- Lack of iris tissue

What are the steps in placement and orientation of the AC IOL?

- Power:
  - AC IOL has a lower power than PC IOL.
  - The A constant for the AC IOL takes this into account, so if the IOL printout includes an AC IOL A constant, use that IOL power after checking that the A constant is correct (usually written on the lens box).
  - Power is roughly 3 D less than that power of the PCIOL (in the bag).
- Determine the AC IOL diameter
  - Measure the limbal white-to-white (WTW) diameter on the axis of IOL placement (usually horizontal) and add 1 mm to this measurement.
  - The AC IOL length should be 1 mm greater than the measured WTW diameter.
- Induce miosis
- Perform a peripheral iridectomy (PI)
- May or may not use a sheets glide to insert the ACIOL.
- Kelman–McPherson forceps grasp the lens by the trailing haptic and about a third of the optic and insert it into the AC.
- Kelman Multiflex ACIOL is specifically designed to be placed in the correct orientation according to its vault.
- The haptics should form the bottom half of a reverse Z.

What are the complications of ACIOLs?

- Pseudophakic bullous keratopathy (endothelial decompensation)
- Glaucoma
- Peripheral anterior synechiae
- Uveitis-glaucoma-hyphema syndrome (UGH syndrome)
- Cystoid macular edema (CME)

Identify and describe the following IOL.

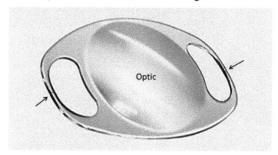

- Iris claw IOL
- PMMA material
- Usually in the shape of one side being convex and the other concave (concave side toward iris) with enclavation slits on either side
- Haptic design: Spherical
- Size varies from 5.5 mm × 8–9 mm

Identify and describe the instrument.

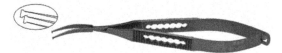

- Iris claw holding forceps
- Holds the optic of the iris claw lens during implantation

Identify and describe this instrument used in iris claw IOL insertion.

- Enclavation rod
- Enclaves the iris tissue in haptics of iris claw lens

What are the indications and contraindications for insertion of the iris claw IOL?

- Indications:
  - Absence of PC support
  - Zonular dialysis
  - Intracapsular aphakia
- Contraindications:
  - Absence of adequate iris support
  - Uveitis
  - Psuedoexfoliation

What are the types of Iris claw IOL? Mention their advantages and disadvantages.

- Anterior chamber iris claw IOL: Enclaving cleft is on superior aspect of the haptics

- Posterior chamber iris claw IOL: Enclaving cleft at 180° away from each other on the terminal ends of the haptics
  - Advantage: Some endothelial cell loss may occur; however, there are less chances of endothelial decompensation than ACIOL
  - Disadvantages:
    - Pupillary distortion
    - Glaucoma
    - CME
    - Iritis
    - Pupillary block
    - IOL dislocation
    - Astigmatism due to large size incision

Identify and describe the IOL.

- Scleral fixated IOL (SFIOL)
- IOLs which have eyelets to facilitate suture fixation
- Alcon: CZ70BD PMMA has eyelets in the haptics
- Bausch & Lomb: Akreos AO60 hydrophilic acrylic lens contains four eyelets for four-point fixation
- Bausch & Lomb: enVista MX60 hydrophobic acrylic IOL contains eyelets at the two haptic-optic junctions

What are the other ways of providing scleral fixation for IOLs?

- Knots tied directly to three-piece IOLs
- Dislocated IOL capsular bag complex can be sutured directly to the capsular bag

What are the various fixation techniques you know of?

- Ab externo suture fixation
  - Sutures are passed from the outside to the inside of the eye.
  - Suture needles: Straight (STC-6), which provides longer range of access, or curved (CIF-4 or CTC-6), which provides a more rigid needle.
- Ab interno suture fixation
  - Suture is passed from inside to outside the eye.

- Sutureless scleral fixation
  - Haptics of the IOL are externalized with a hollow needle or 25G forceps and fixed without the use of sutures.
  - After the haptics are externalized, scleral flaps are closed with 10-0 nylon or fibrin glue.
- Hoffman pockets
  - Make a scleral pocket by making a scleral tunnel from a clear corneal incision.
  - A double-armed suture is then passed through the conjunctiva and scleral pocket.
  - The suture ends can be retrieved through the external corneal incision.
  - The knots are then buried within the pocket.

What are the complications of SFIOLs?

- Corneal edema
- Retinal detachment
- Intraocular hemorrhage (due to the passage of suture through uveal tissue)
- Suture erosion and infection (due to externalized or exposed sutures)
- IOL dislocation or tilt
- Late onset endophthalmitis due to erosion of conjunctival tissue overlying scleral knots
- Breakage of haptic from optics

What are the indications of IOL explantation?

- Preoperative factors: Wrong IOL power calculation
- Intraoperative factors:
  - Broken haptics
  - Posterior capsular rent (PCR)
  - Instability due to zonular dialysis/PCR
  - Suspected IOL dislocation
- Postoperative:
  - For ACIOL: Corneal edema, UGH syndrome, lens propelling (small ACIOL with excessive rotation), globe tenderness due to large size IOL, chronic CME
  - For PCIOL: P. Acne endophthalmitis, IOL decentration/dislocation, refractive surprise, IOL glistening, IOL crack, extensive pitting after YAG CAP, opacification, decentered (sunset, sunrise), exudates in the bag
  - For iris claw IOL: Recalcitrant CME, recurrent uveitis

- Suture fixated IOL: Gross decentration, IOL fixation suture breakage
- Multifocal IOLs: Intolerable glare and halos

7.10 INSTRUMENTS USED IN SMALL-PUPIL CATARACT SURGERY

Identify and describe the device.

- Irrigating: Requires 2.5 mm incision
- Non-irrigating: Requires 1 mm incision
  - Prolene: Disposable
  - Metal: Non disposable, sharp (increased iris damage)
- Adjustable silicone stopper provides a better grip and allows adjustment of pupillary size

What is the difference between iris and capsular hooks?

- Hooks are angled to the plane of the anterior capsule.
- Rounded tip (prevents damage to the capsular bag).
- Silicone lock retains it during surgery.
- Has a larger support area than iris hooks.

What are the various ways to deal with a small pupil during cataract surgery?

- Pharmacological:
  - Intraoperative: Diluted adrenaline (1:10,000) (sulfite- and preservative-free)
  - Epi-Shugarcaine: 9 mL of BSS Plus mixed with 4 ml of 1:1,000 bisulfite-free epinephrine and 3 ml of 4% preservative-free lidocaine
  - Omidria (Omeros, USA): Combination of phenylephrine (1.0%) to dilate and ketorolac (0.3%) to reduce pain
- Surgical:
  - Can commence regular surgery (phacoemulsification with low flow settings, i.e., low vacuum and AFR, reduce the bottle height)

Identify and describe the following:

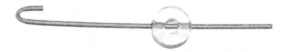

- Iris hook

- Viscomydriasis: Using a highly viscous OVD to dilate the pupil such as Healon 5
- Synechiolysis
- Pupillary stretching using Kuglen hooks, Y hooks
- Iris cutting: Sphincterotomy, iridotomy
- Mechanical pupil expanders

Identify the following device.

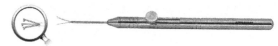

- Beehler pupil dilator
- Straight, active part 10 mm in length
- Has three points of pupil dilatation
- Helps in the mechanical dilatation of the pupil by retracting the iris

Identify and describe this pupil expansion device. Name some other devices you have heard of.

- Malyugin ring
- Manufactured by MicroSurgical Technologies (Redmond, Washington)
- Available in two sizes: 6.25 mm and 7.0 mm in diameter
- Requires 2.5 mm incision to insert
- Eight iris retaining points, which create a round pupillary opening.
- New version of the Malyugin ring (2.0) made of 5-0 polypropylene can fit through a 2 mm corneal incision
- Other devices:
  - Visitec i-Ring pupil expander: Single-use device made of soft, resilient polyurethane that creates a 6.3 mm circular opening.
  - Bhattacharjee pupil expansion ring (B-Hex): Made of 5-0 black monofilament polyamide (nylon), available in square and hexagon shapes in various sizes (6.0, 6.5, and 7.0 mm).
  - Assia pupil expander (APX Ophthalmology in Haifa, Israel): Has two tiny spring-loaded devices that are inserted through 1.1 mm side port incisions opposite each

other. Creates a rectangular pupil opening about 6 × 6 mm.

- Xpand NT iris speculum (Diamatrix Ltd.): Made from titanium alloy nitinol, which is a memory metal. It can be inserted through 2.4 mm incision and creates a circular 6.50–6.75 mm dilatation.

Identify and describe the instrument.

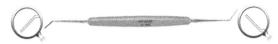

- Iris repositor
- Long narrow flattened extremities with blunt edges
- One end is round and other end is forked
- Uses:
  - To reposit the prolapsed iris tissue during ECCE
  - De-epithelization of cornea during C3R, BSK removal
  - Forked end for reposition of conjunctiva during ECCE

7.11 INSTRUMENTS USED IN THE MANAGEMENT OF SUBLUXATED CATARACTS

Identify and describe the ring. State its use.

- Made of PMMA
- Different sizes (Compressed sizes)
  - 10 mm: Will extend to 12 mm
  - 11 mm: Will extend to 13 mm
  - 12 mm: Will extend to 14–14.5 mm (used in myopes)
- Can be injected or manually inserted
- CTR types:
  - Standard CTR: No eyelets with only two dialing holes
  - CTR ring

- Cionni's Modified (M—CTR) Ring: Has either one or two eyelets
- Ahmed CT Segment (CT—Segment)

What are the various types of Cionni rings?

- There are 3 MCTR models available.
- Model 1-L has a single fixation hook located on the trailing end of the ring.
- Model 2-C has a single fixation hook located on the leading edge of the ring, allowing it to be injected into the bag using a specially designed shooter.
- Model 2-L has two fixation hooks and is used in patients with very significant generalized weakness where two-point fixation is required.

What are the modifications of the CT ring you know of?

- Henderson capsule tension ring
  - Made of PMMA
  - Open, C-shaped loop
  - Difference: Has eight 0.15-mm indentations around its circumference
  - Therefore, helps in easy cortex removal behind the ring

- Ahmed CT segments
  - PMMA ring segment of 120°
  - Use: Severe zonular weakness
  - Advantages over CTR
  - No need for capsulorrhexis
  - Can be inserted with a small PC tear
  - Zonular dialysis >4 clock hours
  - Can be used in progressive zonular dialysis
  - Scleral fixation possible
  - Explantation is easy

What are the indications and contraindications for its use?

- Indications:
  - Subluxation of lens
  - Zonular dialysis:
    - Traumatic
    - Iatrogenic
  - Pseudoexfoliation
  - Marfan's syndrome
  - Weil–Marchesani syndrome
  - Homocystinuria
  - Hypermature cataract
  - Post-vitrectomy
  - Post-trabeculectomy
  - Aniridia
  - Retinitis pigmentosa
  - Intraocular neoplasm
  - Congenital lens coloboma
- Contraindications:
  - Tear in anterior capsule
  - Tear in posterior capsule
  - Incomplete rhexis
  - Extensive zonular damage

What is the mechanism of action of capsule tension rings?

- Intraoperative:
  - Works as a supportive tool during phacoemulsification and increases stability
  - Diameter of CTR is more than the diameter of the capsular bag, so it expands the equator and provides equatorial distribution of support from the remaining zonules
  - Expands the capsular bag
  - Expands the capsular bag and makes PC taut
- Postoperative:
  - Stabilizes the zonular apparatus by redistribution of forces
  - Recenters mildly subluxated bag
  - PC shriveling is decreased
  - Reduced incidence of PCO
  - Reduced incidence of capsule contraction syndrome

What are the complications with the use of capsule tension rings?

- PC rent
- Placement/extrusion into ciliary sulcus

What are the causes of subluxated lenses (ectopia)?

- Simple ectopia lentis
- Ectopia lentis et pupillae
- Ocular disorders associated with the subluxation of the lens:
  - Aniridia
  - Congenital glaucoma
  - Hypermature cataract
  - Pseudoexfoliation syndrome
  - Intraocular tumor
  - Megalocornea
  - Retinitis pigmentosa
  - Axenfeld–Rieger syndrome
- Systemic disorders associated with subluxation of lens:
  - Marfan's syndrome
  - Homocystinuria
  - Weill–Marchesani syndrome
  - Sulfite oxidase deficiency
  - Hyperlysinemia
  - Ehlers–Danlos syndrome
  - Sturge–Weber syndrome
  - Mandibulofacial dysostosis
  - Conradi syndrome

What are the principles of management of subluxated cataracts during surgery?

- Assess degree of zonular weakness in upright and supine positions.
- Local anesthesia preferred.
- Preoperative intravenous mannitol if necessary.
- In cases with zonular weakness less than 3 clock hours, use only capsule retractors to support the bag and slow-motion phacoemulsification.
- In cases with progressive zonular weakness due to PXF, Marfan's syndrome, RP: CTR mandatory for bag fixation also helps stretch the capsular bag.

- In cases with capsular bag dialysis of more than 4 clock hours:
  - CTR augmented by CTS.
  - Cionni's ring can also be alternatively used.
- Incision: Avoid over area of zonulopathy.
- Try to remove as much vitreous as possible prior to starting.
- Capsulorrhexis: Staining with trypan blue if possible to be avoided as the blue may stain the posterior capsule compromising the view. May need to make an eccentric rhexis, with microrhexis forceps.
- Capsular bag hooks and CTR may be needed to support a very subluxated bag prior to commencing phacoemulsification.
- Time of placement of CTR: can be placed before removal of the lens or after removal depending on the severity of the weakness (As early as possible, As late as you can).
- CTS can be used to suture the bag to the sclera to stabilize focal defects.
- Perform slow motion phacoemulsification. Nuclear cracking in the direction of the weakness. Direct chop preferable technique of phacoemulsification.
- Can place a one- or three-piece IOL if bag is well centered and stable

7.12 HISTORICAL INSTRUMENTS

Identify and describe this instrument.

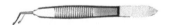

- Arruga's intracapsular forceps
- Curved forceps with cup on inner side
- Holding the lens capsule at lower pole for lens delivery during ICCE
- Indications of ICCE:
  - Anteriorly dislocated lens
  - Extensive subluxation
  - Along with cyclectomy

Identify the instrument and describe the blade and its uses.

- Von Graef's knife
- Sharp blade
- Historical instrument in present day
- Uses:
  - Used earlier, for ab interno sclerocorneal incision during cataract surgery
  - Paracentesis
- Disadvantages:
  - Incision was uncontrolled with anterior chamber collapse with injury to the lens.
  - Hence, universal sclerocorneal scissors came into use.

7.13 FEMTO-LASER-ASSISTED CATARACT SURGERY (FLACS)

Do you know of any newer advances in cataract surgery? Mention some salient features of femtosecond-laser-assisted cataract surgery (FLACS).

- Mechanism of action
  - A femtosecond laser refers to a laser with pulse duration in the femtosecond range (10^{-15}).
  - Principle of photo disruption.
  - Photo disruption is essentially induced by vaporization of target tissues.
  - The focused laser energy increases to a level where a plasma is generated.
  - Plasma expands and causes a shock wave, cavitation, and bubble formation.
  - Bubble expands and collapses, leading to separation of the tissue.
- Steps:
  - Dock the machine onto the cornea—this involves a docking system (patient interface) with a contact lens and suction skirt which distributes pressure evenly on the cornea.
  - Planning parameters include:
    - Location and architecture of corneal incisions/LRIs
    - Size shape and desired center of the laser ablation for the capsule
    - Diameter, patterns, and depth of cuts for lens fragmentation

- Laser is then activated.
- Advantages:
  - Precise and self-sealing corneal incision
  - More circular, stronger capsulorrhexis
  - Reduced ultrasound energy, safer and less technically difficult phacofragmentation
- Disadvantages:
  - Relies on anterior segment imaging for laser pattern mapping; therefore, pupillary constriction poses a problem.
- Relative contraindications are patients with posterior synechiae, intraoperative floppy iris syndrome suspects, phacodonesis, and zonular dialysis.
- Platforms
  - LenSx by Alcon (Fort Worth, Texas, USA)
  - LensAR by LensAR (Orlando, Florida, USA)
  - Catalys by Abbott/Optimedica (North Chicago, Illinois, USA)
  - Victus by Bausch and Lomb (Rochester, New York, USA)
  - LDV Z8 by Ziemer (Port, Switzerland)

Oculoplasty and orbit

8.1 TOPICS

- Probing and syringing instruments
- FAQs on syringing and probing
- Instruments used in DCR (dacryocystorhinos-tomy) and DCT (dacryocystectomy) surgeries
- FAQs on DCR and DCT surgery
- Enucleation and evisceration instruments
- FAQs related to enucleation, evisceration, and exenteration
- Orbital implants
- FAQs on orbitotomy
- Lid-surgery-related instruments
- FAQs on entropion and ectropion
- Ptosis surgery instruments
- FAQs on ptosis
- FAQs on myasthenia gravis
- Proptosis instruments
- FAQs on proptosis
- FAQs on orbital cellulitis

8.2 PROBING AND SYRINGING INSTRUMENTS

Identify and describe the instrument.

- Bowman's Probe.
- Long (~60 mm), round tipped, wire-like probes with central flat plate to enable holding it.

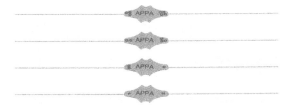

- The plate has various numbers which indicate its diameter.
- Sizes available: 0000, 000, 00, 0, 1, 2, 3, 4, 5, 6, 7, and 8.
- Size 0000 is the thinnest.
- Size 8 is the thickest.
- There is a 5–10° angulation which is for the direction of the NLD (nasolacrimal duct).

8.3 FAQs ON SYRINGING AND PROBING

What are the uses of a Bowman's probe?

- For NLD probing in infants with congenital nasolacrimal duct obstruction (CNLDO)
- To identify the lacrimal sac during DCR, DCT
- Treat lacrimal stenosis
- Canalicular identification and assessment in canalicular injuries or surgery

What are the sizes of probes in metric system?

- Sizes of the probes
  - 0000 = 0.7 mm
  - 000 = 0.8 mm
  - 00 = 0.9 mm
  - 0 = 1.0 mm
  - 1 = 1.1 mm
- Clinical pearls
  - Baby with a wet eye and wet nose unlikely to be NLD block
  - Baby with a wet eye and dry nose may be NLD block
  - Baby with mucoid discharge along with watery discharge likely to be CNLDO

What is the initial management of congenital NLD block?

- Conservative therapy with topical antibiotics/ointment
- Hydrostatic massage using index finger stroke (crigglers massage)
- Sac compressions

What is the timing of NLD probing?

- Between 10 and 12 months
- Revised guidelines above 18 months

What are the indications for early (neonatal) probing (<6 months)?

- Congenital dacryocele
- Prior to intraocular operation
- Recurrent acute dacryocystitis under 18 months of age

What are the advantages and disadvantages of early probing?

- Advantages of early probing:
  - Better success rates
  - Reduced risk of acute dacryocystitis
- Disadvantages of early probing:
  - Anesthesia-related difficulties
  - Spontaneous resolution of the NLD obstruction in known to occur

What are the disadvantages of late probing?

- Chronic infection or recurrent infection
- Intracystic/pericystic fibrosis
- Increase failure rate

What are the steps in NLD probing?

- Punctum dilatation.
- Probe is passed vertically for 2 mm (to follow the vertical path of the canaliculus).
- Followed by horizontal rotation along the eyelid margin while stretching the lateral canthus to enter the horizontal part of the canaliculus.
- On further advancement a hard stop should be felt, indicating the medial wall of the lacrimal sac and adjacent bony lacrimal fossa.
- Then do a second syringing to confirm patency.
- If block is at 10 mm, it may indicate NLD atresia.

What are the complications of NLD probing?

- Bleeding
- Failure
- False passage
- Pericystic abscess/periorbital cellulitis/orbital cellulitis
- Damage to puncta and canalicular mucosa

What are the special precautions for NLD probing under general anesthesia?

- If the patient is intubated with a throat pack, syringing can be done at end of probing.
- If the patient is not intubated, do not perform syringing or do suction at the end of procedure.

What are some of the precautions or tips prior to probing one must know as a resident?

- For NLD probing, prefer to use upper punctum as the lacrimal sac and the NLD are more in continuation with the superior canaliculus allowing easier entry and rotation of the probe. Additional advantage is to safeguard the lower punctum from any iatrogenic trauma which is physiologically more important for drainage.
- Diagnostic irrigation should always precede probing (if sac is patent, avoid probing).
- If syringing is contemplated, always intubate with cuffed tube.
- Mark probe before probing, insert from upper punctum, and rotate it along the supraorbital margin and enter the NLD.
- Start with smaller size probe (00 size).
- Keep the probe in the canal for at least 45 seconds each.
- The older the child, the higher the size of initial probe chosen.
- Avoid size 2 probe in children as it can cause canalicular damage.
- Can use diluted fluorescein to syringe the lacrimal system at end of probing. If fluorescein appears in nose (checked with blue light), it indicates patency.

What are the types of stops during probing?

- Soft stop: Site of block is either canalicular or common canalicular.
- Hard stop: Tactile sensation of medial wall beyond the lacrimal sac is felt during probing.

8.4 INSTRUMENTS USED IN DCR (DACRYOCYSTORHINOSTOMY) AND DCT (DACRYO-CYSTECTOMY) SURGERIES

What is the list of instruments used in a DCR/DCT surgery?

Useful to look out for these on a viva table as all of the further viva questions will be directed toward this particular surgery:

- Nasal packing forceps
- Thudichum's nasal speculum
- Nettleship punctum dilator
- Lacrimal cannula
- No. 15 blade with Bard–Parker handle
- Bowman's probe
- Muller's self-retaining hemostatic retractor
- Cat's paw retractor
- Hemostatic artery forceps
- Lacrimal dissector with curette
- Periosteum elevator
- Bone punch
- Bone mallet and osteotome
- Lacrimal sac protector
- Pigtail probe
- Lacrimal intubation set
- Lester Jones tube
- Balloon catheter

Identify and describe the following instrument.

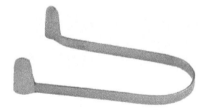

- Thudichum nasal speculum
- Two 45 mm long nasal flanges with inner concavities
- U-shaped handle
- Flanges separate the inner nasal soft tissues in an atraumatic manner
- Uses:
  - OPD procedures like rhinoscopy
  - DCR surgery during nasal packing
  - Maybe used to retract orbital fat during orbital foreign body removal
  - Nasal surgeries

Identify the following forceps.

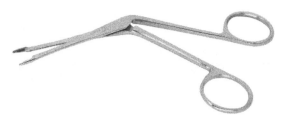

Figure 8.3 Tilley nasal packing forceps

- Tilley nasal packing forceps
- Horizontal serrations near the ends
- The angular bend helps visualize the nasal cavity during packing
- The slender limbs facilitate maneuvering in deep spaces of the nasal cavity
- Uses:
  - Packing the nose prior to DCR surgery (sponges or rolled gauze maybe used)
  - To remove bone during DCR surgery
  - To remove foreign bodies in the nasal cavity

What are the uses of packing the nose before DCR?

- Helps in anesthesia and hemostasis of the nasal mucosa
- Helps in bulging of nasal mucosa for easy identification
- Helps to prevent excess fluid/blood/bone fragments entering nose/throat

What are the precautions while packing?

- Counseling the patient.
- Packing is done up to the middle meatus
- Gauze is soaked with Lignocaine (4% drops or gel) with adrenaline.

Identify and describe the following instrument and state its uses.

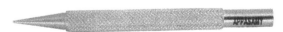

Figure 8.4 Nettleship/wilder punctum dilator

- Nettleship/wilder punctum dilator
- Castroviejo double-ended punctum dilator
- Size 1 = Fine taper
- Size 2 = Medium taper
- Size 3 = Heavy taper

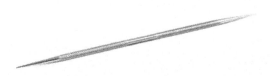

Figure 8.5 Castroviejo double-ended punctum dilator

- Uses:
  - Therapeutic: To dilate the punctum in punctal stenosis
  - Diagnostic: To dilate the punctum prior to syringing or probing
  - As an adjunct in surgeries like puncto-plasty, canaliculoplasty, and NLD probing in CNLDO

Identify and describe the following instruments and state uses.

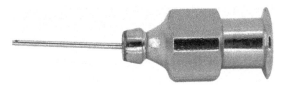

Figure 8.6 Shahinian's lacrimal cannula

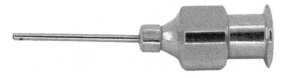

Figure 8.7 Bailey's lacrimal cannula

- Commonly used 23G/25G/27G cannula
- Smooth atraumatic tip with tapered edges so as not to damage the epithelial lining of the lacrimal canaliculus
- Shahinian's lacrimal cannula = 11 mm with tapered ends
- Bailey's lacrimal cannula = 7 mm with a bottle necked end
- Uses:
  - Sac syringing
  - For sac syringing to check patency of the opening between the lacrimal sac and nasal mucosa at the end of DCR procedure
  - At the end of NLD probing in a child to confirm patency

- After canalicular trephination to confirm the patency of the canalicular opening

How does one do lacrimal sac syringing?

- Anesthetize with 0.5% proparacaine hydrochloride eyedrops.
- After upper/lower punctum dilatation, introduce the lacrimal cannula attached to a syringe containing normal saline into the punctum.
- Direction of insertion: Downward, backward, medially (in that order).
- Inject saline.
- Observe five things:
  - Resistance while introducing the cannula
  - Resistance while injecting
  - Regurgitation from the opposite punctum
  - Swallowing movement
  - Taste of the fluid
- If fluorescein-tinged saline is used, check for the presence of fluorescein in the nose using a cobalt blue filter

Identify and describe the following instrument.

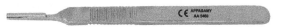

Figure 8.8 Bard–Parker blade handle with no. 15 blade

- Bard–Parker blade handle with no. 15 blade
- One of the most common ophthalmic instruments
- Cylindrical end with longitudinal grooves for attaching the scalpel blade
- Inclined edge at the proximal end has a gap that provides stability to the blade
- Use: To mount and handle surgical blades used to make the skin incision medial to medial canthus

What are the advantages and disadvantages of 3 mm vs. 10 mm incision in DCR surgery?

- 10 mm (medial to medial canthal angle)
  - Medial (avoids angular vein which lies 8 mm medial to the medial canthal angle)
  - Cosmetically good scar
  - Access to sac difficult
- 3 mm (medial to medial canthal angle)
  - Lateral
  - Bowstringing (pseudoepicanthal fold)

- Easy access to sac
- Preferred in re-surgeries

Identify the following instrument.

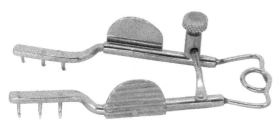

Figure 8.9 Mueller lacrimal sac retractor

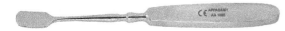

Lacrimal sac protector

- Mueller lacrimal sac retractor
- Spring action with screw lock
- 3 × 3 semi-sharp prongs
- Blade spread = 28 mm

Mention some other self-retaining hemostatic retractors.

- Stevenson's lacrimal sac retractor
  - Curved with 3 × 3 semi-sharp prongs
  - Screw-controlled spread
  - Blade spread = 20 mm

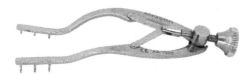

Stevenson's lacrimal sac retractor

- Goldstein's lacrimal sac retractor
  - 3 × 3 semi-sharp prongs
  - Blade spread = 30 mm

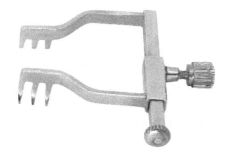

Goldstein's lacrimal sac retractor

Mention their uses?

- Retract muscle and skin during DCR surgery (external)
- During incision biopsy/dermoid cyst excision to retract soft tissue

What are the advantages and disadvantage of the self-retaining hemostatic retractor?

- Advantages:
  - Good exposure
  - Hemostatic
  - Doesn't require assistant to retract
- Disadvantages: The claws can be traumatic.

Identify the instrument and mention its uses?

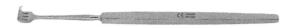

Figure 8.11 Knapp's cat's paw retractor

- Knapp's cat's paw retractor
- Non-self-retaining
- Requires assistant to retract
- 3–5 prongs
- Small, medium, large sizes
- Blunt tipped and claw shaped
- Uses:
  - Retract skin and muscle during DCR surgery, during orbitotomy surgeries, etc.
  - To compress bleeder during DCR surgery
  - To retract skin and muscle during fascia lata harvesting from the thigh in sling surgery for ptosis correction

What are the other ways to retract skin for exposure?

- Taking linen sutures

Identify and describe the following instrument and mention its uses.

- Hartman hemostatic (mosquito) artery/clamps
- 20 mm serrated jaws
- Ratchet lock

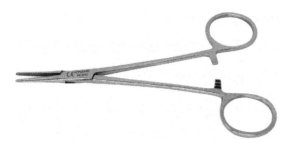

Figure 8.12 Hartman hemostatic (mosquito) artery/clamps

- Uses
  - Clamp bleeder vessel to maintain hemostasis
  - To crush/clamp NLD before cutting in DCT
  - Holding stay sutures
  - To crush tarsal plate during eyelid tumor excision
  - To crush lateral canthal tendon during lateral canthotomy
  - To hold a cyst or mass to provide traction during biopsies
  - To hold needles towel clamps etc.
  - To crush extraocular muscles during enucleation
  - Curved artery forceps are used to crush the optic nerve during enucleation as well as in Fasanella–Servat ptosis surgery where two curved artery forceps are used at the superior end of the tarsal plate

What are the common sources of bleeding during a DCR surgery?

- Angular vein
- Periosteum and bone
- Nasal mucosa
- Ethmoidal vessels

What are the ways to control bleeding during DCR?

- Angular vein: Clamp → crush → ligate → cauterize
- Bone: Use bone wax and cauterize
- Mucosa: Pressure pack (adrenaline) and cauterize
- General bleed: Keep the head high; give hypotensive anesthesia

Identify and describe the following. Mention their uses.

- Lacrimal sac dissectors with NLD curette

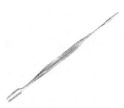

Figure 8.13 Lacrimal sac dissectors with NLD curette

- Double-ended with sharp dissector and curette
- Double-ended with sharp gouge and blunt dissector
- Use: The dissector end is used to gently dissect the lacrimal sac from the lacrimal fossa.

Identify and describe the following instruments.

- Freer's double-ended periosteum elevator

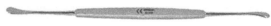

Figure 8.14 Freer's double-ended periosteum elevator

- Double-ended
- Curved
- 6 mm wide by 30 mm long
- Blade with sharp and blunt tips
- Sharp tip—cutting
- Blunt tip—lifting and blunt dissection
- Serrated shaft for better grip

- Traquair's periosteal elevator

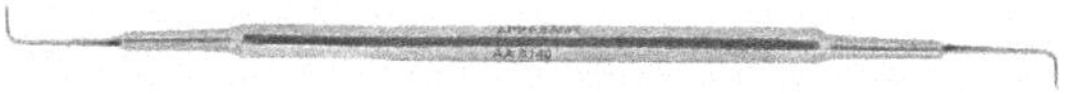

Figure 8.15 Traquair's periosteal elevator

- Double-ended
- Blunt angled tips
- Hexagonal handle

What are the uses of a periosteal elevator?

- To elevate the periosteum off the maxillary bone after incising it and stripping it off the underlying bone to obtain bare bone for bone punching in DCR surgery
- Reflect the lacrimal sac during DCR surgery

- To dissect periosteum off the medial wall of the sac in DCR surgery
- In orbital exenteration surgeries and repair of orbital fractures
- Blunt soft tissue retractor
- Endonasal DCR to lift the mucoperiosteum

Identify and describe the following instrument.

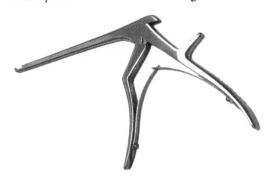

Figure 8.16 A Kerrison bone punch sizes

- Bone punch/bone rongeur or punch/bone rongeur
- Tip of upper arm has a U-shaped sharp cutting edge
- Lower arm is extended and fixed and has a depression to allow for the bone which has been cut
- Longer armed bone punches are used for endonasal DCR for access within the longer, narrower nasal cavity
- Kerrison bone punch sizes:
  - 1.5 mm wide
  - 2.0 mm wide
  - 2.5 mm wide
  - 3.0 mm wide
  - 4.0 mm wide

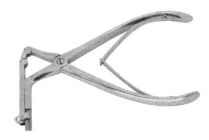

Figure 8.16 B Citelli bone punch sizes

- Citelli bone punch sizes:
  - 2.0 mm wide
  - 3.0 mm wide
  - 4.0 mm wide

- Uses:
  - To punch out bone during DCR surgery to create the bony ostium
  - Enlarge bony openings during floor fracture repair
  - During osteotomy for better access to the lateral and superior tumors
  - To take biopsy in bony tumors

Identify and describe the instrument.

- Bone mallet and chisel

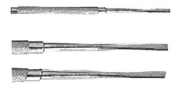

Figure 8.17 Bone mallet and chisel

- Mallet is a hammer, which is heavy and bi-headed
- Chisel is 20 × 6 mm a single-bevel blade
- Sharp and produces linear impact when struck on bone

What are the uses of bone mallet and chisel?

- Can be used instead of bone punch, especially for thicker bones
- Osteotome double edge with square handle blade width: 3, 4, 5, 6 mm
- Osteotome has both sides cutting edge, while chisel has single cutting edge

What are the other instruments for making an osteotomy?

- Arruga's trephine
- High speed burr
- Bone trephine marker with center drill, for marking, with handle
- Available in various sizes

What are the bones forming lacrimal fossa?

- Lacrimal (thin papery)
- Frontal process of maxilla
- Maxillary process of frontal bone

Which bone mainly forms the lacrimal fossa?

- Frontal process of maxilla

Which bones are punched?

- Frontal process of maxilla
- Maxillary process of frontal bone

Which bones are removed?

- Lacrimal (thin papery)
- Frontal process of maxilla
- Maxillary process of frontal bone

What are the limits of osteotomy?

- Anteriorly: As far as the bone punch can be introduced between the nasal mucosa and the bone
- Posteriorly: Posterior lacrimal crest
- Superiorly: Approximately 1 mm above the fundus of the sac
- Inferiorly: Until you partially deroof the NLD

What are the types of canalicular stents and classify them?

- Used primarily in cases of obstruction or laceration of one or more parts of the tear drainage system
- Small diameter tubes placed within the NLD to maintain patency
- Temporary procedure staying in place for a few months
- Canalicular stents can be organized based on the different parts of the nasolacrimal drainage system they intubate.
- Two main types are bicanalicular and monocanalicular.
- Bicanalicular stents pass through both the upper and lower canaliculus to typically create a closed circuit.
- Monocanalicular stents only intubating either the upper or lower canaliculus.

Identify and describe the instrument.

- Catalano/Crawford lacrimal intubation set

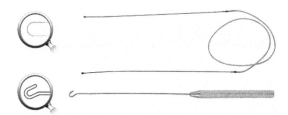

Figure 8.18 Catalano/Crawford lacrimal intubation set

- Bicanalicular stent
- Two blunt stainless steel malleable probes
- 0.7 mm in diameter × 140 mm long
- Attached to long silicone tubing

- Probes and attached stents are passed through the superior and inferior canaliculi and retrieved in the nose via a retrieval hook (Nasolacrimal Stents: An Introductory Guide; https://webeye.ophth.uiowa.edu/eyeforum/tutorials/Stents/index.htm)
- Probes are cut and stents are tied in the nose

Identify and describe the instrument and mention its uses.

- Ritleng canalicular intubation set.

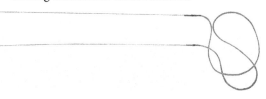

Figure 8.19 Ritleng canalicular intubation set

- Ritleng intubation system consists of a silicone (or PVP) tube connected at each extremity to a PolyEtherEtherKetone (PEEK) thread guide.
- Utilizes an introducer with a hollow lumen and stylet.
- The introducer, loaded with the stylet for rigidity, is used to enter the nasolacrimal system.
- Once inside, the stylet is removed, and one end of a bicanalicular stent is advanced through the hollow lumen of the tube.
- Uses:
  - Epiphora
  - Canalicular pathologies
  - Congenital lacrimal duct obstruction and
  - Dacryocystorhinostomy (DCR)

Identify the probe and mention its uses.

- Modified Worst's pigtail lacrimal probe with eyelet

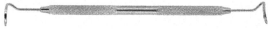

Figure 8.20 Modified Worst's pigtail lacrimal probe with eyelet

- 8 mm diameter
- Knurled shaft with pigtail-shaped probes at two ends
- Round atraumatic tips with eyelets at the ends
- Identification of right and left side is necessary—one side is for the superior punctum of right side and inferior punctum of left side and vice versa

- Uses:
  - Identification of the cut end of the canalicular tear during repair
  - To pass silicon stent or suture from lacerated end of canaliculus to the intact end

How is the pigtail/donut stent used in canalicular laceration repair?

- Stent is used for bicanalicular intubation.
- Probe is passed through one punctum, then retrieved via the opposite punctum
- Eyelet at tip allows passage of a guide-wire suture through the canalicular system
- A piece of hollow silicone tubing (25 mm) is passed over the guide wire to intubate the canal.
- The suture is then cut and tied
- One can distinguish between a Crawford and a pigtail stent by the presence or absence of a black nylon or blue Prolene suture within the stent lumen versus no suture or a white silk suture in the Crawford stent.

Identify and describe the instrument and mention its uses.

- Monoka monocanalicular intubation silicon tube

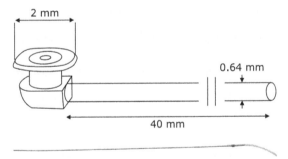

2 mm

0.64 mm

40 mm

Figure 8.21 Monoka monocanalicular intubation silicon tube

- For only stenting a single canaliculus
- Silicone stent is anchored at the punctum by a plug/cap
- Mini Monoka stent is a smaller version and is used to treat lacerations or obstructions in the canaliculus

What are the uses of intubation stents?

- Intubation stents
- Complicated DCR with lot of scarring
- Re-DCR surgery

- Pediatric DCR surgery
- Inability to form nasal/lacrimal flaps
- Canalicular tear

8.5 FAQs ON DCR AND DCT SURGERY

What is dacryocystorhinostomy surgery (DCR)?

- It is a surgery to create a passage from lacrimal sac into middle meatus of nose and bypasses block at lower lid of sac or NLD (**Table 8.1**)

What is DCT surgery?

- Dacryocystectomy, or DCT, refers to a complete surgical extirpation of the lacrimal sac

Which is better DCR or DCT?

- DCR surgery as it by passes the block and relieves patient of epiphora

What is the commonest site of block?

- Lower end of nasolacrimal duct

Where does NLD open?

- In the inferior meatus

Where does the lacrimal sac open after DCR surgery?

- In the middle meatus

What are the bones broken during DCR?

- Lacrimal bone
- Frontal process of maxillary bone
- Ethmoid bone partially

Table 8.1 DCR Surgery Approach

Without Canalicular disease	With Canalicular disease
External DCR	Canaliculo-DCR with silicon intubation: If proximal 8 mm of functional canaliculus present
Endonasal DCR Surgical Laser Combined	Conjunctival-DCR with Lester Jones tube: If extensive canalicular involvement

What are the indications of DCR?

- Chronic dacryocystitis due to primary or secondary NLDO
- Mucocoele
- Repeatedly failed probing
- Bony atresia of Nasolacrimal canal

What are the contraindications of DCR?

- Local:
  - Acute dacryocystitis
  - Tuberculosis (TB) of the sac
  - Tumors
- Focal:
  - Atrophic rhinitis (absolute contraindication)
  - Deviated nasal septum (DNS)
  - Nasal polyp
  - Rhinosporidiosis
  - Inferior turbinate hypertrophy
- General:
  - Uncontrolled HTN
  - Bleeding disorders
  - Very old patients

What are the preoperative evaluations to be done before DCR?

- Evaluation of sac and nasolacrimal passage function to know level and type of block
  - Sac syringing
  - Jones dye test
  - Dye disappearance test
  - DCG/imaging if needed
- ENT evaluation—nasal endoscopy
- Systemic evaluation to rule out
  - Bleeding pathologies
  - Hypertension
  - Anemia
  - HIV

What are the important anatomical landmarks during DCR surgery?

- Medial canthal tendon which is firmly attached to the superior end of the anterior lacrimal crest, important as the fundus of the lacrimal sac lies underneath it.
- Angular vessels which lie 5–8 mm medial to medial canthus

What are the complications in DCR surgery?

- Anesthesia-related:
  - Allergy to lignocaine
  - Raised BP due to Adrenaline
- Intraoperative:
  - Bleeding occurs from:
  - Angular vein: Cautery, clamp, ligate
  - Bone: Use bone wax
  - Nasal mucosa: Pack, cautery
  - Improper identification of lacrimal sac
  - Improper flaps
  - Damage/loss of mucosa
  - Osteotomy too small
  - CSF leak
  - Damage to ethmoid sinus
  - Injury to cornea, injury to orbital septum
- Postoperative:
  - Incision: Pseudoepicanthal fold, keloid tendencies, granuloma formation
  - Failure of DCR
  - Infection, orbital cellulitis
  - Epistaxis
  - Facial ecchymosis

What are the causes of failure in DCR surgery?

- Preoperative:
  - Incorrect evaluation; e.g., missing canalicular block
  - Undetected nasal pathology (polyps, atrophic rhinitis, deviated nasal septum, etc.)
  - Tuberculosis of the sac
- Intraoperative:
  - Excessive bleeding
  - Wrong identification of sac and nasal mucosa
  - Incomplete opening in sac and nasal mucosa
  - Very small osteotomy or incorrect placement
  - Sac filled with polyps, mucous plugs, cicatricial bands, and dacryoliths
  - Loss of nasal mucosal flap, small, contracted flap, improper suturing of flap
  - Failure to recognize anterior ethmoidal air cells
- Postoperative:
  - Excessive bleeding can be early or delayed
  - Infection
  - Retained gauze, cotton in wound
  - Collapse of sac due to tight post-op dressing
  - SUMP syndrome: Surgical opening in the lacrimal bone is too small and high; thus,

secretions collect in the lacrimal sac as they are unable to reach the ostium and hence the nasal cavity)

What are the precautions during re-DCR surgeries?

- Preoperative evaluation with DCG
- Anesthesia preference: GA vs. LA
- Primary aim is exposure and extension of oste-otomy site
- Identification and protection of nasal mucosa
- Identify the lacrimal sac with help of probe
- Lacrimal silicon tube intubation
- Mitomycin C application

What are the special postoperative instructions to tell patient?

- No blowing of nose for at least a week to pre-vent bleeding and emphysema
- Avoid sneezing

What are the indications of DCT?

- Blocked NLD where DCR is contraindicated
- To get rid of septic focus
  - Prior to any urgent intraocular surgery
  - If elderly patients having corneal ulcer/abscess
- Suspected tumor of sac
- Suspected TB of sac

What are the contraindications of DCT?

- Acute dacryocystitis
- Skin infections
- Uncontrolled hypertension

What are the complications of DCT?

- Incomplete removal of the sac
- Injury to orbital septum temporally and inferi-orly in orbit
- Bleeding
- Infection
- Postoperative irregular scar with a resultant pseudoepicanthal fold

What are the modifications of DCR?

- DCR with lacrimal intubation
- Conjunctivo-DCR
- Caniculo-DCR
- Endoscopic DCR
- Laser-assisted DCR

What is conjunctivo-dacryocystorhinostomy?

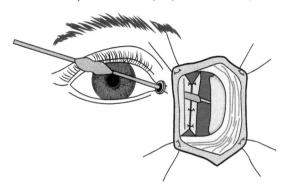

- Performed like DCR
- Lester Jones tube is inserted from lacrimal lake to osteotomy site
- Nasal mucosa and lacrimal flaps then sutured
- Indications:
  - Pump failure
  - Obliteration of canaliculi with more than 8 mm of canaliculus left
  - Lester Jones Tube with Kirschner wire with sharp trephine with styll

What is caniculo-dacryocystorhinostomy?

- Lacrimal sac fundus dissected free, and cana-liculus sutured directly to sac and intubated
- Prerequisite: At least 8 mm of canaliculus should be available

What are the other techniques of DCR?

- Endonasal DCR:
  - Surgical
  - Endolaser
  - Combined
- Advantages:
  - No external scar
  - Nasal pathology can be treated in same sitting
- Disadvantages:
  - GA needed
  - Cannot effectively treat canalicular block
  - Higher failure rate because of a smaller ostium size

Discuss the advantages and disadvantages of external DCR as against endonasal DCR?

- External DCR:
  - Advantages:
  - Better exposure

- Higher success rates
- No need of sophisticated equipment
- Larger osteotomy
- Intra sac pathologies can be seen and treated
- Better for repeat surgeries
- Canaliculo-DCR and conjunctivo-DCR can be done
- Fracture of lateral and nasal wall can be handled better
- Disadvantages:
- SUMP syndrome
- Scar formation
- Endonasal DCR:
  - Advantages:
  - No scar formation
  - No Sump syndrome
  - Intranasal pathology can be treated
  - Disadvantages:
  - Dependence on ENT surgeon
  - Need for silicon intubation (at least 5 weeks)
  - Costly
  - Lower success rate possibly due to smaller ostium size
- Laser DCR:
  - Holmium:YAG
    - 2100 nm
    - Works well in water
    - 0.4 mm penetration
  - KTP:Nd YAG
    - Potassium titanyl phosphate
    - 532 nm, pulsed, frequency doubled laser
    - 4 mm penetration
  - Advantage: Can be used to cut bone and mucosa
  - Disadvantages
    - Cost
    - Charring of nasal mucosa
    - Protection required for users

What are the surgical steps of endoscopic endo-nasal DCR (EEDCR)?

- Identify the sac area
- Create an opening in the nasal mucosa and in the bones forming the lacrimal fossa
- Stenting the rhinostomy opening
- Removal of sialastic lacrimal stents later

Who discovered DCR surgery?

- Dupuys-Dutemps

8.6 ENUCLEATION AND EVISCERATION INSTRUMENTS

Mention the list of instruments used in enucleation.

- Speculum
- Tenotomy scissors
- Muscle hooks
- Hemostatic artery forceps
- Enucleation spoon
- Enucleation scissors
- Post-enucleation orbital implant

Describe the following and mention how they are used in enucleation surgery.

- Muscle hooks
- Uses in enucleation: To hook the extraocular muscles before cutting

What are the identifying characteristics of muscle hook?

- The tip is in same plane as the shaft
- Can be with or without eyelet at the tip
- Do not confuse this instrument with:
  - Lens expressor: Tip is rounded; the shaft is right angled to the tip.
  - Lid hook: The tip is acutely angled.

What are the different types of muscle hooks?

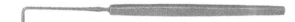

Figure 8.24 Muscle hook - von Grafe

Figure 8.25 Chavasse muscle hook

Figure 8.26 Jameson muscle hook

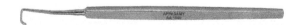

Figure 8.27 Green muscle hook

What are the other uses of muscle hooks?

- Squint surgery
- Scleral buckle
- Enucleation
- IOFB removal via scleral route
- Globe exploration
- Blowout fracture
- Pterygium surgery in order to differentiate the medial/lateral rectus from the pterygium

Describe the instrument and mention its uses in enucleation surgery.

- Hartman hemostatic artery forceps

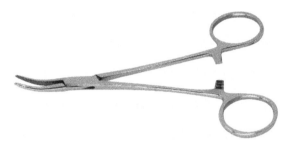

Figure 8.28 Hartman hemostatic artery forceps

- Serrated jaws with ratchet lock
- Uses:
  - Used to clamp and crush the extraocular muscle before cutting
  - Used to help in lifting the globe out of the orbit

Describe the following instrument and mention its uses.

- Wells enucleation spoon

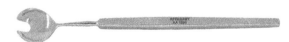

Figure 8.29 Wells enucleation spoon

- Curved with concave hemispherical end
- Available in 15–21 mm diameter for phthisical and staphylomatous globes respectively
- Has optic nerve notch, which is 10 × 5 mm
- Uses:
  - To hold the eyeball before cutting the optic nerve in enucleation surgery
  - Central notch accommodates the optic nerve
  - Do not confuse with evisceration scoop

Describe the following instrument and state its uses.

- Metzenbaum enucleation scissors

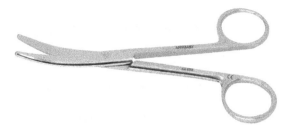

Figure 8.30 Metzenbaum enucleation scissors

- Length (overall length = 135 mm): Helps reach the optic nerve
- Blunt tip: Prevents damage to surrounding orbital structures
- Stout blades: Helps provide adequate force to cut the optic nerve
- The curve of the scissors follows the curve of the globe
- Usually, the scissors are introduced from nasal or temporal side
- Do not to confuse with tenotomy scissors which are comparatively narrower
- Uses:
  - To cut the optic nerve to complete the enucleation
  - Can be used to carry out blunt dissection
  - Can be used to perform full-thickness eyelid incisions in emergency situations
  - Can be rarely used to perform lateral canthotomy

Describe the following instrument and mention its uses.

- Foster enucleation snare

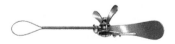

Figure 8.31 Foster enucleation snare

- Fine stainless-steel snare
- Within a stout pipe
- Uses:
  - To perform enucleation when a long optic nerve stump is required
  - Can be used in contracted sockets for enucleation of the eyeball

Identify the following implant introducer.

- Carter sphere holder and introducer

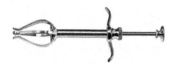

Figure 8.32 Carter sphere holder and introducer

- Proximal broad cavity with distal plunger
- Pushes the implant into the intraconal space
- Uses:
  - To place orbital implants in the intraconal space
  - Maybe used in contracted sockets for implant placement
  - Maybe used in high volume centers in place of disposable plastic introducers

What are the instruments used in evisceration?

- Corneal scissors
- Evisceration scoop
- Post-evisceration orbital motility implant

Describe the instrument and mention its use.

- Mule evisceration scoop
- Bunge evisceration scoop
- Stout curved spatulated scoop

Figure 8.33 Mule evisceration scoop

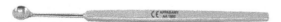

Figure 8.34 Bunge evisceration scoop

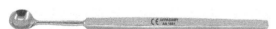

Stout curved spatulated scoop

- Uses:
  - To scoop out the uveal tissue and intraocular contents of the eyeball
  - Scrape the uveal tissue off during evisceration
  - Maybe used for blunt dissection around orbital lesions

8.7 FAQs RELATED TO ENUCLEATION, EVISCERATION, AND EXENTERATION

What is enucleation?

- Enucleation is the surgical removal of the entire eyeball with a portion of the optic nerve
- Extended enucleation or limited exenteration: Removal of conjunctiva, some orbital fat, and portions of EOMs along with standard enucleation

What are indications of enucleation?

- Eyeball donation post-death
- Severe trauma with unsalvageable vision
- Intraocular tumors with unsalvageable eye
- Painful blind eye
- Phthisis Bulbi
- Cosmetically disfigured eyes

What are the contraindications of enucleation?

- Expulsive choroidal hemorrhage
- Panophthalmitis (because there is risk of spread of infection via the cut optic nerve to the brain)

What are the contraindications for eyeball donation?

- Systemic:
  - Death due to unknown cause
  - Transmittable/infectious or potentially infectious disease (CJ disease, HIV/AIDS, hepatitis B/C or active hepatitis A, septicemia, rabies)
  - Central nervous system disorders of unknown etiology (multiple sclerosis, ALS, Alzheimer's disease, Parkinson's disease)
  - Leukemia, lymphoma, lymphosarcoma, Hodgkin's disease (most other types of cancer are acceptable for donation)
- Local:
  - Corneal opacity/pseudophakic bullous keratopathy (PBK)
  - Intraocular malignancy
  - Recurrent uveitis
  - Advanced glaucoma
  - History of refractive surgery
  - Congenital eye disorders
  - Any ocular infection

What are the storage media for eyeball preservation?

Table 8.2 Storage Media for Eyeball

	Medium	Preservation Limit
Immediate	Normal saline/ Ringer lactate	24-hour refrigeration
Short Term	McCarey–Kaufman medium	4 days (96 hours)
Long Term	Optisol and organ culture medium	15 to 30 days

What is length of optic nerve to be cut?

- As long as possible
- At least 10 mm in cases of intraocular tumors

What special precautions to take during enucleation?

- Take care not to perforate sclera, especially in retinoblastoma to avoid seeding
- Avoid orbital implant in case of tumor as it can mask a recurrence

What are the surgical steps of enucleation?

- Get consent.
- Technique: GA, LA.
- Check correct eye.
- 360° conjunctival peritomy.
- 360° blunt dissection, 1.5 mm behind the limbus, in the sub-tenons plane.
- Isolation of recti and oblique muscles and then cut them.
- Cut the optic nerve.
- Pressure pack to achieve hemostasis.
- Place orbital implant in the intraconal space.
- Reattach the muscles.
- Suture the wound in two layers.
- Place conformer and make a temporary tarsorrhaphy.

What special precautions are to be taken during enucleation?

- Check if it is the correct eye of the correct patient.
- Take care not to perforate sclera, especially in retinoblastoma to avoid seeding.
- Avoid Orbital implant in case of tumor.
- Hydroxyapatite not preferred if postoperative radiotherapy has to be given as it prevents vascularization.

What is evisceration?

- Removal of contents of eye, keeping scleral shell intact

What are the indications of evisceration?

- Panophthalmitis
- Expulsive hemorrhage
- Bleeding anterior staphyloma with no PL (perception of light)
- Absolute glaucoma

What are the contraindications of evisceration?

- Seeing eye
- Any of the indications of enucleation

What are the complications of evisceration?

- Bleeding
- Extrusion of implant
- Theoretical risk of sympathetic ophthalmitis of other eye (if the uveal tissue is not removed completely)
- Infection

What are the steps of evisceration?

- Remove the corneal button
- Remove iris, lens, vitreous, retina, choroid
- Make radial cuts and scleral window
- Insert the orbital implant
- Close sclera (absorbable suture with 6-0 Vicryl)
- Close the conjunctiva and tenon's in layers in opposite directions (absorbable suture with 6-0 Vicryl)
- Conformer placed of appropriate size

What is frill evisceration?

- Frill excision (only a frill of sclera around the optic nerve is kept intact)

What is exenteration?

- Removal of eye with all the orbital contents

What are the indications of exenteration?

- Orbital malignancies
- Primary:
  - Rhabdomyosarcoma
  - Neuroblastoma
- Secondary:
  - From the globe: Retinoblastoma, multiple myeloma

- From the adnexa: Lacrimal gland adenocarcinoma
- From the nose and sinuses
- Fungal infections:
  - Mucor
  - Aspergillosis

What are the various approaches to orbital exenteration along with their pros and cons?

- Anterior exenteration:
  - Indications: Conjunctival Malignancy
  - Contents removed:
    - Globe
    - Posterior lamella of eyelids
    - Conjunctival sac
  - Contents preserved:
    - Periorbita
    - Posterior orbital contents
  - Final appearance: A shallow socket lined with skin
  - Complications:
    - Delayed healing
    - Hematoma behind the flaps
    - Immobile, ill-fitting prosthesis
- Subtotal exenteration sparing the lids
  - Indications:
    - Primary orbital malignancy without involving lids
    - Secondary malignancy, spread from globe or conjunctiva, not involving lids
  - Contents removed: The contents of orbit including periosteum of orbital wall
  - Contents preserved: Some or all of the skin and orbicularis muscle of eyelids
  - Final appearance: A deep orbit with residual lid, skin, and orbicularis sutured together
  - Complications:
    - Granulation and delayed healing of wound
    - Hematoma behind the flaps
    - Ill-fitting, immobile prosthesis
    - Ptosis, entropion, ectropion of the lids
- Total radical exenteration, including the lids
  - Indications:
    - Primary orbital malignancy
    - Secondary orbital malignancy spreading from lids, conjunctiva, globe, PNS
    - Mucormycosis or orbit
    - Advanced stage of pseudotumor of orbit for relief of pain

- Contents removed:
  - The contents of orbits
  - Periosteum of orbital wall
  - Lids
  - Sometimes combined with radical craniofacial surgery or radical sinus surgery
- Contents preserved: Orbital bare bones with or without a primary split skin graft
- Final appearance: When healing is completed, a spectacle mounted prosthesis (or) prosthesis fixed with titanium pegs placed in the orbital rim
- Complications:
  - CSF leak
  - Fistula into PNS
  - Delayed healing by granulation tissue
  - Hematoma formation
  - Keratinization of skin graft
  - Malodorous socket
  - Infection
  - Recurrence of malignancy
  - Poor cosmetic appearance
- En bloc orbitectomy or super exenteration
  - Indications:
    - Primary or secondary malignancy of orbit involving the adjacent bones
    - Multidisciplinary procedure involving orbital surgeon, neurosurgeon, faciomaxillary reconstructive surgeon
  - Contents removed: Fronto-temporal-sphenoidal craniectomy
  - Contents preserved: Subfrontal dura reflected and mobilized posteriorly, frontal bone is replaced, anastomosis of superficial temporal artery to a myocutaneous vascular flap
  - Final appearance:
    - Primary bony reconstruction using posterior plate of frontal craniotomy, or rib graft
    - Orbitectomy cavity can be filled with a delto-pectoral myocutaneous vascular flap
    - A spectacle-mounted prosthesis
  - Complications:
    - All the aforementioned complications
    - Exposure of intracranial contents
    - Extremely poor cosmetic appearance

8.8 ORBITAL IMPLANTS

Describe the post-enucleation implant.

- Orbital implant covered with Vicryl mesh

- Implanted after enucleation with help of injector
- Vicryl mesh acts as scleral shell and helps in ingrowth of blood vessels

Describe the post-evisceration orbital implant?

- Orbital implant introduced with injector
- Not covered with Vicryl mesh as scleral shell is already present

Classify the various types of orbital implants?

- Nonintegrated: No integration of the implant with the structure of the orbit; e.g., PMMA or silicone implant
- Semi-integrated: Mechanical integration of the implant with the structures of the orbit, without a prosthesis; e.g., Allen implant
- Integrated implant: Mechanical integration of the implant with the structures of the orbit and with a prosthesis; e.g., Cutler's implant
- Bio-integrated implant: Biological integration of natural or synthetic implant with structures of the orbit with or without integration with a prosthesis; e.g., hydroxyapatite implant, porous polyethylene implant, aluminum oxide implant
- Biogenic implant: Biological integration of the orbital structures with an autogenic or allo-genic implant of natural tissue; e.g., dermis fat graft, cancellous bone

What are the advantages of orbital implants?

- Cosmetically fuller appearance of the orbit
- Gives motility to the artificial prosthesis
- Acts as a stimulus for bony growth in children

What are the disadvantages of implants?

- Extrusion
- Reaction
- Infection
- Masking recurrence of malignancy

What are the properties of ideal orbital implant?

- Non-toxic
- Resists infection
- Suture material can be placed through it.
- Inexpensive
- Should maintain volume

What materials are commonly used in orbital implants?

- Biological: Dermis fat graft
- Non-biological:
  - High-density polyethylene (Medpor)
  - Acrylic
  - Hydroxyapatite
  - Other: Glass, plastic, and gold
- Options of material for covering the implant
  - Sclera
  - Mersilene mesh/Vicryl mesh/Dacron mesh
  - Amniotic membrane

What are the advantages and disadvantages of non-biological implants?

- Integrated:
  - Made of porous material (tissues can grow into the implant)
  - Examples:
    - Hydroxy-apatite
    - Polyethylene (Medpor)
    - Aluminum oxide (Alumina)
  - Advantages:
    - Excellent mobility
    - Rarely migrates
    - Pegging of the implant is possible
  - Disadvantages:
    - Infections
    - Extrusion is higher than non-integrated implants
    - Expensive
- Semi-integrated:
  - They have large gaps through which the muscles are pulled and tied
  - Example: Allen implant
  - Advantages:
    - Inexpensive
    - Good mobility
  - Disadvantage: Risk of exposure is higher due to the irregular surface rubbing against the artificial eye
- Non-integrated:
  - Acrylic
  - Often encased in a capsule of tissue
  - There is little or no contact with the muscles
  - Example: Acrylic ball implant
  - Advantages: Inexpensive; very low risk of exposure
  - Disadvantages: Less movement; can migrate within the orbit

What are the advantages and disadvantages of biological implants?

- Advantages:
  - No risk of extrusion
  - Infection is easy to treat as it does not require removal of the implant
  - Graft provides volume (fat) and lining
- Disadvantage: Unpredictable volume replacement as variable resorption

What are the causes of a contracted socket?

- Chemical burns or radiation injury
- Poor initial surgical technique with excessive sacrifice of conjunctiva and tenons tissue
- Cicatrizing conjunctival diseases
- Implant migration or exposure or an ill-fitting prosthesis

What is the classification of a contracted socket?

- Gopal Krishna classification
  - Grade 1: Shallow lower fornix
  - Grade 2: Loss of upper and lower fornices
  - Grade 3: Loss of upper, lower, medial, and lateral fornices
  - Grade 4: Loss of all four fornices along with reduction of vertical and horizontal palpebral aperture
- Grade 5: Recurrence of socket contraction

8.9 FAQS ON ORBITOTOMY

What are the surgical approaches to the orbit? (Table 8.3)

What are the common indications for performing an orbitotomy?

- 1 year: Dermoid, hemangioma, retinoblastoma (only if the retinoblastoma tumor has extra-ocular extension)
- 1–5 years: Dermoid, retinoblastoma, rhabdomyosarcoma
- 5–10 years: Pseudotumor, dermoid, optic nerve glioma, RMS, lymphangioma, lymphoma
- 10–30 years: Peripheral nerve sheath tumor (schwannoma), dysthyroid ophthalmopathy, pseudotumor
- 30–70 years: Lacrimal gland tumors (pleomorphic adenoma, adenoid cystic carcinoma), cavernous hemangioma, dysthyroid orbitopathy, pseudotumor, meningioma

Table 8.3 Surgical Approaches to the Orbit

1. Stallard–Wright incision	For superior/lateral orbitotomy
2. Byron Smith lid-splitting incision	
3. Benedict's incision	
4. Berkes–Kronlein incision	
5. Lynch incision	For medial orbitotomy
6. Gull wing incision	
7. Subciliary Incision	For inferior orbitotomy
8. Infraorbital Incision	
9. Transconjunctival incision for medial/lateral orbitotomy	
10. Forniceal approach for superior/posterior/lesion at orbital apex	For transconjunctival orbitotomy
11. Transnasal endoscopic approach for medial posterior lesions	
12. Transantral approach for inferior lesion/blowout fractures	

- 70 years: Melanoma, metastatic orbital tumors, basal cell carcinoma, mucocoele
- Orbital foreign body removal

8.10 LID-SURGERY-RELATED INSTRUMENTS

Identify and describe the instrument.

- Meyerhoefer chalazion curette

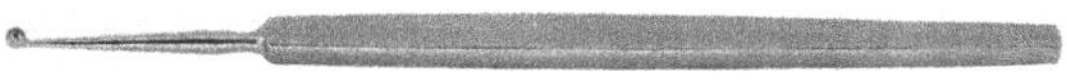

Figure 8.35 Meyerhoefer chalazion curette

- Small round scoop-like end with a long shaft
- Edges of the curette maybe sharp or serrated
- Uses:
  - Helps in non-traumatic curetting of chalazion
  - Residual uveal tissue during evisceration maybe removed using this

Identify and describe the instrument.

- Lambert chalazion forceps

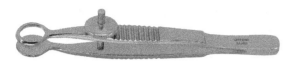

Figure 8.36 Meyerhoefer chalazion curette

- Plate and ring at one end with a screw lock
- Various types are present:
  - Lamberts: Round plate
  - Desmarres: Oval plate
  - Hunt: Angulated limbs
  - Cauer: Serrated inner plate surface
- Uses:
  - During incision and curettage of a chalazion it helps in localization of the lesion and achieving hemostasis
  - Hemostasis during biopsy of small eyelid lesions

Identify and describe the instrument.

- Desmarres eyelid retractor

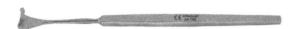

Figure 8.37 Desmarres eyelid retractor

- C-shaped blades with blunt edges
- Depending on the width of this blade, it comes in various sizes:
  - 0 = 11 mm wide
  - 1 = 13 mm wide
  - 2 = 15 mm wide
  - 3 = 17 mm wide
- Uses:
  - Double eyelid eversion to search for superior fornicial foreign bodies
  - To evert the eyelids to wash off debris after chemical injuries
  - To open the eyelids in uncooperative patients or in patients with blepharospasm
  - Retract eyelids, muscle and fat in orbital surgeries

What is a chalazion?

- Chronic inflammatory granuloma of the Meibomian glands

How is the chalazion clamp used?

- The plate is placed on the cutaneous side and ring on the conjunctival side and the screw is tightened.

Why is the incision vertical?

- Injury to the adjacent meibomian glands is minimized
- Minimum injury to conjunctival and tarsal blood vessels, which are vertically placed

What is your approach to recurrent chalazion after surgery?

- Rule out diabetes.
- Rule out sebaceous gland carcinoma in the elderly.
- Treat anterior blepharitis and meibomian gland disease.

Identify and describe the following instrument.

- Epilation forceps

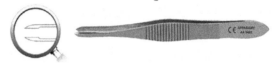

Figure 8.38 Epilation forceps

- Stout handle with round or tapered angulated tips
- Use: Manual epilation of trichiatic lashes
- Disadvantage: Recurrence of trichiasis
- Other alternatives to epilation
  - Electrocautery (2 milliamp current is used to burn the hair follicle permanently)
  - Cryotherapy of hair follicle (not advisable in pigmented races as depigmentation of the skin may occur)

What is trichaisis? What are its causes?

- Trichiasis is the inward turning of the eyelashes
- Etiology:
  - Thermal/chemical burns/radiation
  - Herpes zoster ophthalmicus (HZO)
  - Trachoma
  - Chronic blepharitis; post-ulcerative blepharitis
  - Benign mucosal pemphigoid
  - Stevens–Johnson syndrome
  - Lid malignancies

Identify and describe the following instrument.

- Jaeger/Berke–Jaeger/Khan–Jaeger eyelid plate

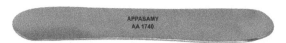

Figure 8.39 Jaeger/Berke–Jaeger/Khan–Jaeger eyelid plate

- Slight convex surface
- 100 mm long plate life
- Available in pediatric and adult sizes
- Two surfaces:
  - Convex = Dull surface
  - Concave = Touches the cornea
- Uses:
  - Lid surgeries: Entropion, ectropion, ptosis correction to provide stability while making incisions and incising the tarsal plate
  - Protects globe from needles or silicone rods during ptosis surgery
  - Provides support
  - Helps in creating dissection planes during orbitotomy when used as a fat retractor

Identify and describe the following instrument.

- Snellen entropion clamp

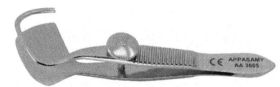

Figure 8.40 Snellen entropion clamp

- U-shaped superior rim
- D-shaped inferior plate acts as a flat base
- Screw mechanism to tighten the limbs
- Uses:
  - Plate design supports the lid
  - Protects the globe
  - Hemostasis

How do you determine which eye and which lid the instrument has to be used for?

- Hold the clamp in such a way that:
  - Handle faces the temporal side
  - Screw faces anteriorly
  - Plate is on the posterior side
  - Ring is on the anterior side
- This hold determines which sides upper lid it belongs to. (This position will be the position for the opposite eye lower lid.)

8.11 FAQs ON ENTROPION AND ECTROPION

What is entropion?

- Inward turning of the eyelid margin (trichiasis is the inward turning of a lash)
- Types:
  - Congenital
  - Involutional or senile entropion is commonest in the lower lid
  - Cicatricial entropion is commonest in the upper lid (Commonly due to Trachoma)
  - Spastic
- Degree (snap test)
  - Mild
  - Moderate
  - Severe
- Sequelae:
  - Chronic conjunctivitis
  - Corneal ulcer non-healing
  - Persistent FB sensation
  - Tearing

What is the difference between congenital entropion and epiblepharon?

Table 8.4 Differences between Congenital Entropion and Epiblepharon

Congenital Entropion	Epiblepharon
Lid margin and tarsal plate both turn in	Only lid margin turns in
Very rare	Common
No spontaneous resolution	Spontaneous resolution can occur
Lid crease absent	Lid crease present
Treatment: Hotz procedure	Treatment: Hotz procedure

- Congenital entropion is rather rare, but one should rule out epiblepharon which is inward turning of lid margin and not tarsal plate.

What are the points to note while evaluating entropion?

- Check for conjunctival scarring, check the rest of the ocular surface for foreign bodies, dry eyes, trichiasis, or any anterior or posterior blepharitis.
- Check for transverse ridge due to overriding of preseptal muscle on pretarsal muscle.

- Tests to be performed: Syringing, Jones' test, Schirmer's test.
- Check horizontal lid laxity—pinch test.
  - Horizontal eyelid distraction.
  - Hills test: Pinch and pull lower lid from center.
  - If cornea and posterior lid margin distance is >8 mm, then it is abnormal.
- Check lid elasticity—snap test:
  - Put finger at the center of lower lid and pull lower lid.
  - Ask patient not to blink and leave the lid and look for:
  - Quick snap—no laxity (<2 seconds)
  - Slow snap—mild laxity
  - Needs a blink to come back to normal—moderate laxity
  - In spite of blinking, the lid does not come back to normal—severe laxity
- Canthal Tendon Laxity: Pull the medial or lateral canthus in the opposite direction, look at the movement of the canthal angle toward closest limbus on the lateral side and visualize movement of the punctum (inferior) on the medial side.
  - It should not pull >1–2 mm.
  - If you can pull more than 1–2 mm, then it is abnormal.
  - Rounding of the lateral canthus is abnormal.

What is the management of entropion?

- Non-surgical:
  - Lubricants and taping of the eyelids
  - Botulinum toxin injection
  - Bandage contact lens over the cornea
- Surgical: Management per type of entropion:
  - Congenital entropion: Hotz procedure (ellipse of skin and orbicularis muscle excision from medial two thirds of the lower lid and lower lid crease creation, skin is fixed to the lower tarsal edge)
  - Acquired/involutional
  - Temporary procedures
    - Transverse sutures: Used to prevent the upward movement of the preseptal orbicularis muscle
    - Everting sutures: Placed obliquely to shorten the lower lid retractors, in mild cases and the effect is temporary (approximately lasts for 18 months)
  - Permanent procedures
    - Tightening of canthal tendons

  - Weiss procedure: Transverse lid split with everting sutures, in those cases with minimum horizontal lid laxity
  - Quickert procedure: Vertical lid split and everting sutures along with horizontal lid shortening in cases with additional horizontal lid laxity (effect is longer lasting)
  - Jones procedure: In recurrent lower lid involutional entropion (possibly after Quickert procedure) wherein plication of lower lid retractors is performed (effect is longer lasting)
- Acquired/cicatricial
  - Tenzel procedure: Tarsal fracture and margin rotation (lid retraction <1.5 mm from limbus)
  - Everting sutures with posterior lamellar graft with tarsal split
  - Tarsal wedge resection (cases with scarring due to trachoma)
  - Posterior lamellar grafting (lid retraction >1.5 mm from limbus)
  - Eyelid lengthening with free tarsoconjunctival, scleral, or cartilage graft

What is ectropion? Classify it.

- Definition: Outward turning of the eyelid margin
- Classification:
  - Involutional
  - Cicatricial: Look for scar/generalized tightening
  - Paralytic due to seventh-nerve palsy
  - Mechanical
  - Congenital
- Degrees:
  - 1st: Punctum of lower lid seen (normally not seen)
  - 2nd: Conjunctiva immediately behind inter-marginal strip
  - 3rd: Inferior fornix seen; check for horizontal lid laxity

What are the tests for diagnosing ectropion?

- Pinch test
- Snap test
- Orbicularis muscle tone
- Lower lid retractor disinsertion
- Canthal tendon integrity
- Also check the lacrimal apparatus, corneal sensations, and whether there is lagophthalmos or not

What are the procedures in the management of ectropion?

- Involutional/paralytic
  - Non-surgical: Lubricants along with antibiotics if required.
  - Sutures: From inferior border of tarsus emerging through skin at infraorbital rim used in bed ridden patients as a temporary procedure.
  - Electrocautery: Deep burns are placed at the junction of conjunctiva and lower border of the tarsal plate.
  - Medial spindle procedure: Diamond-shaped tarsoconjunctiva is excised below the punctum.
  - Medial canthus laxity: Medial canthal ligament is attached it to the posterior lacrimal crest.
  - Lateral canthal laxity: Lateral canthal sling procedure is performed.
  - Pentagon wedge resection: In case of horizontal lid laxity, a horizontal lid shortening with pentagon skin excision is performed.
  - Smith's modification of Kuhnt-Szymanowski Procedure: Done when there is horizontal lid laxity with excessive redundant skin
  - It has two components:
    - Lid shortening
    - Blepharoplasty
  - Lazy T: It is done when there is excessive horizontal lower lid ectropion with punctal ectropion. Tarsoconjunctival diamond excision with horizontal lid shortening with medial wedge resection is performed in this procedure. Usually done in seventh nerve palsies.
- Cicatricial ectropion:
  - Linear scar: Z-plasty
  - Generalized contraction: Full-thickness skin graft (most commonly used is post-auricular skin)

8.12 PTOSIS SURGERY INSTRUMENTS

Identify and describe the instrument.

- Berke's ptosis clamp
- L-shaped blades with transverse serrations on the inner surface

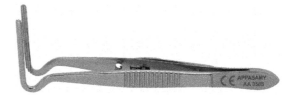

Figure 8.41 Berke's ptosis clamp

- Tips of blades point nasally and slide lock should be kept superiorly
- Two different ptosis clamps for the right and left side lid depending on the side of the tips of the blades
- Uses:
  - To support and clamp the levator muscle during its dissection
  - Helps achieve hemostasis
  - Can be used in LPS resection, disinsertion, and advancement

Identify and describe the following.

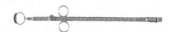

Figure 8.42 Fascia lata stripper

Figure 8.43 Wright's fascia needle

- Needle tip bent at 90°
- Large eye for passing harvested fascia lata

What are the types of sling materials?

- Permanent:
  - Fascia lata
  - Autologous dura
  - External digiti minimi tendon
- Temporary:
  - PTFE suture (Gore-Tex)
  - Nylon
  - Silicone band
  - Mersilene mesh

Identify and describe the following.

- **Putterman clamp**

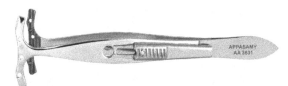

Figure 8.44 Putterman clamp

- Uses:
  - Müller's muscle–conjunctival resection (MMCR) blepharoptosis repair
  - Can be used to correct mild ptosis (2 mm) with good levator function (>10 mm) and positive response to pheylephrine test
- Role in surgery:
  - Putterman Müller's muscle–conjunctival resection clamp is placed at the border of the superior tarsus and clamped shut, sandwiching the conjunctiva and Müller's muscle.
  - It has three needles to penetrate through the squeezed conjunctiva and Müller's muscle so that they do not slip out of the clamp, thereby ensuring the correct desired amount of tissue is resected.

8.13 FAQs ON PTOSIS

What are the important points to remember during ptosis examination?

- Head posture: Chin up in severe ptosis.
- Refraction must be done to rule out amblyopia or astigmatism.
- Iris color is hypochromic in Horner's syndrome.
- Pupil anisocoria is present in Horner's syndrome and third-nerve palsy.
- EOM examination to check for SR weakness, aberrant third-nerve palsy.
- Orbicularis function must be tested.

What is the classification of ptosis?

- The difference between the MRD1 between two sides or the difference from normal (in bilateral cases) gives the amount of ptosis:
  - Mild: ≤2 mm
  - Moderate: 3 mm
  - Severe: ≥4 mm

What are the tests done and measurements taken prior to ptosis surgery?

- MRD 1: Distance from light reflex to center of upper lid margin (CULM)
  - Normal: 4–5 mm
  - Positive value if it is above the light reflex and negative value if it is below the central corneal light reflex
  - In U/L cases: MRD1 normal—MRD1 ptotic lid
  - In B/L ptosis = 4.5 mm—MRD1
  - Amount of ptosis
    - Mild: 2 mm
    - Moderate: 3 mm
    - Severe: 4 mm
- MRD 2: Distance from corneal light reflex to the center of the lower lid margin
- MRD 3: Alternate to MLD2 in cases of vertical squint (normal = 7 mm)
- Levator function evaluation:
  - Presence of lid crease
  - Berke's method: Excursion of upper lid from extreme downgaze to upgaze after blocking the action of the frontalis muscle
    - Poor: ≤4 mm
    - Fair: 5–7 mm
    - Good: ≥8 mm
    - Normal: 15 mm
  - Putterman's method: MLD is the distance between center of upper lid margin to the inferior limbus while patient is looking in extreme upgaze
    - Normal MLD: 9 mm
    - In unilateral ptosis: Difference in MLD of two eyes is measured
    - In bilateral Ptosis: Difference from normal is measured
    - And that MLD × 3 = Amount of levator resection
  - Indirect methods are used (in children):
    - Presence of lid fold and if it increases/decreases with lid movements.
    - Abnormal head posture.
    - In young children <1 year of age, evert the upper lid. If the levator function is good, the lid reverts on its own.
  - Illiff test: Upper lid is everted in downgaze on looking up lid should return to normal.
- MCD
  - Distance from the CULM to the central upper lid skin crease in downgaze.

- The most prominent lid crease is taken and compared on the normal side.
- It is the cutaneous insertion of the levator aponeurosis.
- Normal: 5–7 mm
- Essential in planning position of lid crease in Skin approach levator resection surgery.
- Absent lid crease suggests poor levator function with high lid crease suggests aponeurotic dehiscence.
- MLD1: Same as MRD 1 instead inferior limbus is used instead of the corneal reflex measured in primary gaze.
- MLD 2:
  - CULM to 6 o'clock limbus in extreme upgaze
  - Gives degree of loss of function rather than LPS function
  - In U/L ptosis = MLD2 Normal—MLD2 ptotic lid
  - In B/L ptosis = 9—MLD2
  - Putterman and Urist formula = Amount of LPS resection (in mm) = Difference in LPS function × 3
- Palpebral aperture:
  - Measure in all positions gives an idea of the etiology of ptosis
  - Width of the palpebral aperture at maximal separation in primary gaze
    - Normal: 9–10 mm in primary gaze
    - In unilateral ptosis difference in palpebral aperture of two eyes gives the degree of ptosis
    - In bilateral ptosis difference in palpebral aperture from normal amount
  - Disadvantage: Alteration in lower lid position can alter the measurements, such as in Horner's syndrome where there is reverse ptosis of the lower lid.
  - Congenital ptosis: Palpebral aperture in ptotic eye in downgaze will be equal or larger than the normal contralateral eye.
  - Aponeurotic ptosis: Palpebral aperture in ptotic eye in downgaze will be smaller than the normal contralateral eye.
- Pretarsal show: Distance between the lid margin and the skin fold with the eyes in primary position
- Check for ocular movements, cover-uncover test to rule out squint, third-nerve palsy
- Bell's phenomenon:
  - Disappearance of Cornea under upper lid on attempted eye closure
  - Good: >2/3rd disappears
  - Fair: 1/3rd–2/3rd disappears
  - Poor: <1/3rd disappears
- Marcus Gunn jaw winking phenomenon: 5% cases of congenital ptosis
  - Mild = <2 mm lid lift
  - Moderate = 2–5 mm lid lift
  - Severe = >5 mm lid lift
- Schirmer's test
- Corneal sensations and fluorescein staining
- Lagophthalmos
- Pupils: In Horner's syndrome, third-nerve palsy
- Old photographs
- Fatiguability: Look up for 30 seconds without blinking
- Cogan lid twitch: Overshoot of the upper lid on saccade from downgaze to primary position in myasthenia
- Pharmacological test:
  - 2.5% phenylephrine test: For Muller's muscle function, if ptosis reduces then a mullerectomy surgery can be done
  - Tensilon test: For myasthenia gravis
- Manually elevate the ptotic lid to check for dropping on the opposite side as increased innervation to the LPS muscle particularly in upgaze on the ptotic side may cause increase in innervation to the contralateral normal levator resulting in lid retraction.

What are the indications of surgery in ptosis?

- Visual:
  - Prevention of deprivation or anisometropic amblyopia especially in unilateral moderate to severe ptosis in a baby
  - Bilateral congenital ptosis—in moderate to severe ptosis to prevent long term structural neck changes
  - Severe aponeurotic ptosis in elderly
  - Post traumatic
  - Complete third-nerve palsy after management of strabismus
- Cosmetic

What are the contraindications of ptosis surgery?

- CPEO
- Reduced or absent Bell's phenomenon

- Myasthenia gravis
- Strabismus fixus
- Mechanical ptosis

How does one decide when to operate?

- Severity: Severe ptosis covering the pupil requires early surgery.
- Age: Babies with severe ptosis require early surgery.
- Laterality: Unilateral ptosis requires early surgery if risk of developing amblyopia is high.
- For bilateral/severe condition, the ideal time is as early as possible for amblyopia prevention.

What are the factors that determine the choice of surgery?

- Cause of ptosis: Congenital, traumatic, aponeurotic
- Laterality: Unilateral/bilateral
- Severity
- Levator function
- Associations such as squint/amblyopia/ blepharophimosis/aberrant third nerve
- Decision makers: Levator function and degree of ptosis
  - If levator function (LF) is more than 4 mm, then levator resection can be done for mild/moderate or severe ptosis.
  - If levator function is good (>10 mm) and ptosis mild (<2 mm), then the surgery done is Fasanella–Servat operation.
  - If levator function is poor (<4 mm), a brow suspension surgery is performed.

What is the treatment of ptosis?

- Non-surgical:
  - Crutch glasses
  - Treatment of myasthenia
  - Guanithidine eyedrops: In Horner's syndrome
- Choice of operations per LPS function:
  - LPS function 8–10 mm: Fasanella–Servat surgery
  - LPS function 4–8 mm: Levator resection surgery
  - For LPS function <4 mm: Brow suspension/tarso-frontal sling surgery
  - Crawford technique
  - Fox procedure

- Repair and exploration of an aponeurotic defect, especially if there is excess of skin: Levator aponeurotic repair
- Choice of operation as severity of ptosis:
  - Mild ptosis (2 mm of upper lid covering limbus) + Good LPS action
  - Positive phenylephrine test: Fasanella– Servat operation
  - Negative phenylephrine test:
    - LPS resection (small: 0–13 mm)
    - Fair LPS action: LPS resection (moderate: 14–17 mm)
  - Moderate ptosis (2–4 mm of upper lid covering limbus) +
    - Good LPS action: Moderate LPS resection
    - Fair LPS action: Large LPS resection
    - Poor LPS action: Sling/max LPS resection
  - Severe ptosis (>4 mm of upper lid covering limbus):
    - Bilateral:
      - Fair LPS action: Max resection of LPS
      - Poor LPS action: Tarso-frontal sling surgery
    - Unilateral: LPS action:
      - Fair LPS action: Maximal resection of the LPS
      - Poor LPS action
      - Beards method: Levator excision of that eye with bilateral sling
      - Callahan's method: Only bilateral sling
      - Supramaximal resection of LPS
- If associated with Marcus Gunn phenomenon
  - Mild MG phenomenon: Treat per the protocol
  - Moderate/severe MG Phenomenon: Levator excision with bilateral sling

What should the lid level be at the time of the surgery?

- 1–3 mm from upper limbus
- Likely to change in first 6 weeks
- Will rise by 1–2 mm if LPS action >7 mm
- Will drop by 1–2 mm if LPS action <7 mm

What should the time of surgery be?

- Congenital ptosis: 3–4 years
- Severe ptosis leading to amblyopia: Temporary sling (especially if unilateral can be done in infancy)

What are the various types of ptosis surgeries?

- Muller's muscle surgery: If levator function is >8–10 mm
  - Fasanella–Servat procedure
  - Tarsomullerectomy—Mullers muscle conjunctival resection (MMCR)
- Levator muscle surgery: If levator function is 4–8 mm
  - LPS resection
  - Levator aponeurosis advancement
  - Levator aponeurosis repair
- Tarso-frontal sling: If levator function is < 4 mm

What are the complications of ptosis surgery?

- Overcorrection
- Undercorrection
- Asymmetry after bilateral levator resection
- Exposure keratopathy
- Lid lag/lagophthalmos
- Entropion/ectropion
- Lid contour deformity
- Loss of lashes
- Lid crease improper/absent
- Conjunctival prolapse
- Orbital hemorrhage

What are the principles of levator surgery in ptosis?

- Levator resection less than 10–12 mm is not effective.
- Amount of levator resection:
  - Small = 10–13 mm
  - Moderate = 14–17 mm
  - Large = 18–22 mm
  - Maximum = 23
- Overcorrection is easier to correct (by massage) than undercorrection that requires re-surgery.
- In all congenital ptosis, lid will come down by 0.5 mm after 6–8 weeks.
- In all acquired ptosis, lid will lift by 0.5 mm after 6–8 weeks.

What is the Life Placement as per Levator Function?

Table 8.5 Lid Placement According to Levator Function

Levator Function	Lid Placement
2–4 mm	1 mm above the limbus
5–7 mm	1 mm below the limbus
More than 8 mm	2 mm below the limbus

What are the various approaches of levator (LPS) resection surgery and their pros and cons?

Table 8.6 Approaches of LPS Resection Surgery

	Anterior	Posterior
Name	Everbush	Blascovick
Approach	Skin	Conjunctiva
Orientation	Direct	Upside down
Speed and localization of levator	Better	Tougher
Access to tarsus and advancement	Easy	Difficult
Large resection	Possible	Difficult
Adjusting lid margin curves	+	-
Risk of injury to lacrimal gland	Less	More
Skin scar	+	-

What are the indications and contraindications of sling surgery?

- Indications for sling surgery:
  - Moderate or severe ptosis with poor LPS action
  - Moderate or severe ptosis with Marcus Gunn phenomenon
  - Blepharophimosis syndrome
  - Misdirected third-nerve/total third-nerve palsy
  - Failed previous ptosis operation
  - Temporary sling in children
- Contraindications:
  - Poor Bell's phenomenon
  - Reduced corneal sensations
  - Unilateral ptosis

8.14 FAQs ON MYASTHENIA GRAVIS

What is myasthenia gravis?

- Autoimmune disorder of postsynaptic neuromuscular junction characterized by weakness of muscle

What are the types?

- Can be:
  - Ocular
  - General
  - Bulbar

- Systemic
- Neonatal
- Can be:
  - Primary (autoimmune)
  - Secondary (paraneoplastic syndrome)

What are its associations?

- Thymoma
- Thyroid disorder
- Vitiligo
- SLE
- Pernicious anemia
- Less common:
  - Ulcerative colitis
  - Aplastic anemia
  - Kaposi's sarcoma
  - Sjogren's syndrome

Describe the clinical feature.

- Pathology: Deficiency of acetyl choline receptors due to auto antibodies
- Clinical features:
  - Onset at any age
  - Peak at third decade
  - Females > Males
  - Variable and fluctuating symptoms
  - Recovery with rest/sleep
  - May mimic any muscle palsy
  - On upgaze, there is increased droop due to fatigue
  - Lower lid droop
  - Increased droop on repeated up and down movements
  - Does not involve pupil
  - Complaints of double vision
- Signs:
  - Levator signs:
    - Curtain sign: Lift one lid, other droops
    - Cogan lid twitch: Re-fixation from down to primary gaze causes over elevation of upper lid
  - Orbicularis signs:
    - Eyelash sign: Eyelashes cannot be buried on forced lid closure
    - Eye peek sign: Lid drifts open slowly after closure
  - Other:
    - Variability in signs and symptoms
  - Pupils normal

What are the investigations for diagnosis of MG?

- Sleep test

- Ice pack test
- Edrophonium test: 0.2 mg test dose, then 0.8 mg IV
- Neostigmine test
  - Pretreat with atropine
  - 1.5 mg for adults or 0.04 mg/kg for children
- Pyridostigmine test: 60 mg three times/day to be tapered per response
- For aforementioned tests: Pre- and post-injection photographs to be taken
- ACh receptor antibodies: Normal <0.7 nmol/liter
- Orbicularis is most frequently involved
- Investigations of MG with orbicularis involvement is highly suggestive of MG
- Nerve conduction study: Abnormal decremental response
- Single fiber EMG: Impaired impulses
- CT chest and thyroid function to r/o associated disorders

Which are the drugs with aggravate MG?

- Aminoglycosides, clindamycin
- Anesthetics
- B blockers
- Chloroquine
- Tranquilizers
- Lithium, magnesium
- Penicillamine

What are the treatment options?

- Anticholinesterase:
  - Usually pyridostigmine (60 mg three times/day tapered per response during day)
  - Side effects: Salivation, sweating, palpitations, diarrhea (patient should be made aware of it)
  - Maximum dose: 120 mg every × 3 hourly
- Immunosuppressants:
  - Steroids:
    - 60–100 mg/day of prednisolone
    - Indications: No response to anticholinesterase
  - Azathioprine, cyclosporine, cyclophosphamide
  - Plasmapheresis
    - For MG crises
    - Pre-op before thymectomy
  - Thymectomy
    - For thymoma
    - <55 years with generalized MG

- – Not controlled with pyridostigmine
- – Response seen after 2–3 years most of the time
- Temporary ocular treatment
  - – Diplopia treated with patching or prisms
  - – Avoid squint surgery

What is the prognosis?

- 40% remain ocular
- 10% remission
- 50% progress to generalized MG

What is the differential diagnosis?

- Myotonic dystrophy
- Thyroid ophthalmopathy
- CPEO
- Botulinum
- Lambert–Eaton MG:
  - Presynaptic defect (calcium channel)
  - Negative tensilon test
  - Associated with small cell carcinoma of the lung
  - Treatment with guanethidine
- GBS
- Precautions in dealing with MG patients:
  - Inform anesthetist to avoid curare like agents
  - To differentiate between myasthenic crises and cholinergic crises

8.15 PROPTOSIS

Identify the instrument.

How does one clinically measure proptosis?

- Inspection methods:
  - Naffziger's method: Standing behind the seated patient, the observer gazes tangentially toward the chin from the forehead (asking the patient to tilt head slightly back), to assess the relative protrusion of the eye beyond the orbital rim

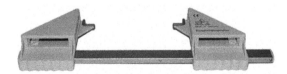

Figure 8.45 Hertel's exophthalmometer

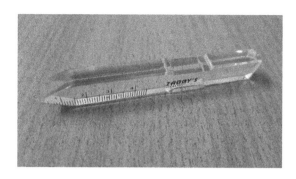

Figure 8.46 Leudde's exophthalmometer

- Worm's eye view: Like above, but observer is in front of patient looking form below upward, while the patient tilts head back.
- Palpation using special equipment:
  - Exact measurement of proptosis can be performed using exophthalmometer or proptometer of various types. These special devices measure the distance from the lateral orbital rim to the apex of the cornea while the patient is in primary gaze.
  - Optical devices:
    - Plain transparent ruler (not recommended)
    - Leudde's exophthalmometer
      - Transparent elongated rectangular box with one end tapered with a notch for fitting at the lateral orbital rim and a scale from 0–40 mm.
      - To measure, patient is seated and the procedure is explained to them.
      - The scale is placed at right angles to the lateral wall, snugly fitting the notch at the orbital rim.
      - Patient is asked to fixate at a target in the primary position.
      - The observer positions one eye from the lateral side of the patient in such a way that the rectangular ends of the Leudde's scale exactly overlap to remove parallax.
      - The apex of the cornea is assessed and reading taken directly off the scale.
      - A variation using twin Leudde's on a transparent scale is also used, which can measure IPD and horizontal dystocia directly along with bilateral exophthalmometry

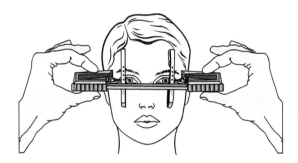

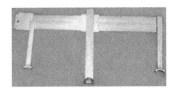

Figure 8.48 Gormaz exophthalmometer

– Hertel's exophthalmometer examination
  – Consists of two horizontally adjustable stands with prisms having a scale (0–40 mm) and a red mark (to ensure no parallax) along with mirrors at each end and a calibrated scale (70–120) for noting the base intercanthal value connecting the two. The adjustable stands at each end have a narrowed notch to be placed at the lateral orbital rim
  – To measure, the patient is seated, and the procedure is explained to them.
  – The examiner should be at eye level of the patient, while the patient is fixating in primary gaze at the examiner's eye while the other eye is occluded.
  – Place the device such that the angled mirrors are above the connecting calibrated rod and the intercanthal distance is adjusted by placing each the notch at the lateral orbital rim at each end, at the level of lateral canthi. (Calibrated scale gives the reading denoted as base.)
  – The examiner closes one eye (usually the right for patient's right side) and tilts head slightly to ensure no parallax, confirmed by aligning the red marks on the scale and base.
  – Note distance from the lateral orbital rim to the corneal apex by checking where the mirror image of the patient's anterior-most corneal curvature falls along the mirror's millimeter ruler. Repeat for the other side.
  – Each side's reading along with base is mentioned.
– Naugle exophthalmometer:

– It uses fixation points slightly above and below the superior and inferior orbital rims (cheekbones and forehead).
– Measures the difference in proptosis between the two eyes rather than absolute measure with the Hertel method
– Gormaz exophthalmometer
  – This is a metal device having essentially two rulers, one horizontal (0–130 mm) and one vertical (0–40 mm), which is movable on the horizontal scale, connected via metal bars. Each end further has metal resting bars, one fixed at 0 mm, with a notch at end to align with the lateral orbital rim.
  – To measure, the patient is seated, and the procedure is explained to them.
  – The fixed vertical bar is kept at right orbital margin, while the mobile one is adjusted to rest at the left side. Distance between the two is the lateral orbital margin distance in mm
  – The patient is then asked to lie down supine at fixate straight above in primary position and cornea is anesthetized
  – The vertical scale is adjusted such that it lies gently on the cornea and the reading on the central connecting bar gives the exophthalmometry for that side. Repeated on the other side.

8.16 FAQs ON PROPTOSIS

Mention the dimensions of the adult orbit?

- Volume: 30 cc
- Shape: Pyramid
- Entrance height: 3.5 cm
- Diameter: Horizontal
- Entrance width: 4 cm

Table 8.7 Contents of the Following Anatomical Parts

Name	Site	Content
Optic canal	Lesser wing of sphenoid	Optic nerve, ophthalmic artery, sympathetic fibers
Superior orbital fissure	Lesser and greater wing of sphenoid	Third, fourth, and sixth ophthalmic of the fifth SOV, anastomosis of recurrent lacrimal and middle meningeal artery
Inferior orbital fissure	Greater wing of sphenoid, palatine and maxillary bone	Infraorbital zygomatic nerve, parasympathetic branches of pterygopalatine ganglion, IOV
Anterior ethmoidal canal	Frontal and ethmoid	Anterior ethmoidal nerve and artery
Post-ethmoidal canal	Frontal and ethmoid	Posterior ethmoidal nerve and vessels
Nasolacrimal canal	Lacrimal and maxillary bone	Nasolacrimal sac and duct

- Distance between posterior globe to optic foramen: 18 mm
- Length of optic nerve in orbit: 25 mm

What are the bones of the orbit?

- Ethmoid
- Frontal
- Lacrimal
- Maxillary
- Palatine
- Sphenoid
- Zygomatic

What bones form the roof?

- Frontal
- Lesser wing of sphenoid

What bones form the medial wall?

- Frontal process of maxilla
- Lacrimal
- Ethmoid
- Body of sphenoid

What bones form the floor of the orbit?

- Maxillary
- Zygomatic
- Palatine

What bones form the lateral wall?

- Zygomatic
- Greater wing of sphenoid

What are the surgical spaces in the orbit?

- Sub-periostial
- Peripheral orbital
- Central intraconal
- Tenon's space

Name the contents of the following anatomical parts?

What do the following sinuses drain?

Table 8.8 Sinus Drainage

Sinus	Drainage
Sphenoid	Spheno-ethmoid recess
Posterior ethmoid	Superior meatus
Anterior and middle ethmoid and frontal	Middle meatus
Nasolacrimal duct	Inferior meatus
Maxillary sinus	Middle meatus

When did the following sinuses appear?

Table 8.9 Sinus Development

Sinus	Age of Development
Ethmoid	Present at birth
Frontal	At 6 years
Maxillary	After 6 years
Sphenoid	Rudimentary at birth develops at puberty

What is proptosis?

- Definition: Abnormal protrusion of the eye
- More than 21 mm is abnormal
- Hertel: >18 mm is abnormal
- Krahn: >19 mm is abnormal
- More than 2 mm asymmetry in protrusion of two eyes is abnormal

What are the common causes of proptosis in an adult?

- Thyroid related ophthalmopathy (TRO)
- Cavernous hemangioma
- Orbital inflammatory syndrome (OIS)
- Lymphocytic lesions
- Meningioma
- Lacrimal gland tumors
- Dermoid and epidermoid cysts

What are the common causes of proptosis in children?

- Orbital cellulitis
- Rhabdomyosarcoma (most common primary orbital malignancy in children)
- Capillary hemangioma and lymphangioma (most common primary benign orbital tumor in children)
- Dermoid and epidermoid cyst
- Optic nerve glioma
- Leukemia
- Orbital pseudotumor
- Neurofibroma
- Metastatic neuroblastoma (most common to metastasize to orbit in children)
- Retinoblastoma

What are the causes of bilateral proptosis?

- Inflammatory:
  - Thyroid-related ophthalmopathy
  - Orbital inflammation
  - Wegner's granuloma
- Neoplastic:
  - Lymphoma and leukemia
  - Metastatic neuroblastoma
  - Diffuse optic nerve glioma in neurofibromatosis
  - Midline fibrous dysplasia
  - Sinus carcinoma

- Structural: Craniofacial dysostosis
- Degenerate: Myopia
- Vascular:
  - AV shunt
  - Bilateral varices
  - Cavernous sinus thrombosis

What are the causes of bilateral enlargement of the lacrimal gland?

- Lymphoma
- Sarcoid
- Sjogren's
- Idiopathic inflammation
- Cysts

What are the causes of pulsatile proptosis or lesions, which vary with position, or Valsalva maneuver?

- Congenital absence of sphenoid wing (NF)
- Meningoencephalocoele
- Post-traumatic/surgery bone defects
- Bone destruction due to:
  - Massive frontal mucocoele
  - Aneurysmal bone cyst
  - Xanthoma
  - Dermoid
  - Cystic metastasis
  - Histiocystosis
- AV shunt
  - High flow
  - Capillary hemangioma
- Vascular tumors
  - Thyroid carcinoma
  - Nephroblastoma
  - Prostatic cancer
- Varices

What is Pseudoproptosis? What are the causes?

- Pseudoproptosis is because of asymmetries of bony orbit/globe/lid fissure
- Causes:
  - Globe:
    - Myopia
    - Buphthalmos
    - Anisometropia
  - Lid position:
    - Ptosis
    - Lid retraction
    - Surgical recession of muscle

- Structural:
  - Facial asymmetry
  - Contralateral enophthalmos

What are the causes of enophthalmos?

- Horner's syndrome
- Duane's retraction syndrome
- Blowout fracture of orbit
- Phthisis bulbi
- Atrophic bulbi
- Sphenoid wing absent
- Orbital fat atrophy:
  - Post-radiation
  - Post-traumatic
  - Varices
- Scleroderma
- Nystagmus retractorius
- Lypodystrophy

What are the causes of non-axial displacement of the globe?

- Superior:
  - Maxillary sinus tumor
  - Lymphoma
  - Lacrimal sac lesions
  - Metastatic tumors
- Inferior:
  - Thyroid-related ophthalmopathy (TRO)
  - Neurofibromatosis (NF)
  - Frontal mucocoele
  - Subperiosteal hematoma
  - Medial dermoid
  - Fibrous dysplasia
  - Neuroblastoma
  - Lymphoma
  - Schwannoma
- Lateral:
  - Ethmoidal mucocoele
  - Nasopharyngeal tumor
  - Lethal midline granuloma
  - Large intraconal mass
  - Lacrimal sac tumor
  - Metastatic
- Medial:
  - Lacrimal gland tumor
  - Sphenoid wing meningioma

What are the common causes of the following on X-ray/CT scan?

- Isolated circumscribed legion:
  - Benign

  - Cavernous hemangioma
  - Schwannoma
  - Neurofibroma
  - Fibrous histiocytosis
  - Sub-acute inflammation
  - Hemangiopericytoma
  - Malignant:
    - Lymphoma nodule
    - Carcinoid
    - Rhabdomyosarcoma
    - Metastasis
- Cystic lesions
  - Dermoid cyst:
  - Encephelocoele/meningocoele
  - Mucocoele
  - Sweat gland cyst
  - Microphthalmos with cyst
  - Lacrimal cyst
  - Parasitic cyst
  - Abscesses
  - Cystic degeneration in rapidly growing tumor like rhabdomyosarcoma, melanoma, metastasis
  - Cystic or mucinous degeneration in neo-plasms like lymphangioma, benign mixed lacrimal gland tumor, schwannoma, NF
- Infiltrative orbital legions:
  - Benign:
    - Plexiform from NF
    - Lymphangioma
    - Capillary hemangioma
  - Malignant:
    - Metastasis
    - Lymphoma
    - Leukemia
    - Fibrous histiocytosis
- Inflammation in the orbit:
  - Amyloid deposit
- Diagnosis of enlarged muscles:
  - TRO: Tendons not involved
  - Myositis: Tendons involved and irregular involvement
  - Orbital pseudotumor
  - Metastasis: Commonest CA breast with nodular enlargement and next most common is leukemia
  - Lymphoma mainly involves LP (Levator Palpebralis) & SR (Superior Rectus), superior rectus, and medial rectus
  - AV shunt
  - Amyloid deposit: Smooth enlargement
  - Wegner's granulomatosis

- Rhabdomyosarcoma
- Trichinosis
- Hyperostotic legions of the bones of orbit:
  - Carcinoma prostate
  - Meningioma
  - Osteomyelitis
  - Primary bone tumor: Fibrous dysplasia, osteoma, osteosarcoma
- Destructive bone legions:
  - Solid:
    - Reparative granuloma
    - Sinusitis
    - Osteomyelitis
    - Metastasis
    - Aneurysmal bone cyst
    - Ewing's tumor
    - Wegener's granuloma
    - Osteogenic carcinoma
    - Histiocytosis
  - Cystic:
    - Dermoid
    - Mucocele
    - Xanthoma
- Calcification in the orbit:
  - With bone destruction:
    - Fibro-osseous tumors
    - Dermoid
    - Epidermoid

- Mucocele
- Without bone destruction:
  - In the eye:
    - Drusen
    - Phthisis bulbi
    - Retinoblastoma
  - In the orbit:
    - Trochlea
    - Dystrophic phlebolith
    - Varix
    - Lymphangioma
    - AVM
    - Old hemorrhage
    - Neoplastic
- Epithelial tumor of the lacrimal gland
- Meningioma
- Chondrosarcoma
- Neuroblastoma
- Osseous and cartilaginous tumor
- Dermoid cyst

What is the difference between a dermoid and meningoencephalocele?

How does one differentiate microphthalmos with cyst from congenital cystic eye?

How does one differentiate between optic nerve glioma and optic nerve sheath Meningioma?

Table 8.10 Differences between a Dermoid and Meningoencephalocele

Dermoid	Meningoencephalocele
Upper outer angle	Upper inner angle
Immovable fixed	Immovable
No bony hole felt	Bony hole felt
No pulsations	Pulsations synchronous with respiration
Valsalva—no change	Valsalva—increases
Non-fluctuant	Fluctuant
Pressure—same size	Pressure—decreases in size
Exploratory puncture—sebaceous material	CSF
Translucency—absent	Translucency—present
Ectodermal cells pinched off at suture line	Either brain parenchyma or meninges or both

Table 8.11 Differences between Microphthalmos and Congenital Cystic Eye

Microphthalmos with Cyst	Congenital Cystic Eye
Failure of fetal fissure to close and proliferation of neuroepithelium	Arrested development of primary optic vesicle
Occurs around the fourth week of embryonic life	Earlier than the fourth week of embryonic life
Mainly the lower lid with orbit is involved	Upper lid with orbit is involved
Small rudimentary eyeball is present	No visible ocular structures

Table 8.12 Differences between Optic Nerve Glioma and Optic Nerve Sheath Meningioma

Features	Optic Nerve Glioma	Optic Nerve Meningioma
Origin	Low grade pilocytic astrocytoma	Proliferation of meningoendothelial cells of arachnoid villi
Age	First decade (75%)	Middle aged (mean 42 years)
Sex	Females > Males (slightly)	Females > Males (significantly)
Laterality	Bilaterality pathognomonic for Von Recklinghausen's disease	Nil
Classification	Isolated vs. diffuse (in Von Recklinghausen's—multifocal)	Angioblastic—rare (3%), recurs and metastasizes Sarcomatous—in younger age group; more pleomorphic
Association	With Von Recklinghausen's—up to 50%	Nil
Clinical		
1. Vision	Lost, disproportionately in comparison to proptosis	Maybe better preserved than glioma
2. Proptosis	Mild to moderate	Moderate to severe
3. Opticociliary Shunt vessels	Absent	Present, characteristic
4. ON head invasion	Rare	Maybe invaded
5. Pupil RAPD	Present	Present
6. Optic nerve changes	Atrophy: Primary type	Edema followed by atrophy: Usually secondary type
7. Strabismus	Present	Present
CT Scan		
1. Margin	Smooth: Dura intact	Irregular: Dura invaded
2. Shape	Mostly fusiform	Diffuse with apical bulbous enlargements
3. Optic nerve	Central remnant of ON maybe present	Seen as railroad track
4. Optic nerve	Kinking, cystic degeneration frequent and characteristic	Straight or splinted
5. Calcification	Rare	Typical—Fine present in psammomatous lesions
6. Bony changes	Rare	Present at apex
7. Density	Same as optic nerve	
8. Contrast		
Tumor blush	Absent	Present
Railroad track	Absent	Present
9. Optic canal	Uniform Enlargement	Irregular enlargement/erosion
10. HPE	Astrocytic filaments Rosenthal fibers Arachnoid hyperplasia	Meningoendothelial cell proliferation Psammoma bodies Intranuclear vacuoles
11. Growth	Does not invade dura	Depends on site
2. Glioblastoma progress to blindness and fatality, unaffected by any mode of treatment	Intrinsic: Increases thickness of optic nerve Extra neural—in arachnoid space	Intracranial Optic canal Optic nerve Orbit

Table 8.12 (*Continued*) Differences between Optic Nerve Glioma and Optic Nerve Sheath Meningioma

Features	Optic Nerve Glioma	Optic Nerve Meningioma
12. Diagnosis of progression	Vision Fields Proptosis Optic nerve appearance Optociliary shunts	Vision Fields Proptosis Optic nerve appearance Optociliary shunts
13. MRI	Important in diagnosis if in optic canal	
14. Management	Observe: Chiasmal involvement, stable, diffuse types Excision: Limited to optic nerve or orbit, large, progressive Radiotherapy or shunt or both if diffuse type and progresses, chiasmal involvement	

8.17 FAQs ON ORBITAL CELLULITIS

Why sinus infection commonly spreads to the orbit?

- Since medial orbital wall is thin and incomplete
- Multiple foramina interconnecting
- Valveless venous system
- Origin:
  - Sinuses
  - Continuous spread: Lids, face, conjunctivitis, H. zoster, lacrimal sac/gland panophthalmitis
  - Pyemic
  - Foreign body such as an orbital implant

What are the predisposing factors?

- Diabetes Mellitus
- Chronic alcoholic
- Immunocompromised state
- Inter current other chronic infection

What are the causes of orbital cellulitis?

- Extension from periorbital structures, PN sinuses, Face and lids, dacryocystisis, dental infection, Intracranial infection
- Exogenous
  - Trauma (always rule out foreign body)
  - Post-surgery (orbital/periorbital)
- Endogenous: Bacteremia with septic embolization
- Intraorbital
  - Endophthalmitis
  - Panophthalmitis

What are the types of proptosis in orbital cellulitis?

- Axial: Orbital cellulitis
- Non-axial: Subperiosteal abscess

What are the causes of visual loss in cellulitis?

- Increased intraorbital tension
- Direct optic neuritis
- Vasculitis

What are the complications of orbital cellulitis?

- Non-ocular:
  - Cavernous sinus thrombosis
  - Intra cranial abscess
  - Subdural empyema
- Ocular:
  - Visual loss
  - Exposure and neurotrophic keratitis
  - Conjunctival prolapse
  - Secondary glaucoma
  - Septic uveitis
  - Retinitis
  - Exudative retinal detachment
  - Optic neuropathy
  - Panophthalmitis

What is Chandler's classification?

- Group 1: Preseptal cellulitis
- Group 2: Orbital cellulitis: Sterile/bacterial
- Group 3: Subperiosteal abscess
- Group 4: Orbital abscess
  - Intraconal
  - Extraconal
- Group 5: Cavernous sinus thrombosis

What are the clinical features?

- Ocular:
  - Swelling of lids because of obstruction to the venous flow
  - Conjunctival congestion
  - Painful proptosis
  - Ophthalmoplegia
  - Decreased visual acuity
  - Palpable mass
- General:
  - Malaise
  - Fever
  - Headache
  - Nausea, vomiting
  - Altered consciousness

What is the role of CT in orbital cellulitis?

- To know extent, staging, and location of inflammation
- Diagnosis of sinus pathology
- Diagnosis of retained foreign body
- Diagnosis of ocular involvement: Increased thickness of sclerouveal coat
- Diagnosis of orbital abscess: Capsule enhanced with contrast, which may be homo/hetero or ring enhancement
- Diagnosis of enlargement of superior ophthalmic wing
- Involvement of muscles
- Types:
  - Coronal: Good for subperiosteal abscess under roof
  - Axial: Good for subperiosteal abscess under medial wall

What is the role of ultrasonography?

- In orbital cellulitis, fat intensity altered
- In orbital abscess, medium to low reflectivity form the legion
- In cavernous sinus thrombosis, SOV enlarged and muscle size increased

What is the role of plain X-ray?

- Diagnose sinus involvement
- Air fluid level

How does cellulitis of the orbit differ in a child from an adult?

- History:
  - URTI in children
  - Allergy, sinus, dental extraction in adults
- Signs and symptoms:
  - Axial proptosis is more common in children, and non-axial is more common in adults
  - General symptoms like fever and malaise more in children
- Site of origin:
  - Ethmoid and pan sinusitis common in children
  - Fronto-ethmoid common in adults
- Bacteriology:
  - No growth or *H. influenzae* or *S. aureus* in children
  - Positive cultures more common in adults: *S. aureus* and mixed anaerobes
- Treatment:
  - Drainage rarely required in children
  - Frequently required in adults
- Outcome: Recovery with few complications in children
- Complications are more common in adults

Why hospitalize?

- Prevention of complications
- Careful monitoring

What are the investigations you will request for?

- Culture: Direct aspirate from sinus or abscess
- Blood culture
- CSF culture if CNS signs present, bilateral involvement, meningeal signs present
- CT scan
- Evaluation of sinuses
- USG

What are the treatment options?

- Specific: Antibiotics
- Surgical
  - Sinus drainage
  - Subperiosteal abscess drainage
- Symptomatic for pain and fever
- Miscellaneous: Corneal protection
- For prevention of conjunctival prolapse: Frost stitch
- Aggressively treat if vision decreases, or pupil gets affected

9

Strabismus and orthoptics

9.1 TOPICS

- Muscle hooks
- FAQs on muscle hooks
- Scissors, forceps, and retractors
- FAQs on strabismus surgeries
- Orthoptics

9.2 MUSCLE HOOKS

Mention the various types of muscle hooks?

1. Jameson Muscle hook

- Hook (6 mm) with bulbous tip
- Uses:
  - Holding the recti at their insertions
  - Minimal damage or distortion to the muscles

2. Stevens Muscle/Tenotomy hook

- Bunt angled tip (4 mm)
- Use: Retracting muscles during squint surgery

9.3 FAQs ON MUSCLE HOOKS

What are the uses of muscle hooks?

- To hook the extraocular muscles in squint, scleral buckling surgeries, pterygium surgery, sclerocorneal tear repair, IOFB removal (scleral approach)

- The tip is in same plane as the shaft
- Can be with or without eyelet at the tip
- Surgeries in which muscle hooks can be used are:
  - Squint surgery
  - Scleral buckle
  - Enucleation
  - IOFB removal via the scleral route
  - Globe exploration
  - Blowout fracture
  - Pterygium surgery in order to identify the medial rectus

How do you differentiate between a muscle hook and a lens expresser?

- Muscle hook: To hook the extraocular muscles, the shaft is in the same plane as that of tip.
- Lens expressor: Tip rounded, the shaft is right angled to tip.
- Lid hook: The tip is acutely angled.

9.4 SCISSORS, FORCEPS, AND RETRACTORS (USED IN STRABISMUS SURGERIES)

Identify the instrument and describe its use.

Steven's tenotomy scissor

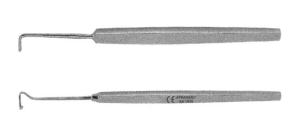

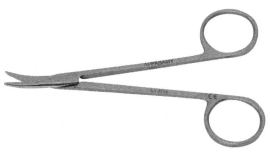

- Tenotomy scissor designed for tenon's dissection, usually having blunt tips, stout blades, lap joint with ring handles
- It is theorized that the crushing effects of its stout blades help in hemostasis
- Uses:
  - To perform tenotomy and tenon's dissections, especially near muscle insertion and between the recti
  - Blunt dissection of orbicularis oculi and orbital septum
  - To cut skin, muscle soft tissues during oculoplasty procedures
  - To dissect between sclera and episclera and create planes, especially during enucleation, evisceration, and orbital surgeries
  - May be used to cut thicker sutures (3-0, 4-0) silk or Vicryl

Identify the instrument and describe its use.

Muscle resection clamp

- Toothed (taumatic)/non-tooth (atraumatic): Muscle to be tagged to prevent muscle loss
- Used in muscle resection to provide appropriate measurement (of resection) and some degree of hemostasis
- Advantages: Correct amount of resection can be done
- Disadvantages: Muscle can be lost if clamp is prematurely loosened

What is the difference between a lost muscle and a slipped muscle?

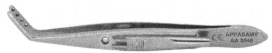

Figure 9.4 Muscle Resection Clamp

- Lost muscle: Lost muscle is characterized by the absence of any attachment of the muscle tendon or its sheath to the sclera, the muscle along with its sheath recoil posteriorly through the tenon's capsule.
- Slipped muscle: The tendon retracts posteriorly within the muscle sheath; the sheath remains empty and attached to the sclera at the chosen insertion site.
- A lost muscle will typically have a marked degree of under-action, whereas a slipped muscle and muscle with elongated scar will usually show some force.

How do you differentiate between lost versus slipped muscle?

- One must do a CT scan/MRI to differentiate between the two to identify position of muscle in relation to sclera.
- Dynamic orbital imaging is preferred.

Identify the instrument and describe its use.

Moody's fixation forceps

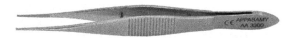

Figure 9.5 Moody's fixation forceps

- To fix muscle insertion
- To fix globe and give good exposure
- Avoid keeping the slider ends together, as they can brush against each other during retraction and lead to loss of the lock

Identify the instrument and describe its use.

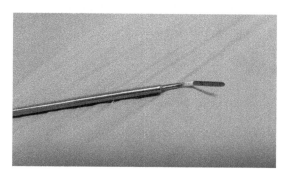

Figure 9.6 Scleral ruler

- Used to measure arc distances on sclera from limbus
- Important for measurements over sclera above 7–8 mm as curvature of the globe causes an error in measurements if straight caliper or ruler is used
- Alternate option is to use a piece of suture and mark it at either end of measurement to be taken, then place it against a straight ruler to find the exact distance

Identify the instrument and describe its use.

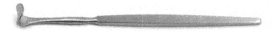

Figure 9.7 Conway lid retractor

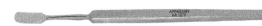

Figure 9.8 Helveston Barbie retractor

- Used to retract conjunctiva, tenons, and lids
- Especially useful during oblique muscle surgery, scleral buckling surgery

Identify the instrument and describe its uses in squint surgeries.

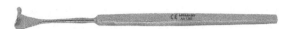

Figure 9.9 Desmarre's retractor

- Available in various sizes, having blunt curved edge overturned on itself to engage the lid margin with tarsus, which helps in eversion as well as double version of lids.
- Uses:
  - Retraction of conjunctiva and tendons during oblique muscle surgery
  - Double eversion of lid for removing chemical particles/deeply embedded foreign bodies
  - For examination of the eye under anesthesia in children and uncooperative patients

Identify and describe the instrument.

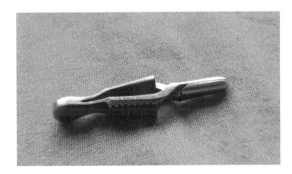

Figure 9.10 Dieffenbach–Serrafine bulldog forceps

- Self-retaining forceps
- Serrated jaws, which are interlocking
- Overall length: 35–38 mm
- Uses:
  - To clip long end of sutures
  - Squint surgeries, ptosis surgery, used in scleral buckling surgery before final typing of sutures
  - To hold on to suture threads during lid surgeries

- Can be used to hold the superior rectus suture during SICS surgery/ECCE/keratoplasty

9.5 FAQs ON STRABISMUS SURGERIES

What is the basic principle of squint surgeries?

- Two basic approaches—weaken a strong muscle and strengthen a weak muscle
- Recession is the commonest method to weaken a muscle:
  - Usually involves moving the insertion closer to origin of muscle along the same plane altering the torque and producing a slack in the muscle.
- Resection or plication are usually preferred to give a "strengthening effect"
  - Shortens the effective length of the muscle while continuing to act from the same insertion, leading to shortening of the length—tension curve.

Which are the weakening surgeries?

- Recession (Including hang-back procedures)
- Myotomy: Partial/complete
- Tenotomy

Which are the strengthening surgeries?

- Resection
- Advancement
- Plication

What is the unit in which measurements are made?

- $1° \approx 2 \Delta$ or PD (prism diopters) or sometimes denoted simply as "D" (for angles smaller than 45°)

What is the principle of correction of AV phenomenon in squint?

- If associated with oblique muscle dysfunction, manage that first.
- If vertical gaze incomitance is not due to oblique muscle issues, then simple offset or slanting of the horizontal recti can be done.
- The principal for the same is—MALE for offset.
- Medials to apex:
  - Laterals to extremity
  - 1/2 width of muscle shift if vertical difference of deviation 15–20 PD
  - Full width of muscle shift if vertical difference of deviation >20 PD

Table 9.1 Bilateral Recession versus Unilateral Recession and Resection

Bilateral Recession	Unilateral Recession and Resection
Reversible	Resection is irreversible
No additive effect	Additive approximately 25%
	Good in amblyopic eye/poor vision
No palpebral aperture disparity	Palpebral aperture disparity may occur

Table 9.2 Pros and Cons of Fornicial versus Limbal Incisions

	Fornicial	Limbal
Technique	Difficult to learn	Easy to learn
Postoperative comfort	Better	Less comfortable
Risk of Dellen formation	Nil	Possible
Surgical field exposure	Limited	Broad
Age >40 years	More difficult as conjunctiva is thin but can be done in all ages	Possible
Approach to 2 recti	Possible	Not possible

- For slanting:
  - The margin of the muscle where greater weakening is desired is recessed more
  - Slightly easier to perform
  - Be careful; problems are encountered in:
    - LR recession → IO inclusion syndrome
    - SR recession → SO can get damaged
    - IR recession → Ligament of Lockwood and IO can get damaged

What are the pros and cons of bilateral recession versus unilateral recession and resection (R&R)? (Table 9.1)

What are the pros and cons of fornicial versus limbal incisions? (Table 9.2)

What are the disadvantages of excessive recession?

- Palpebral aperture abnormalities
- Medial rectus and lateral rectus: Widening of palpebral aperture
  - Inferior rectus: Lower lid ptosis
  - Superior rectus: Retraction of upper lid
- Under-action of muscle
- Decreased excursion of globe

What is the minimum and maximum amount of resection and recession that can be done for each rectus? (Table 9.3 and Table 9.4)

Table 9.3 Recession Limits from Insertion

	Minimum (mm)	Maximum (mm)
MR	2.5 mm	5.5–6 mm
LR	4 mm	8–9 mm
SR	2.5–3 mm	5 mm
IR	2.5–3 mm	5.5 mm

Table 9.4 Resection Limits

	Minimum (mm)	Maximum (mm)
MR	4 mm	5.5–6 mm
LR	5 mm	8–9 mm
SR	2.5–3 mm	5 mm
IR	2.5–3 mm	5 mm

- SR recession and resection limited to 5 mm (Exception: Large recessions of SR are done for DVD)
- Care of LL retractors while resecting IR

What is the Harada Ito procedure?

- To correct the extorsion by tightening anterior SO fibers.
- Full tendon tuck not appropriate as it causes hypotropia and iatrogenic Brown's.

- The anterior 4 mm of SO tendon are disinserted and sutured 8 mm posterior to superior pole of lateral rectus.
- If placed anterior to 8 mm, there are chances of esodeviation.
- Note: For the superior oblique muscle:
  - Anterior 1/3rd fibers are responsible for intorsion.
  - Posterior 1/3rd fibers are responsible for depression and adduction.

What is the Harada Ito plus procedure?

- Harada Ito procedure that also includes few mm of the SO posterior tendon and improves its function.
- This procedure can correct small hypertropias in addition to the excyclotropia.
- Advantage of the Harada Ito procedure is that it is reversible if done within 24–48 hours.
- Adjustment of torsion: By examining the retina before and after procedure, usually by fundus examination.

How do you test for torsion on fundus examination?

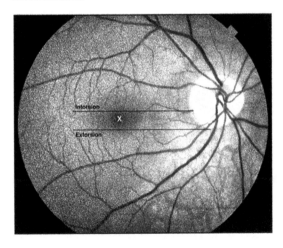

Figure 9.11 Fundus Tortion

- Normal eye alignment on fundus examination with indirect ophthalmoscopy and patient asked to fix at center of examiners light:
  - Horizontal line from fovea should intersect inferior half of disc (classification by Dr. Kushner is from lower 1/3rd of the optic disc, i.e., normally the line should be between the lower margin of the optic disc and the lower 1/3rd of the optic disc)

- Shift of ½ DD is 10° of torsional change
- Fundus torsion diagrammatic view

What is full tendon SO tuck?

- Used in SO palsy
- Disadvantage: Iatrogenic Browns

What are the indications of transposition procedures?

Common indications for transposition procedures in strabismus are:

- Third-, fourth-, and sixth-nerve paresis
- Duane's retraction syndrome
- Lost muscle
- AV pattern
- Small vertical tropia
- Certain torsional squint
- Double elevator palsy

What are the types of transposition procedures?

The common transposition procedures in strabismus are:

- Knapp procedure:
  - Full tendon transfer to paralyzed muscle
  - Complications: Anterior segment ischemia
- Jenson procedure:
  - Split tendon transfer with adjacent muscle and tied together but not disinserted
  - So less risk of anterior segment ischemia
- Hummelsheim procedure:
  - Split tendon transposition by disinserting and sutured to paralyzed muscle
  - Procedure of choice for lost muscle
  - Least changes of anterior segment ischemia
- Augmented Hummelsheim procedure:
  - 4 to 6 mm of transposed rectus muscle is resected, thus increasing the leash effect
  - Muscle union modification: The transposed and paretic muscle are sutured together for 4–5 mm at insertion

What are the advantages of use of adjustable sutures in squint surgery?

- Good fine-tuning of alignment of deviation in postoperative cases in select patients

What are the indications for using adjustable sutures in squint surgery?

Common parameters and indications to keep in mind for adjustable sutures in strabismus surgery

- Cooperative adults
  - Best with rectus muscle surgeries
  - Best with recessions
- Vertical squint
- Thyroid-related orbitopathy
- Brown syndrome
- Sixth-cranial-nerve palsy
- Repeat surgeries

What are the contraindications for use of adjustable sutures in squint surgery?

- Childhood squint
- Uncooperative patients
- Oblique muscle dysfunction
- DVD
- Concomitant squint

How does one decide if a patient will cooperate for suture adjustment in the postoperative period?

- Q-tip test: Touch the bulbar conjunctiva with Q-tip without topical anesthesia
- If the patient permits this, select patient for adjustable suture surgery

What is the best time to adjust sutures?

- Within 24–48 hours as later becomes difficult
- Avoid strong sedation
- Under topical anesthesia
- During surgery avoid bupivacaine and adrenaline (due to its prolonged duration of action)

What are the techniques for using adjustable sutures?

- Limbal sliding noose technique
- Fornix
  - Sliding noose technique
  - Bow tie technique

What are the complications associated with any squint surgery?

- Anesthesia complications:
  - General anesthesia:
    - Bradycardia
    - Hypothermia/hyperthermia
    - Malignant hyperthermia
    - Respiratory distress
    - Asphyxia
    - Cardiac arrest
  - Local anesthesia:
    - Retrobulbar hemorrhage
    - Globe perforation
    - Optic nerve injury
- Surgical complications: MAD mnemonic
  - Intraoperative complications
- Malignant hypertension
- Muscle loss
- Muscle slippage
- Muscle hematoma
  - Early postoperative complications
- Alignment
- Anterior segment ischemia
- Muscle Adherence syndrome
- Allergy
  - Late postoperative complications
- Dellen
- Diplopia
- Droopy lids
  - Strabismus-surgery-related complications:
  - Intraoperative complications:
    - Surgery on wrong patient
    - Surgery on wrong eye/wrong surgery on wrong muscle
    - Split muscle
    - Slippage of muscle
    - Sagged muscle
    - Lost muscle
- Inadvertent cutting
- Breaking of suture
- Slippage from clamp
- Spontaneous disintegration
- Do CT scan: Important to identify lost/slipped muscle position
- If found, reattach even if after months/ transposition suture
    - Muscle hemorrhage/hematoma
    - Globe perforation is more common with Faden procedure, so hang-back procedure is better
    - Vitreous loss
    - Vitreous hemorrhage
    - Retinal detachment
    - Oculocardiac reflex
    - Misidentification of SR as SO

- Orbital hemorrhage: Due to damage to the vortex veins, or due to blood dyscrasias
- Postoperative complications:
- Alignment:
  - Undercorrection
  - Overcorrection
- Mild to moderate overcorrection can be corrected by giving prisms, botulinum toxin, or repeat surgery.
- If excess, keep in mind slipped muscle and explore immediately.
  - Dellen
  - Suture granuloma
  - Infection
  - Endophthalmitis
  - Panophthalmitis
  - Orbital cellulitis
  - Suture abscess
  - Anterior segment ischemia:
    - More common in transposition surgeries
    - Fornicial incision better than limbal incision
    - Early: Onset in 24 hours: Presents with corneal edema, KPs, flare
    - Late: Presents with iris atrophy, distorted pupil, cataract
    - If all four recti are operated in a single eye, the chances of anterior segment ischemia are present throughout the duration of the patient's life, irrespective of how long back the surgery was performed.
  - Fat adherence syndrome (when posterior tenons is violated in inferior oblique surgery)

- Conjunctival cysts
- Inferior oblique complications:
  - Fat adherence
  - Anterior orbital hemorrhage
  - Pupillary dilatation
  - Damage to lateral rectus
  - Macular hemorrhage
  - Persistence of IO over action
  - Anti-elevation syndrome
- Superior oblique complications:
  - Residual superior oblique over action
  - SO palsy
  - In case of silicon expander, limitation of depression
- Complications of Faden surgery:
  - Lack of effect
  - Muscle necrosis due to tight suture
  - Scleral perforation
  - Retinal tears
  - Violation of orbital fat
- Lid fissure abnormalities

9.6 ORTHOPTICS

How does one measure the inter-pupillary distance (IPD)?

- The distance between the two pupil centers
- Performed for all patients undergoing orthoptic exam
- Average in adults is 65 mm and in children 50 mm
  - Methods to measure:
  - By an ordinary metric scale
  - Pulzone–Hardy rule
  - Synaptophore
  - Automated devices for IPD

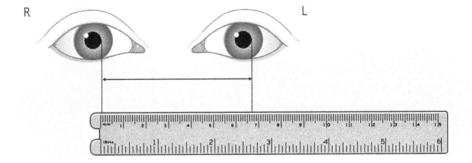

Figure 9.12 IPD measurement diagram

- Most modern auto refractometers have IPD measurements
- Subjectively, by adjusting fine stereopsis under a microscope and reading the distance of the scale of microscope
- Using a straight ruler
  - Patient seated in front of examiner, 33 cm in front and in the same vertical plane of eyes.
  - The ruler is placed on the nasal bridge of the patient in the spectacle plane.
  - The examiner closes his right eye and asks patient to look at his left eye with the patient's right eye (patient's left eye may be closed).
  - The scale reading bisecting the pupil is aligned to zero.
  - Cover other eye, and ask patient to look with left eye to examiners right eye.
  - Reading bisecting the pupil of left eye of patient is taken.
  - The addition between the two readings is taken and give IPD.
  - To repeat measurement with the patient looking at distant target also.

Identify and describe the instrument.

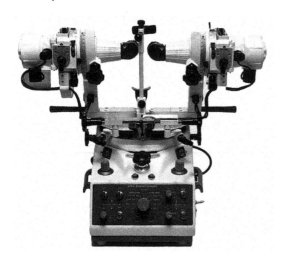

Figure 9.13 Synaptophore

- It is a haploscopic device for evaluation of sensory and motor state of patient having squint.

- Haploscopic principle: Division of physical perception into two separate areas of visual space, each of which is visible to one eye only. Mechanical dissociation of two eyes by two optical tubes.
- Parts:
  - Eyepiece with 6.5 D lens
  - Slide carrier at focal point of eyepiece. Hence, parallel rays emerge and patients' accommodation is relaxed
  - Two optical tubes
  - A base, chin rest and head rest
  - Various scales for horizontal, vertical, and torsional deviations
  - IPD scales
  - For Hardinger brushes, on and off switches

What are the various uses of the synaptophore?

Common uses of the synaptophore are:

- Diagnostic:
  - To check grade of binocular vision:
    - Simultaneous macular perception (SMP)
    - Fusion
    - Stereopsis (fine stereopsis has special slides available)
    - There are simultaneous paramacular, macular, and foveal perception slides
  - Measure of angle of deviation in all nine gazes:
    - Objective angle of Squint
    - Subjective angle of Squint
  - Normal retinal correspondence: If objective = subjective
  - Abnormal retinal correspondence (ARC):
    - If objective > subjective, then the difference between objective and subjective = angle of anomaly
    - If angle of anomaly = objective → harmonious ARC
    - If angle of anomaly < objective → non-harmonious ARC
    - Bielschowsky's after-image test slides are used to diagnose ARC
  - Maddox slides (circle and plus) are used to measure torsion
  - Range of suppression scotoma
  - Measurement of angle kappa (angle between optic axis and visual axis, rarely exceeds 5–7°)

- – Positive: When visual axis cuts nasal to optic axis
- – Negative: Opposite
- – For this, slides with number and alphabets (43210 ABCDE) and animal pictures are put
- – When patient looks at the light, examiner looks at the corneal reflections
- Measurement of IPD
- To measure eccentric fixation (special slides are available)
- Range of fusion or version:
  - – To measure convergence, tubes are moved toward each other.
  - – Fusion breaks when diplopia present.
  - – Arms are moved back so that fusion is regained.
  - – Similarly, range of divergence is estimated.
  - – To check the amplitude for near—3D lens is placed before each eye.
  - – Similarly vertical and torsional range of fusion estimated.
- Therapeutic:
  - Anti-suppression exercises
  - Fusional (for heterophorias and Intermittent exotropia) exercises
  - Treatment of amblyopia
  - In treatment of eccentric fixation, entoptic phenomenon of Haidinger brushes (because polarized light is used)

What are the disadvantages of the synaptophore?

- Time consuming
- May accommodate
- Very small children may not cooperate
- Suppression may prevent superimposition of pictures especially in subjective test
- Patients with abnormal head posture can have difficulty and alterations in measurement

How do you detect and measure eccentric fixation?

- Visuscope (fixation ophthalmoscope) is used to measure eccentric fixation.
- These are usually available as an in-built filter in most modern direct ophthalmoscopes.
- It is used to assess fixation in cases of amblyopia, manifest strabismus and even orthophoric subjects.

- The instrument incorporates a four-pointed star with a central clear area as the fixation target (some use rings).
- A green filter is occasionally used to produce a red-free image of the retina.
- The normal eye is assessed first, to ensure patient understanding.
- The position of fixation is recorded in relation to the foveola (central, parafoveal, macular, peripheral) and according to the state of fixation (steady/unsteady, central/eccentric, maintained/wandering)

Identify the lens and state its uses?

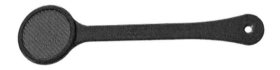

Figure 9.14 Maddox rod

- Red-colored disc with several parallel grooves
- Converts a point source of light into a line perpendicular to the grooves
- Principle: Dissociation of vision in two eyes
- Uses:
  - Measures deviation in combination with prism at any distance or in any direction of gaze
  - Commonly used for the diagnosis of phoria for far
  - Can be used for double Maddox rod test for torsion

How does one use the Maddox rod?

- The patient fixes a small light, and a rod is placed in front of the deviating eye.
- The distances used are 6 m and 33 cm.
- Grooves are placed horizontally to measure horizontal deviation.
- The patient sees vertical line.
- Two eyes see dissimilar images and are dissociated, allowing muscle imbalance to become manifest.
- The instrument is made of multiple cylindrical lenses which are red in color and hence white light appears as red line
- Vertically placed grooves will create horizontal line for measuring the vertical deviation
- The Maddox rod can be used in conjunction with the Maddox tangent scale instead of prisms.

What is a Maddox tangent scale?

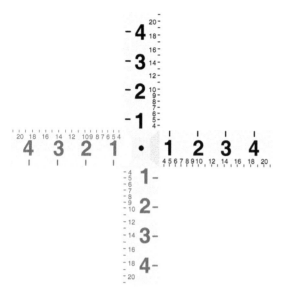

Figure 9.15 Maddox tangent scale

- Made of two wooden beams set at right angles to each other, marked in degrees with a spotlight in the center.
- The amount of deviation is measured by asking the patient to observe the number on the scale where the red line traverses.
- The tangent scale is calibrated at 5 m distance.
- It can also be used to measure and quantify eccentric fixation using foveo-foveal test of Cuppers

How does one interpret the results of the Maddox rod test?

- If no deviation, then the line passes through light.

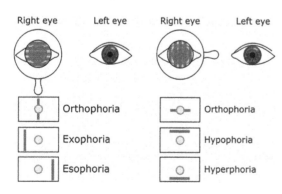

Figure 9.16 Interpretation of the Maddox rod test

- Test only measures deviation present and does not differentiate between heterotropias and heterophorias.

Identify and describe the instrument.

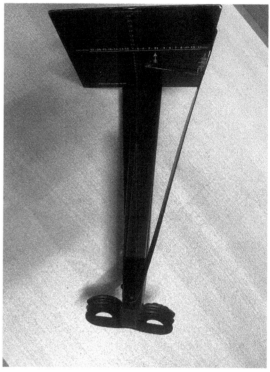

Figure 9.17 Maddox wing

- Aim: To diagnose and measure heterophorias at near in prism diopters.
- The metal screen has markings in prism diopters for horizontal and vertical deviations.
- The other end has two apertures for the eyes and a nose slot.
- Two metal septae, which are wing-like, dissociate the view of the two eyes so that scales are read by the left eye and the white vertical and horizontal arrows are seen by the right eye.
- It cannot differentiate between heterophorias and heterotropias.
- Principle: Dissociation of vision in two eyes; i.e., the right eye sees arrows, and the left eye sees the scales.
- Has three scales: Horizontal, vertical, and torsional scales.
- Method:
  - Put corrective lenses.

- Patient is asked to indicate the position of the vertical arrow on the horizontal scale to record the horizontal deviation.
- Position of horizontal arrow on the vertical scale to measure vertical deviation.
- Torsion: Indicated if the horizontal arrow is not parallel to the horizontal measurement scale, the arrow must be adjusted until patient sees it parallel
- Interpretation:
  - On horizontal scales:
    - Even number: Exophoria
    - Odd number: Esophoria
  - On vertical scales:
    - Even number: Left hypertropia
    - Odd number: Right hypertropia
  - Red arrow (cyclophoria)
    - Tilted superiorly: Incyclophoria
    - Tilted inferiorly: Excyclophoria
  - 1 line = 2° Incyclophoria

What is the double Maddox rod test?

- Vertical diplopia will see white line above the red line indicating right hypertropia.
- Red Maddox rod is rotated until the two lines appear parallel this gives us the quantity of extorsion.
- Used to detect and measure torsion.
- Requisites: Two differently colored Maddox rods (red and white). Some prefer to use both red in order to remove subjective bias.
- Method: Maddox rod with grooves placed vertically to form a pair of horizontal lines when patient looks at spotlight.
- Distance: Both near and far can be ideally done.
- Patient is asked if lines are parallel or not.
  - If parallel: No torsion.
  - If either one or both lines appear tilted: Torsion present.
  - Patient is asked to adjust position of rods until lines appear parallel.

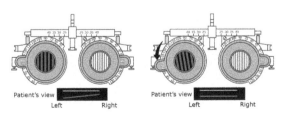

Figure 9.18 Double Maddox rod test

- Results:
  - Amount of axis change read off scales
  - If lines are tilted toward nose: Excyclotorsion
  - 10° excyclodeviation: Bilateral SO paresis
  - <10° excyclodeviation: Unilateral SO paresis

Identify and describe the following instrument.

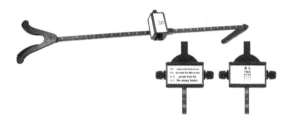

Figure 9.19 RAF ruler

- The Royal Air Force binocular gauge or RAF near point rule is designed for the measurement of convergence and accommodation.
- It has the observer end splayed out in such a manner that the two wings straddle the patient's nose and rest upon cheekbones.
- At this position, the calibrated scale directly reads values from the anterior surface of cornea.
- The scale is mounted with a rotating box, about 6 cm wide, with each side having different chart:
  - Vertical black line with central dot for convergence
  - Alphabets for accommodation,
  - Near vision chart for N series measure and
  - running near script for Near vision
- The sides of the scale give values in centimeters, age in years and diopters for direct measurement and comparison

What is the near point of convergence? What is the method used to measure it?

- Method: Objects moved toward the patient in the midline from about 50 cm away
- Apparatus: Interesting object, RAF rule
- Results:
  - When near point of convergence has been reached and fusion is lost, one eye will diverge.

- Patient may or may not indicate when object appears double.
- If they suppress, it may indicate a long-standing convergence problem.
- Recording:
  - E.g., convergence to nose or left eye breaks at 10 cm, common symptom is diplopia
  - Normal: 8–10 cm or less

How does one measure the near point of accommodation?

- Apparatus: RAF rule
- Method:
  - Tested binocularly and uniocularly
  - Appropriate optical correction is given for distance
  - Reading target that patient can see clearly at the end of the rule is moved toward the fixing eye until the patient first notices that the print is blurred
  - Usually, N series near target is used on RAF rule
  - NPA to be recorded for individual right and left eyes as well as with both eyes open

What is the Prince rule?

- It is used to measure the near point of accommodation.

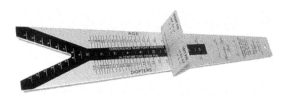

Figure 9.20 Prince rule

- Uses a 24 inches rod that has a sliding target with 20/30 target and different marking on all four sides:
  - First side—centimeter marking
  - Second side—inch marking
  - Third side—age in years marking
  - Fourth side—diopter marking
- Each eye is tested separately the other eye is occluded and the ruler is rested against the cheekbone.
- Move the 20/30 target till the vision blurs.

- That reading in cm measures the NPA in cm, the reading in diopters is the amount of accommodation left, and age for which the accommodation is normal.

What is difference between amplitude of accommodation, range of accommodation, and relative accommodation?

- Amplitude of accommodation: The difference in diopters between the near and far points of accommodation (between the minimum and maximum amount of accommodation).
- Range of accommodation: It is the distance over which accommodation is effective; the distance between the near and far points.
- Relative accommodation: It is the amount by which accommodation can be increased or relaxed while convergence remains constant.
- One diopter has a focal distance of 1 meter, and hence, accommodation is calculated in terms of diopters or the reciprocal of the fixation distance.
- The near point of accommodation (NPA) is measured using the RAF rule while the patient fixates at N series target both uniocularly and binocularly.
- It can also be measured using Prince's ruler, trial lenses, synaptophore, etc.

Identify and describe the following instrument.

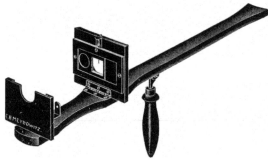

Figure 9.21 Bishop–Harman diaphragm test

- Uses:
  - To detect the strength of fusion response usually
  - Used as a screening test in pilots
- Card holder with a row of letters (ABCDEFG) or numbers (12345467)
- Viewed through adjustable diaphragm

- Method:
  - Adjust IPD.
  - Gradually close aperture while subject is reading.
  - He will indicate when there is loss of binocularity.
- Results:
  - Bar response/exophoric: A dividing bar separates numbers into two groups.
  - Esophoric response: Crowding of central numbers.
  - Hyperphoric response: Numbers separate, one being higher than the other.
  - Unicolor response: Numbers at one end disappear.
  - Reading on ocular poise scale is recorded and anything above 4 is considered abnormal binocular function.

Identify the following:

- The prism bar is a linearly arranged set of prisms of increasing dioptric power
- Two bars, one for vertical and one for horizontal needed along with a 30 D and 40 D loose prism for larger deviations.
- Loose prisms are available in glass or plastic and must be held in Prentice (perpendicular to the line of sight) or frontal plane

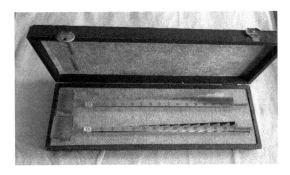

Figure 9.22 Prism bars and loose prisms

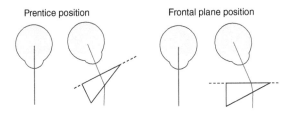

Figure 9.23 Prentice position for prisms

(parallel to the infra orbital margin) positions, respectively.
- Here the plastic prism is held such that its back surface is parallel to the frontal position of the patient's face.
- Other types of prisms: wafer, clip-on, Fresnel; prisms on trial scale mount are also useful for finer adjustments.

What is Hirschberg's test (corneal reflections test)?

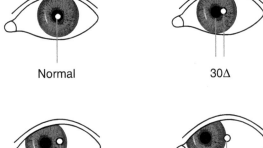
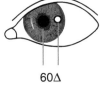
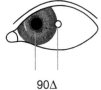

Figure 9.24 Hirschberg's test

- Distance: Near fixation
- Method:
  - Spotlight held in front of the patient at 33 cm from his eyes.
  - Examiner must be directly behind the light.
  - Position of light's reflection on each cornea checked
  - 1 mm displacement = 7° of strabismus (deviation estimation has variability in recent literature and is fraught with controversy, at best Hirschberg is only an approximation, and like any screening test should not be solely relied upon for surgical planning)
- Pitfall: Slight displacement from the center nasally (positive angle kappa) or temporally (negative angle kappa) may occur, giving the impression of a strabismus when in fact the eyes are correctly aligned as test is for near only.
- Use: Rough estimate of angle of deviation.

What is the Krimsky test?

 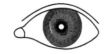

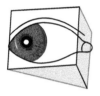 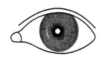

Figure 9.25 Krimsky's test

- Krimsky's test or prism reflex test
- Carried out in the same way as Hirschberg.
- Prisms are used to move the corneal reflection in the deviating eye to a position similar to that of the fixing eye.
- Apex of prism in direction of squint.
- Right esotropia: Base out prism right eye.

What is the modified Krimsky's test?

- If squinting eye is densely amblyopic or blind, then the prism is placed in front of fixing eye until corneal deviation in the deviating eye becomes central.

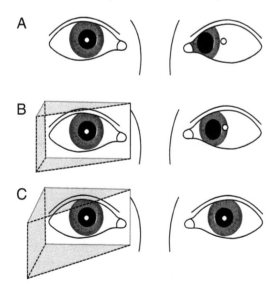

Figure 9.26 Modified Krimsky test for estimating deviation: The decentered corneal reflex in the left eye (A) is brought to the center by placing progressively stronger prisms in front of the fixating right eye (B, C)

- Modified Krimsky cannot be done if squinting eye has resistance of movement.
- Disadvantages:
  - Krimsky underestimates in deviation >15 PD (compared with PBCT).
  - It measures only near deviation.
  - Uncontrolled accommodation and wrong interpretation in presence of angle kappa.
- Recording: E.g., Krimsky's: 45 PD RET

What is the prism bar cover test (PBCT) or the prism cover test (PCT)?

- It is the gold standard for measuring deviation.
- Prerequisite is to have good vision, central fixation, no abnormal head posture (or neutralize head posture), and cooperation along with appropriate eye level target.
- Can be done with loose prisms or a prism bar (called PCT or PBCT, respectively).
- Test performed at a distance of 1/3 m, 6 m, and if possible, greater than 6 m.
- Alternate cover test is used when patient is fixating at accommodative target (to control accommodation) with and without glasses (to confirm if any change with accommodation); also, +3 DS can be put in front of distance correction to confirm if equal measurement between near and far.
- Prisms of increasing strength are added till no re fixing movement occurs.
- For complete dissociation of fusion, use post-patch test measurement.
  - After at least 1 hour of patching, ensure that while removing and measuring no fusion is occurring.
- The test is performed in all nine gazes and with either eye fixating to rule out incomitance.

What is the simultaneous prism introduction and cover test?

- Also called prism cover-uncover test
- Measures the manifest strabismus only
- Used in cases of microtropia associated heterotropia
- Prism should be placed before the deviating eye at the same time as the fixing eye is covered
- Allows the measurement of the deviation with the minimum of dissociation of two eyes, i.e., deviation in as much possible physiological viewing

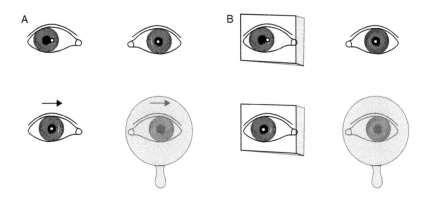

Figure 9.27 Prism cover test

Simultaneous prism cover test ET10$^\triangle$

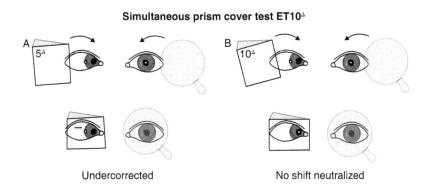

Figure 9.28 Simultaneous prism cover test

- Essential to do this part of the test before doing the prism and cross-cover test in the monofixation syndrome and accommodative esotropia
- Also useful for DVD and other dissociated measurements
- Simultaneous prism cover test tells us whether intervention is needed (physiological measurement) while alternating PCT indicates what to intervene with

What is the prism and cover-cross-cover test (alternating cover test)?

Alternating cover test

- Measures manifest and latent component of squint as well as total deviation
- Distance: Near and distance
- Target: Use a toy or the Snellen chart (accommodative target)
- Method:
  - Patient fixes on chosen target
  - Prism placed in front of deviating eye
  - Fixing eye covered and eye behind the prism is watched to see if it makes any movement to take up fixation
  - Strength adjusted until no movement is detected
  - Apex of prism in the same direction as the squinting eye is pointing
  - E.g., right esotropia: Base out prism in front of right eye
- Prerequisites and cautions:
  - Central steady fixation
  - Vision should be enough to see the target
  - EOM must be normal

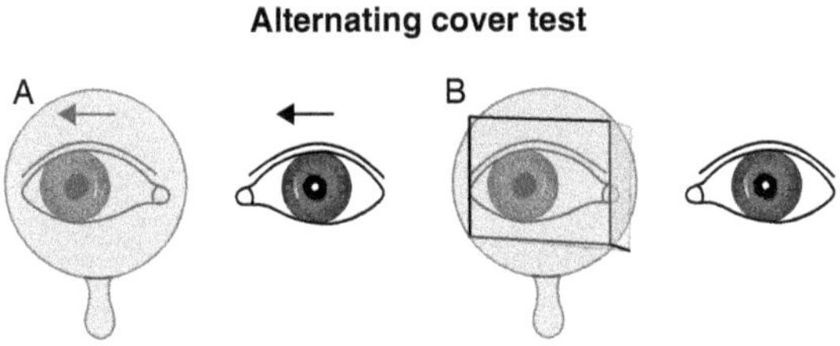

Figure 9.29 Alternating cover test

- Must have a cooperative patient
- Must have a target to control accommodation
- Position of prism held
- Do not stack prisms
- Both eyes should not be uncovered at the same time till deviation is neutralized
- High refractive errors in spectacles can induce prismatic aberrations. Further measurements in PBCT in positive lenses decreases and negative lenses increases the deviation measured on PBCT, especially if lenses have power > ±5 D.
- Advantages:
  - Measures total angle of deviation
  - Most accurate and widely used

What is the 4D prism test?

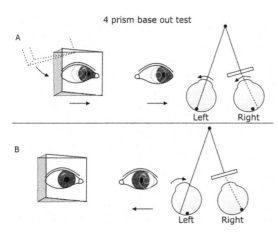

Figure 9.30 4D prism test

- Aim: Confirm presence of monofixation syndrome
- Method:
  - Patient fixes on a penlight or small target for distance.
  - A 4D base out prism is introduced from temporal side in front of the eye suspected of having foveal suppression.
- Results:
  - Positive test: No movement is indicative of foveal suppression shows no movement of the fellow eye.
  - If there is bifoveal fusion and no suppression, the fellow eye makes a small corrective movement.

Identify these and state their uses.

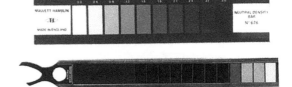

Figure 9.31 Neutral density filtes

- Consists of a ladder or bar of increasing density filters (neutral or red)
- Photographic filters that are used for assessing depth perception
- Also used to grade RAPD
- Uses:
  - Differentiate between organic and strabismic amblyopia. Visual acuity in cases of organic amblyopia is reduced by diminishing the illumination with a neutral density filter, whereas the visual acuity in an eye with strabismic amblyopia remains relatively unchanged.
  - Not useful in cases of anisometropia amblyopia because there is a depression of sensitivity throughout the visual field and not mainly at the macula, as in cases of strabismic amblyopia.
- Grade accurate to neutral filter density
- Neutral density filters come in densities of 0.3, 0.6, 0.9, and 1.2 log units
- Higher densities can be obtained by combining filter
- Density of the RAPD is the density of the filter required to neutralize it
  - Grade I: 0.3 to 0.6 log
  - Grade II: 0.45 to 1.2 log
  - Grade III: 0.75 to 1.5 log
  - Grade IV: 1.5 to 2.7 log
  - Grade V: too dense to measure

Identify the glasses and state the tests they are used in.

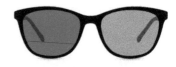

Figure 9.32 Red and green glasses

- Pair of red and green glasses
- Special type known as Armstrong glasses
- Colors are mutually exclusive therefore red light is seen only by a red filter and not the green filter (and vice versa)
- By convention red is used for right eye and green is used for the left eye
- Uses:
  - Diplopia charting: Charts the separation of double vision in nine different positions of gaze
  - Worth four dot test
  - Hess screen testing
  - Lancaster's chart testing
  - Stereoscopic tests of TNO

How are red and green goggles used to measure aniseikonia? What is the Awaya test?

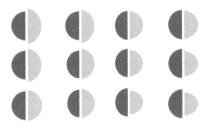

Figure 9.33 Awaya test uses R&G goggles to measure aniseikonia

- It consists of one plate containing two equal sized semicircles, one red and one green.
- If these are perceived to be of same size: No aniseikonia.
- Where a difference is noted, the patient is then shown a series of semicircles, which vary in size and is asked to choose the plate that matches the control.
- Each semicircle changes in 1% size difference steps.

What are the uses of a red filter?

- Red kodaloid filter
- Diagnostic uses:
  - With prism bar to diagnose retinal correspondence
  - For diplopia charting, red glass test
  - Diagnosis of Bielschowsky's phenomenon
  - Worth's four-dot test

- To break fusion
- Therapeutic uses:
  - Diagnosis of eccentric fixation (Kodak Wratten 25)
  - To eradicate suppression
  - To counsel patients preoperatively by showing physiological diplopia
  - Convergence and divergence exercises

Identify and describe the Worth's four-dot test.

- Four circles arranged in a rhombus form
- Two horizontal dots are green the top one is red and the bottom one is white
- Viewed through red/green goggles
- Distance: 6 m/33 cm
- Aim: To diagnose fusion and dominance of eye
- Method:
  - Patient wears red/green glasses and is asked how many lights he sees at 6 meters and 33 cm
  - Very dissociative test
- Responses:

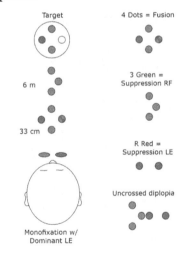

Figure 9.34 Worth's four-dot test—W4DT

- Four lights: one red, two green, one pink or green depending on dominant eye = indicates bifoveal or peripheral fusion
- Five lights: two red, three green = indicates diplopia, which may be crossed (heteronymous) or uncrossed (homonymous)
- Two lights or three lights = suppression of one eye; there may be alternation between

Table 9.5 Normal Fusional Amplitudes

Distance	Convergence	Divergence	Vertical	Incyclotorsion	Excyclotorsion
6 m	14PD	6PD	2.5PD	10–12°	10–12°
25 cm	38PD	16PD	2.6PD	10–12°	10–12°

two or three lights, indicating alternating suppression
- Dissociating tests like Worth's four-dot test can have exceptions. Suppressing patient may sometimes give diplopia response because of disruption of suppression or dissociation caused by red/green glasses.
- Test recorded as fusion, diplopia, or suppression and distance tested.
  - At distance: Four dots cover 1.25° area
  - At near: Four dots cover 6° area (which will cover tiny foveal scotoma)
- For near fusion response positive therefore, monofixation is diagnosed better at distance response

What are the normal fusional amplitudes? (Table 9.5)

- Following can be used to measure fusional amplitudes:
  - Synaptophore
  - Prisms in free space, prism bar, rotational prism
- Endpoint: Diplopia
- Distance: 6 m, 33 cm
- Fixation target which is accommodative
- Gradually increasing strength of prisms until diplopia is experienced subjectively or watch for break in either eye (objectively)
- Uses:
  - Order to keep prisms to measure fusional amplitudes:
    - Base out in esodeviation
    - Base up in hypodeviation
    - Base in in exodeviation
    - Base down in hyperdeviation
  - If manifest squint is present, correct the deviation, then assess amplitudes using additional prisms.

What is retinal correspondence?

- Normal retinal correspondence (NRC): It is a binocular condition in which the fovea and areas on the nasal and temporal side of one

retina correspond to and have, respectively, common visual directional sensitivity with the fovea and temporal and nasal areas of the retina of the other eye
- Abnormal retinal correspondence (ARC): It is a binocular condition in which there is a change in visual directional sensitivity such that the fovea of the fixing eye has a common visual directional sensitivity with an area other than the fovea of the deviating eye. The pairing of all retinal areas is similarly changed.
- Retinal correspondence can be measured using:
  - After-image test
  - Synaptophore
  - Bagolini's glasses

Identify these glasses?

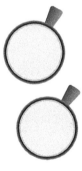

Figure 9.35 Bagolini's striated glasses

- Glass or plastic discs with linear striations
- Two glasses each which are right angles to each other
- Usually mounted in a frame but may be available as individual pieces
- Least dissociative test therefore more physiological dissociative test
- Uses:
  - To assess binocular function
  - Can also be used for measuring torsion, similar to double maddox rod

Various subjective findings obtainable with the striated glasses and their interpretation

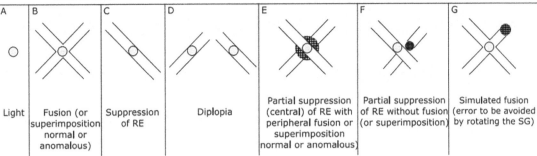

A	B	C	D	E	F	G
Light	Fusion (or superimposition normal or anomalous)	Suppression of RE	Diplopia	Partial suppression (central) of RE with peripheral fusion or superimposition normal or anomalous)	Partial suppression of RE without fusion (or superimposition)	Simulated fusion (error to be avoided by rotating the SG)

Figure 9.36 Bagolini's striated glasses results

- Test of foveal to extra-foveal correspondence in cases of strabismus by providing images that fall on the fovea of the fixing eye and on foveal area of the deviating eye
- Apparatus:
  - Glasses consisting of plane glass marked with fine, parallel striations, which produce a line image of a spotlight at 90° striations.
  - One glass is placed in front of each eye with striations set at angles 45° and 135°.
- Method:
  - Fixes a spotlight 33 cm or 6 m away
  - Patient asked either to draw what they see or tell what they see
  - Ask the patient and document:
    - Number of lines seen with both eyes open
    - Exact position of lines and spot of light
  - Results

What are the tests for suppression?

Suppression can be measured using:
- Synaptophore
- Worth's four-dot test
- Bagolini's glasses
- Four-prism test
- Red filter ladder test:
  - Detects degree of depth of suppression
  - Filters of increasing density kept over seeing eye till its image is degraded to such an extent that it allows the suppressed image in strabismic eye to be perceptible and the patient complains of diplopia

What are the various tests for stereopsis?

- Tests for stereopsis for near (**Table 9.6**)
  - TNO test
    - Principle: Anaglyph
    - Equipment: Contains seven plates and red/green spectacles
    - Stereopsis grade tested: 15–480 seconds of an arc
  - Titmus fly test
    - Principle: Vectrograph
    - Equipment: Polaroid vectograph with polaroid spectacles
    - Stereopsis grade tested
- Fly: 3500 arc seconds
- Graded circle test: 800–40 seconds of arc
- Animal tests: 400, 200, 100 seconds of arc
  - Stereo butterfly test

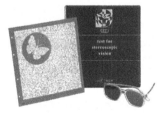

Figure 9.37 TNO test

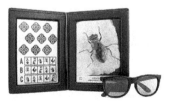

Figure 9.38 Titmus fly test

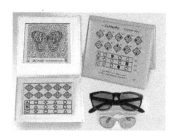

Figure 9.39 Stereo butterfly test

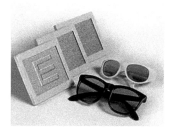

Figure 9.40 Random dot stereogram

- Principle: Vectrograph
- Equipment: Polaroid vectograph with polaroid spectacles
- Stereopsis grade tested
- Upper wings: 2000 seconds of arc
- Lower wings: 1150 seconds of arc
- Abdomen: 700 seconds of arc
  - Graded circle test and animal test is same as titmus fly test
  - Random dot stereogram
    - Principle: Vectrograph
    - Equipment: Polaroid spectacles
    - Stereopsis grade tested: 400–20 seconds of arc
  - Lang test
    - Principle: Panograph
    - Equipment: Test plates—Stereo I, Stereo II
    - Stereopsis grade tested
- Car: 550 seconds of arc
- Star: 600 seconds of arc
- Cat: 1200 seconds of arc
- Moon: 200 seconds of arc
- Truck: 400 seconds of arc
- Elephant: 600 seconds of arc
  - Lang 2 pencil test
    - Principle: Panograph
    - Equipment: 2 pencils only
    - Stereopsis grade tested: 3000–5000 seconds of arc

- Stereopsis slides placed in synaptophore carrier
  - Principle: Haploscopy
  - Equipment: Synaptophore with stereopsis slides
  - Stereopsis grade tested: 720–90 seconds of arc
- Tests for Stereopsis for distance
  - AO Vectographic project-O-chart slide
    - Equipment: Phoropter with polarizing lenses
    - Stereopsis grade tested: 480–30 seconds of arc
  - Mentor B-VAT II SG video acuity tester
    - Equipment: Video system with monitor using random dot E (BVRDE) and Contour circles (BVC)
    - Stereopsis grade tested: 240–15 seconds of arc
  - Frisby Davis Distance Stereopsis (FD2 test)
    - Equipment: Box with four translucent objects at varying distances
    - Stereopsis grade tested: 5–50 seconds of arc at 6m
  - Distance Randot Stereotest
  - Equipment: Three-dimensional polaroid vectograph and polaroid spectacles
  - Stereopsis grade tested: 400–60 seconds of arc

Define stereopsis.

- Depth may be perceived in two forms: Binocular disparity (stereopsis) and monocular depth clues in the absence of binocular single vision.
- Stereopsis is a cortical phenomenon for the perception of the relative depth of objects (true three-dimensional depth) on the basis of binocular disparity, which reflects the slight difference in images presented to each eye.
- Stereoacuity is the angular measurement of the minimal resolvable binocular disparity (this is necessary for the appreciation of stereopsis).
- Normal level of stereopsis being 40 seconds of arc with normal equal visual acuity in each eye; this also indicates normal retinal correspondence.

Table 9.6 Tests for Stereopsis for Near

Stereopsis for Near	Principle	Equipment	Stereopsis Grade Tested (in seconds of arc)
TNO test	Anaglyph	Contains 7 plates and red/green spectacles	15–480
Titmus fly test	Vectrograph	Polaroid vectograph with polaroid spectacles	Fly—3500 Graded circle test—800–40 Animal tests—400, 200, 100
Stereo butterfly test	Vectrograph	Polaroid vectograph with polaroid spectacles	Upper wings—2000 Lower wings—1150 Abdomen—700
Random dot stereogram	Vectrograph	Polaroid spectacles	400–20
Lang test	Panograph	Test plates: Stereo I Stereo II	Car—550 Star—600 Cat—1200 Moon—200 Truck—400 Elephant—600
Lang 2 pencil test	Panograph	2 pencils only	3000–5000
Stereopsis slides placed in synaptophore carrier	Haploscopy	Synaptophore with stereopsis slides	720–90

- The level of stereoacuity decreases with reduction in visual acuity, and there is an age-related deterioration in stereo acuity with a linear correlation between age and stereopsis threshold.

What does one require for stereopsis?

- Horizontal image disparity
- Fusible images, i.e., within Pannum's area (each image should be sharp enough, limited by distance also and near equal to other image)
- Cortical function normal: Binocular correlation

What are the monocular clues to stereopsis?

- Apparent size (larger nearer)
- Overlay (closer object covers the distant one)
- Light shading
- Aerial perspective (distance object appears more indistinct and less color saturated)
- Geometric perspective (the more parallel lines converge, the further they are)
- Motion parallax: When nearer object moves in opposite direction by smaller amount and distance object moves in same direction by larger amount
- Relative velocity

Identify and describe the screen.

Hess and Lees screen
- These charts are used to investigate incomitant strabismus in order to assess paretic or spastic element.
- By using principle of dissociation, it is possible to indicate the position of the non-fixing eye when the other eye is fixing, in specified positions of gaze.
- Hence, these are usually documented with LE placed on initial reading side in Latin script-left.
- Hess chart
  - Tangent scale calibrated at 50 cm, anterior plane of the cornea as the starting point and angle of deviation of eyes projected on a 2D scale calculated by tangent method
    - Black cloth/board
    - Dimensions: 3.5 feet vertical × 3 feet horizontal width

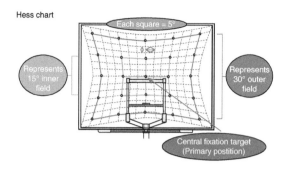

Figure 9.41 Hess chart

- Series of red lines forming squares of 5° each at macula at 1 meter distance (this was the original designed with red lines instead of red bulb lights—Keith and Wyber)
  - Method:
    - Need to wear red/green goggles
    - Show red dots one by one and the subject aligns them with a green pointer
- Lees screen
  - Does not require red/green glasses
  - Mirror is used to dissociate the two eyes
  - Two square translucent screens at 90° to each other
  - In between the two is a mirror spectrum
  - Patient is 50 cm from the other screen

What are the tests for measurement of torsion?

- Torsion may be measured objectively or subjectively
- Objective measurement
  - By observing the fovea–optic disc relationship opthalmoscopically in congenital cases
  - If torsion is present, the disc will appear displaced and either intorted or extorted in relation to the fovea
- Subjective measurements include the following:
  - Synaptophore

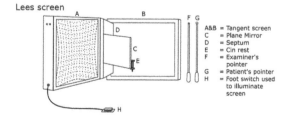

Figure 9.42 Lees screen

- Adapted Lees screen
- Maddox wing
- Awaya cyclo test
- Bagolini glasses
- Maddox double rod

What are the indications for orthoptic exercises and how are they commonly done?

- Indications for orthoptic exercises:
  - To increase control in latent deviations
  - To increase control in intermittent deviations
  - Pre- or postoperative to consolidate the result
  - To achieve good binocular convergence
  - To improve fusional reserves
- Patient's cooperation and motivation is needed
- Methods for orthoptic exercises
  - Synaptophore
  - Bar reading
  - Stereograms
- Methods to overcome suppression
  - Occlusion or monocular reading
  - Red filter drawing
  - Recognition of diplopia
  - Sbisa bar also known as Bagolini's filter bar
  - Synaptophore
  - Septum
  - Vertical prism
  - Cheiroscope
- Fusional exercises: Application of orthoptics for the management of convergence insufficiency and improving control of intermittent exotropia

What is a Cheiroscope?

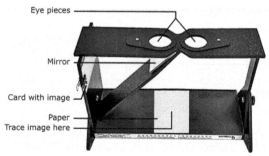

Figure 9.43 Cheiroscope

- Device used for anti-suppression exercise using subjective drawing by the patient based on the principle of haploscopic dissociation (mirror septum used).
- The target is seen by the dominant eye and the drawing surface by the suppressed eye.
- Different levels used for drawing: Crayons, tracings, tic-tac-toe.
- Increasing fusional vergence possible by shifting drawing paper.
- Patient should not be using fast alterations or shifting septum.

What is a Pigeon–Cantonnet stereoscope?

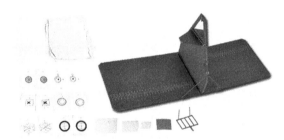

Figure 9.44 Pigeon–Cantonnet stereoscope

- Device used for anti-suppression exercise using subjective drawing by the patient based on the principle of haploscopic dissociation (mirror septum used)
- Similar to cheiroscope but with three flaps, middle having mirror on one side
- Used in two positions:
  - Position 1:
    - Two flaps rest on desk, while middle is vertical
    - Used to train relative convergence and relaxing accommodation, as the subject is made to fuse the two figures with visual axes parallel
  - Position 2:
    - Right flap rest on desk, while left makes an obtuse angle with the first and the middle flap bisects the same
    - This works like the cheiroscope: Ipsilateral flap seen by same side eye

(dominant) and the other eye is used to trace the figure on the other flap

What is convergence insufficiency and how does one diagnose and treat it?

- The inability to obtain and/or maintain adequate binocular convergence without undue effort.
- Convergence insufficiency may be a primary or secondary insufficiency.
- Primary:
  - Predisposing causes include a wide inter-pupillary distance, occupations using mainly distance vision or occupations using mainly uniocular vision.
  - Precipitating causes include illness, ocular fatigue from prolonged close work and poor lighting, school & college examinations, advancing age, drugs, and pregnancy.
- Secondary: Post-trauma or neurological illnesses
- Convergence insufficiency is confirmed by:
  - Near vision affected if accommodation involved
  - An exophoria usually present on cover-uncover testing more of convergence weakness type
  - Good level of monocular accommodation but accommodative amplitude reduced on binocular testing
  - NPC is increased
  - Poor fusional amplitudes
- Convergence sustenance less than 30 s for a 10 cm fixation target is usually symptomatic
- Management:
  - Orthoptic treatment is usually effective for primary type of convergence insufficiency.
  - Correct refractive error, lifestyle, and environment modification.
  - Home-based exercises reduce symptoms while improving near point of convergence and fusional amplitudes.
  - Recognition of pathological diplopia should be taught, if not already appreciated.

- Pen convergence exercises:
  - Binocular convergence is improved with pen convergence exercises.
  - Recognition of physiological diplopia is then taught, and the patient should continue to improve using exercises.
- The range of positive fusional convergence is improved with base out prisms, the synaptophore, dot cards, and stereograms with near fixation.
- Good voluntary convergence is established where possible.

10

OPD instruments and related

10.1 TOPICS

- Instruments in OPD
  - Slit lamp and slit-lamp examination techniques
  - Direct ophthalmoscope
  - Indirect ophthalmoscope
- Cornea
  - Dry-eye investigations
- Glaucoma
  - Tonometry
  - Gonioscopy
  - Other lenses in glaucoma
  - Optic disc evaluation
- Squint and neuro-ophthalmology
  - Pupil
  - Pupillary disorders
  - Confrontation test
- Retina l enses
  - Lenses used for fundus biomicroscopy
  - Lenses used for laser
  - Retina-viewing systems for surgery
- Lasers in ophthalmology

10.2 INSTRUMENTS IN OPD

10.2.1 Slit lamp and slit-lamp examination techniques

Identify the instrument.

Slit lamp is a type of compound microscope having the unique ability of enabling depth perception using slit illumination techniques as well as binocular viewing of various structures of the eye with versatile attachments for associated ophthalmic examination.

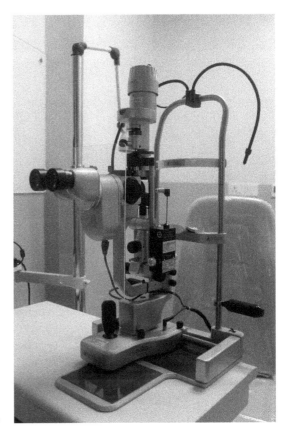

Figure 10.1 Slit lamp (Zeiss type)

What are the parts of a slit lamp?

- Observation system:
  - It is a compound microscope with two optical elements: an objective and an eyepiece.
  - Objective lens: The lens consists of two planoconvex lenses with their convexities put together providing a composite power of +22 D.

DOI: 10.1201/9781003455646-10

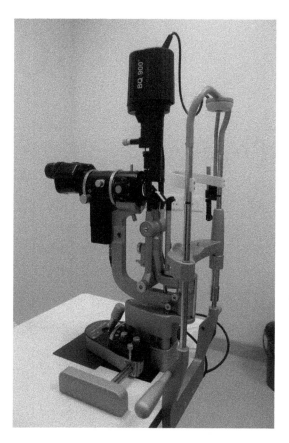

Figure 10.2 Slit-lamp Haag–Streit

- Eyepiece lens: Eyepiece has a lens of +10D, the tubes are converged at an angle of 10–15°.
- To overcome the problem of inverted image produced by the compound microscope, slit lamp microscope uses a pair of prisms between the objective and eyepiece to rein-vert the image.
- Magnification: Range is usually between 6× and 40×
- Illumination system:
  - Based on Gullstrand's illumination system
  - Halogen lamps used provide illumination between 2 × 105 and 4 × 105 lux
- Condenser lens system:
  - Filters
  - Cobalt blue: Produces light of wavelength between 450–500 nm, used in the eye after staining with fluorescein as the dye absorbs blue light and emits green
  - Red-free: Obscures anything that is red, so blood vessels and hemorrhages appear black
  - Neutral density filter: Decreases brightness for photosensitive patients

- Diffuser: General overall observations of the eye and adnexa
- Mechanical support system:
  - Joystick arrangement
  - Up and down movement
  - Patient support arrangement
  - Fixation target

What are the various illumination techniques?

- Diffuse illumination:
  - Diffuse broad beam of light
  - Angle between light and microscope is 45°
  - Slit: Open
  - Filter: Diffusing filter
  - Magnification: Variable (low/high)
  - Examine: Overall view of lid, conjunctiva, cornea, sclera, pupil
- Direct illumination:
  - Observation and illumination system are focused on the same point
  - Angle between light and microscope is 45–50°
  - Magnification: Variable (low/high)
  - Can vary width and height of light source
  - Techniques:
    - Optic section:
      - Tall but narrow slit of focused light (<0.25 mm wide)
      - Uses
      - Evaluate structural layers of cornea and lens
      - Estimate the depth of abnormality in cornea (foreign body) or lens
      - Can estimate depth of AC by Van Herrick's technique
    - Parallelopiped section:
      - Wider beam of focused light (1–2 mm wide)
      - Provides broader view for extensive examination
      - Layered view of cornea and lens
    - Conical beam:
      - Smaller circular or square spot of light formed by reducing the height of the parallelepiped beam
      - Dark room
      - Use: To examine the transparency of anterior chamber for cells and flare
- Indirect illumination:
  - Narrow beam of light (1–2 mm wide)
  - Beam is then focused adjacent to the area to be observed such that the area is

observed in the shadow by virtue of the scattered light
- Foci of light source and microscope are not coincident
- Magnification: Varies (low/high)
- Retro illumination:
  - Visualized using reflecting light of the slit beam from a structure more posterior than the structure under observation so as to place the object of regard against a dark background allowing the object to appear dark or black
    - Retro illumination from iris: Beam is directed to an area of iris bordering the portion just behind the pathology to be observed. This provides a dark background allowing corneal opacities to be viewed with greater contrast.
    - Retro illumination from fundus: Slit beam is at 2–4°. Shorten the beam to the height of the pupil to avoid reflecting bright light off the iris. Magnification is 10×–16×. Focus the beam directly on the pathology, and opacities will appear in the silhouette.
  - Uses:
    - Keratic precipitates (KPs) on corneal endothelium
    - Water clefts and vacuoles in the crystalline lens
    - Corneal edema neovascularization, microcysts, infiltrates
    - Contact lens deposits

- Specular reflection:
  - Formed by separating the microscope and slit lamp beam by equal angles (30° to one side) from the normal to the cornea, i.e., angle of incidence equals angle of reflection
  - Start with low magnification (10× or 16×) to observe the endothelium and direct a narrow beam onto the cornea.
  - Then switch to the highest magnification available.
  - Endothelium maybe best viewed using one ocular (can close one eye)
  - Uses:
    - Irregularities, deposits, excavations in corneal surfaces
    - Endothelial changes
    - Tear film debris, tear film lipid layer thickness
- Sclerotic scatter:
  - Formed by focusing a tall but narrow slit beam (1 mm) on the limbus
  - Magnification: Low
  - Angle between light and microscope is 40–60°
  - Magnification: 10×
  - Halo glow of light around limbus
  - Light is absorbed and scattered through the corneal layers highlighting pathology
  - Principle: Total internal reflection
  - Uses:
    - Central corneal epithelial edema
    - Corneal abrasions
    - Foreign bodies in the cornea

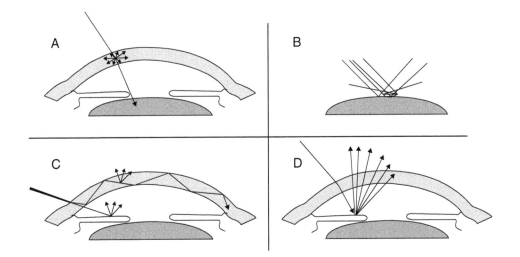

Figure 10.3 Slit-lamp examination techniques

- Tangential illumination:
    - Angle between light and microscope is 70–80°
    - Medium-wide beam width
    - Moderate height
    - Magnification: 10×, 16×, 25×
    - Uses: Anterior posterior cornea, iris, and anterior lens (useful for pseudoexfoliation)
- Oscillation technique of Koeppe
    - Microscope is kept in focus on the structure to be observed, and the illumination beam is oscillated alternately using quick to-and-fro movements resulting in direct and indirect illumination.
- Diagram of how light rays interact with the eye in slit-lamp biomicroscopic examination: (A) direct illumination; (B) specular reflection; (C) sclerotic scatter; (D) retro illumination from iris.

10.2.2 Direct ophthalmoscope

What is this instrument?

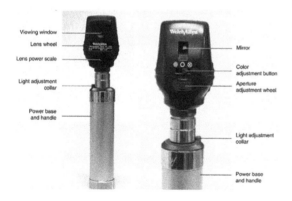

Direct ophthalmoscope

Who invented it?

- Babbage in 1848
- Hermann von Helmoltz revolutionized it in 1850

What is the principle of the direct ophthalmoscope?

- When the fixation point of the observer's retina is coaxial with the patient's eye to be examined, light emanating from an illuminated portion of the retina is refracted on its way to the observer's

retina at the interfaces it passes: vitreous, lens, aqueous, cornea, air, the ophthalmoscope's lens or lenses, and the elements of the eye of the observer; and in emmetropia the image is focused directly on the observer's retina.
- Prerequisites:
    - Illumination of the target area of fundus to be examined
    - Co-axial nature of observer and patient's retina
    - Emmetropia or ametropia corrected with an appropriate intervening lens

State the characteristics of the image formed?

- Image: Virtual erect
- Field of view: 2 DD = 10°
- Magnification: 15×
- Area of fundus seen: 50–70%
- Working distance: 1–2 cm
- Image brightness: 4 watts
- Stereopsis: None

What are the various apertures and accessories for?

- Small aperture: For easy view of the fundus through undilated pupil
- Large aperture: For dilated pupils and general examination of the eye, particularly the red reflex
- Small micro spot aperture: Allows through very small, undilated pupils
- Slit aperture: Useful in determining various elevations like tumors or disc edema
- Fixation aperture: The pattern of open center and thin lines permits easy observation of eccentric fixation without masking macula
- Fixation star: To determine patient's fixation
- Pinhole/half-circle diaphragm: Used to reduce reflections by limiting the illumination beam
- Red-free filter: To see vessels and hemorrhages
- Blue filter: Enhance visibility of fluorescein
- Set of crossed polarized filters: Used to reduce reflections

How does one perform direct ophthalmoscopy?

- Should be done on same side of patient and examiner. For example, for the patient's right eye, use your right hand to hold the DO, and use your right eye on the right side of the patient.

- Stand at approximately one arm's length while illuminating both the patient's eyes using the large aperture to examine the red reflex.
- Select small aperture and while fixing on the red reflex as your target ask patient to look straight ahead.
- Tilt slightly 15–25° lateral to the patient. The optic disc should be within view 1–2 inches from the patient's eye.
- Hypermetropia patients require more plus lenses and myopia patients require more minus lenses if the optic disc is not focused.
- Follow each vessel to the periphery.
- Ask patient to look superior, inferior, nasal, and temporal.
- Last look at the macula, which is approximately 2 DD temporal between superotemporal and inferotemporal vessels.

10.2.3 Indirect ophthalmoscope

Identify the following instrument.

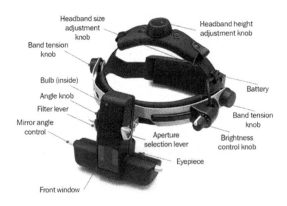

Indirect ophthalmoscope (IDO or IO)

Who invented it?

- Ruete (1852) designed the first monocular indirect ophthalmoscope.
- Marc Antoine Giraud–Teulon invented the binocular handheld indirect ophthalmoscope (1861).
- Charles Schepens (1946) invented the modern binocular indirect ophthalmoscope.

What is the principle of IDO?

- Involves making the eye highly myopic
- By placing a powerful convex lens in front of the eye
- So a real, inverted, laterally reversed image is formed close to the principle focus of the lens between the lens and the observer.

What are the factors which affect the field of view?

- Pupil size
- Power of condensing lens
- Overall size of the condensing lens
- Refractive error (to a small extent)
- Distance of the condensing lens form the eye

What are the factors that affect the magnification?

- Dioptric power of the convex lens
- Position of lens in relation to eye
- Refractive state of the eye

What is the procedure?

- Dark room.
- Patient may be supine.
- Dilate and anesthetize preferably both eyes if indentation is planned.
- Ask patient to fixate on his/her thumb.
- Keep arm-length distance, writing hand usually holds depressor initially, but later ambidexterity should be incorporated subconsciously.
- Focus light on outstretched thumb to check your own binocularity.
- Adjust the pupillary distance and height of the beam so you can see a full beam with each eye.
- The medium light gives an 8-mm-diameter illuminated view when in focus with the 20 D lens.
- Viewing must be coaxial: Maintain axis: All in one line
  - Viewing system
  - Condensing lens center
  - Patient's pupil
  - Area of retina to be visualized
  - Depressor tip (if being used)
  - Eyepiece must be perpendicular to pupillary axis

- Illuminate patients' pupillary area.
- Interpose condenser lens close to the eye.
- Hold with more convex side toward observer (usually silver ring toward patient).
- Pull back lens till the image fills the lens.
- Stand 180° away from quadrant to be examined.

What are the contraindications of scleral indentation?

- Recent penetrating injury
- Orbital injury
- Intraocular surgery (<8 weeks)

What are the advantages and disadvantages of IDO?

- Advantages:
  - Larger field of view
  - Less distortion of retinal images
  - Easier to examine during patient's eye movements
  - Easier to examine in patients with high spherical power or astigmatism
  - Stereopsis
  - Can be used intraoperatively
  - Useful in hazy media
  - Peripheral retinal evaluation
  - Dynamic examination
  - Camera recording possible
  - Laser delivery possible
- Disadvantages:
  - Long learning curve
  - Less magnification
  - Difficult in small pupils

What are the differences between direct and indirect ophthalmoscopy? (Table 10.1)

Table 10.1 Differences between Direct and Indirect Ophthalmoscopy

Direct Ophthalmoscopy (DO)	Indirect Ophthalmoscopy (IDO)
Monocular view	Binocular view
Limited field of view (10–15°)	Wide field of view (35°)
Poor view in hazy media	Better view in hazy media

Table 10.1 *(Continued)* Differences between Direct and Indirect Ophthalmoscopy

Direct Ophthalmoscopy (DO)	Indirect Ophthalmoscopy (IDO)
Less working distance	Working distance about 35–40 cm
Illumination: 0.5–2 watts	Illumination: 15–18 watts
Magnification: 15×	Magnification: 2–5×
Virtual erect image	Real and inverted image
No teaching aid	Teaching aid
No scleral indention	Scleral indentation possible

10.3 CORNEA

10.3.1 Dry eye

Identify this strip.

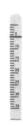

Figure 10.6 Schirmer strip

- Special (Whatman No. 41) filter paper is used
- 5 mm wide × 35 mm long
- Test can be performed with anesthetic (Schirmer 1) or without anesthetic (Schirmer 2)
- Theoretically Schirmer 1 evaluates baseline secretion whereas a Schirmer 2 measures baseline plus reflex secretion of tears

What is the definition of dry eye?

- Dry eye disease is a multifactorial disease of the ocular tear film and ocular surface that results in symptoms of ocular discomfort, visual disturbance, and tear film instability with potential damage to the ocular surface.
- It is usually associated with increased osmolarity of the tear film and subacute inflammation of the ocular surface (Table 10.2).

Table 10.2 Composition of Normal Tear Film

	Lipid Layer (Outer)	Aqueous Layer (Middle)	Mucin Layer (Inner)
Source	Meibomian glands	Lacrimal glands	• Conjunctival goblet cells • Crypts of Henle • Glands of Manz
Function	• Decreases evaporation of aqueous layer • Decreases surface tension of tear film • Lubrication	• Provides oxygen to the cornea • Antibacterial (IgA, lysozyme, lactoferrin) • Decreases irregularity of anterior corneal surface • Washes away debris and toxic agents	• Wets cornea by converting hydrophobic corneal epithelium to hydrophilic • Lubrication
Dysfunction	Evaporative dry eye	Hyposecretive dry eye	Evaporative and hyposecretive

Table 10.3 Tear-Deficient (Hyposecretive)

1. Sjogren's		2. Non-Sjogren's
Primary Autoimmune with dry mouth	Secondary Systemic autoimmune associations • Rheumatoid arthritis • SLE • Wegener's granulomatosis • Systemic sclerosis • Dermatomyositis • Polymyositis • Relapsing polychondritis • Primary biliary cirrhosis	• Senile • Lacrimal gland destruction (inflammation, sarcoidosis, thyroid, radiation, malignancy) • Scarring of lacrimal gland ductules (trachoma, cicatricial pemphigoid, chemical burns, radiation, erythema multiforme) • Alacrimia • Riley–Day syndrome • Reflex (seventh-nerve palsy, fifth-nerve palsy, chronic contact lens wear) • Post-LASIK

- Average tear flow is 1.2 µl/min.
- Average blink rate is once per 5 seconds (10–12 per minute).

What is the classification of dry eyes? (Tables 10.3 and 10.4)

What are the signs and symptoms of dry eye disease?

- Symptoms:
  - Excess mucous strands
  - Foreign body sensation
  - Irritation

Table 10.4 Tear-Sufficient (Evaporative)

Oil deficiency	Because of Meibomian gland dysfunction, meibomitis, blepharitis, distichiasis
Defective tear resurfacing	Abnormal blink rate, defective lid-to-globe congruity, xerophthalmia
Miscellaneous	Chronic contact lens wear

- Paradoxical excess watering
- Note: Symptoms worsen in air-conditioned environment, windy situations
- Symptoms improve with increased humidity
- Signs
  - Reduced blink rate
  - Excess mucous strands
  - Marginal tear meniscus thin/concave
  - Froth on lid margin especially in Meibomian gland dysfunction
  - Keratopathy
    - Punctate epithelial erosions
    - Filamentary keratopathy
    - Mucous plaques

What are the investigations to diagnose dry eyes?

- Tear film break-up time (TFBUT)
  - Determined after instillation of unpreserved (BAK can speed up TBUT) fluorescein drops without topical anesthesia using a slit lamp with a cobalt blue filter.
  - After a complete blink, the time to the first break-up of the tear film is measured.
    - <10 seconds is abnormal
- Dye staining:
  - Fluorescein:
    - Most common
    - When epithelial cell desquamate dye rapidly diffuses in intercellular spaces and stains
    - Also penetrates corneal epithelium when mucous layer is lost
  - Rose Bengal:
    - Rose Bengal stains devitalize epithelial cells, as well as epithelial cells that lack a healthy layer of protective mucin coating
    - More sensitive for staining the conjunctiva
    - Causes irritation and reflex tearing
    - Van Bijsterveld grading scale: Scale that involves evaluation of intensity of staining based on a scale of 0–3 in:
      - Nasal conjunctiva
      - Temporal conjunctiva
      - Cornea
  - Lissamine green strip (1%) with small non-preserved saline drop

- Look for conjunctival staining
- Does not irritate conjunctiva like Rose Bengal
- Schirmer test or Schirmer tear test (STT):
  - Place the strip in the conjunctival sac of the temporal third of the lower eyelid with the patient's eyes closed.
  - Wetting is measured, in the form of tears going across via capillary action, measured after 5 minutes.
  - Basic (with anesthesia): Normal >10 mm.
  - Reflex (without anesthesia): Normal >15 mm.
  - If the Schirmer test is performed after nasal stimulation, it is termed the Schirmer II test.
  - Test sometimes criticized for its variability and poor reproducibility.
- Phenol red impregnated thread test (PRT):
  - Cutoff value: 10 mm at 15 seconds
  - Measures basal tear volume
- Corneal sensations:
  - Can be both cause and effect
  - Procedure: Extend a few strands of a cotton swab and gently touch the surface of the cornea and conjunctiva
  - Cochet–Bonnet esthesiometer consists of a nylon monofilament that can be extended in length from 0 to 6 cm and measurements are taken by advancing it toward the center of the cornea, contact is detected by the slightest bend of the nylon. Normal cutoff is 4.5 cm.
- Tear film osmolarity:
  - Increased in dry eye (does not differentiate evaporative/deficient dry eye)
  - Sensitive test not specific for dry eye disease
- Lactoferrin assay
  - Indicator of lacrimal gland function in a relative manner.
  - Tear lactoferrin concentrations are measured by the Lactocard which is a commercially available colorimetric solid phase ELISA technique.
- Delayed tear clearance or fluorescein clearance test (FCT)
  - Method to objectively measure tear turnover from the ocular surface

- Standardized amount of fluorescein is placed in the conjunctival sac and the tear turnover rate is determined by the persistence of fluorescein in the tears at time points specifically measured
  - Can use a Schirmer strip to collect the fluorescein-stained tears
  - Precise method is to use a fluorophotometer
- Tear film meniscus height (meniscometry)
  - Tear meniscus below 0.25 mm is regarded as pathological
  - Can be measured using a slit-lamp beam or by reflective meniscometry
- Interferometry of the tear film lipid layer is useful in screening and evaluating dry eye
- Lysozyme measurement with diffusion in agar plate: Difficult and expensive
- In cases where Sjogren's syndrome is suspected, a thorough review of systems is performed and one or more of the following blood tests may be ordered—anti-SS-A, anti-SS-B, rheumatoid factor, ANA, ESR (sedimentation rate) and C-reactive protein in addition to work-up by a rheumatologist.

What are the criteria for diagnosing Sjogren's syndrome?

- Four of the six criteria must be fulfilled:
  - Subjective description of oral symptoms by the patient.
  - Subjective description of ocular symptoms by the patient.
  - Objective signs of oral dryness.
  - Oral dryness is determined by unstimulated salivary flow rate and/or Saxon test.
  - Objective signs of ocular dryness.
  - Dry eye disease is diagnosed based on a reduced Schirmer test result, reduced tear film break-up time, and/or positive ocular surface staining.
  - Histopathological evidence of infiltrating lymphocytes in minor salivary glands.
  - Evidence of serum autoantibodies, especially antibodies to Ro (SSA) or La (SSB) antigens.

What are the treatment options for dry eyes? (Table 10.5)

- Etiological treatment:
  - Vitamin A: Topical (10,000/20,000 IU orally) increases secretion especially mucin

Table 10.5 Treatment Options for Dry Eyes

Preservation of Tears	Tear Substitutes	Mucolytics	Reduction of Tear Drainage
• Decrease room temperature • Room humidification • Small lateral tarsorrhaphy	• Tear substitutes should ideally be preservative free • Benzalkonium chloride is most epithelio-toxic (BAK) • Newer preservatives: Sodium perborate and purite disintegrate on exposure to light into harmless products —Normal drops without preservatives: § High molecular weight polymers § Polyvinyl alcohol § Cellulose esters § Methylcellulose § HPMC —Gels: Carbomers—ot increases duration of action; Hence, less frequency of instillation —Ointment	5% Acetylcysteine (especially in filamentous keratopathy)	Punctal occlusion • Temporary: Collagen plug • Permanent: Cautery • Reversible Long term: Silicon plugs

- Diet: Fish/flax oil—ω3 fatty acids increases lipid phase
- Treatment of infection:
  - Trachoma: Azithromycin 20 mg/kg single dose
  - Dacryoadenitis: Treat with antibiotics
  - Meibomitis: Cholesterol esters in meibomian secretion is good culture medium for organisms as *S. aureus*. This organism produce lipase, which denatures meibomian secretion and increases evaporation of aqueous serous phase of tears.
- Cyclosporin A:
  - Systemic 1 mg/kg/day
  - Topical 1% aqueous solution
  - Binds cytosolic protein (cyclophilin) inhibits T-cell activation, therefore inhibits liberation of IL-2 and IFN (inflammatory cytokines)
- Surgical management:
  - Occlusion of lower punta
    - Collagen plugs
    - Silicon Plugs
    - Cautery
  - Transplantation of salivary glands: submandibular, parotid (not possible in Sjogren's syndrome)

10.4 GLAUCOMA

10.4.1 Tonometry

Identify the instrument.

- Schiotz tonometer
- Parts:
  - Foot plate radius of curvature: 15 mm
  - Plunger diameter: 3 mm
  - Plunger + needle + hammer weight: 5.5 g
  - Total weight: 16.5 g
  - Additional weights: 7.5 g, 10 g, and 15 g
  - Each scale: 0.05 mm of protrusion of plunger
  - Test block for checking calibration
- AAO standardized Schiotz tonometer
  - The footplate concavity has radius of curvature of 15 mm and weighs 11 g.
  - Plunger diameter is 3 mm, and it weighs 5.5 g.
  - The plunger extends 0.05 mm beyond the footplate curve.

- 0.025 mm radius of plunger edge curvature reduces corneal abrasions.
- IOP estimation by Schiotz tonometry is based on average coefficient of ocular rigidity (E = 0.0245)
- Consists of a concave footplate attached to a shaft enclosing a freely sliding plunger.
- The extent to which the anesthetized cornea is indented by the plunger and a simple lever moves a needle on a calibrated scale.

What is the principle of Schiotz tonometry?

- Indentation tonometry: IOP is measured by correlating the force responsible for deformation of the globe to the pressure within the eye.
- According to Friedenwald the steady state pressure (Po) of the eye is raised to a higher pressure (Pt) due to volume displacement caused by corneal indentation.
- The volume displacement causes some distention of the globe, which is regulated by ocular rigidity (resistance of the eye).
- Thus, calculations include a factor k which is the coefficient of ocular rigidity.
- Friedenwald gave a table after simplifying calculations for the same (k = 0.0215).

Describe this technique of tonometry.

- Patient lies supine.
- Cornea is anesthetized.
- Eyelid separated using fingers.

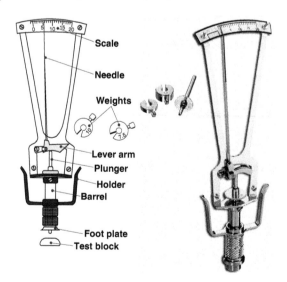

Figure 10.7 Schiotz tonometer

- Patient asked to fixate at distant object.
- Footplate applied to cornea.
- Tonometer must be kept vertical.
- Needle oscillates and midpoint of excursions is used as a reading.
- Additional weights may be used as required.

What are its sources of error?

- Low ocular rigidity underestimates IOP: Myopia, RD surgery, vitrectomy, intravitreal as injections, miotics
- High ocular rigidity overestimates IOP: Extreme myopia, high hyperopia, chronic glaucoma, vasoconstrictor therapy
- Changes in corneal curvature: False high IOP occurs in steep and thicker corneas, which increase the fluid displacement during tonometry
- Errors due to instrument: Due to differences in size and shape of the footplate, difference in weights of different parts of the tonometer, friction between plunger and pointer on the scale
- Accommodation: Contraction of ciliary muscle increases aqueous outflow facility (lowers IOP)
- Error due to extraocular muscle contraction
- Parallax errors from readings of the scale
- Changes due to blood volume alteration
- Moses effect: False high IOP if cornea gets sucked into space between plunger and hole in footplate

How will you disinfect it after use?

- Dissemble and clean with alcohol
- Clean with spirit
- Boiling/autoclave/hot air oven/UV rays
- 2% glutaraldehyde
- Wipe foot plate with isopropyl alcohol

What are the advantages and disadvantages of Schiotz tonometry?

- Advantages: Cheap, simple, portable
- Disadvantages:
  - Falsely low reading in low scleral rigidity
  - Affected by corneal thickness
  - Repeat tension: Low reading
  - Muscle contraction: High reading
  - Needs conversion table
  - Can cause corneal abrasions

Identify the tonometer?

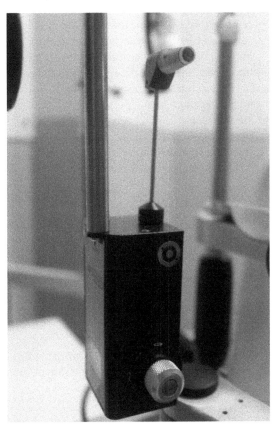

Figure 10.8 Goldmann applanation tonometer

- Goldmann applanation tonometer
- Prism: Area of contact of Prism 7.35 sq.mm
- Diameter of corneal flattening: 3.06 mm
- Force required 0.1 g = 1 mmHg

What is the principle of applanation tonometry?

- Tonometry is based on Imbert Fick's principle or Maklakov–Fick law: For an ideal sphere (perfectly spherical, dry, infinitely thin-walled, and perfectly flexible) the pressure (P) inside the sphere is equal to force (F) required to applanate the surface divided by the area (A) of flattening, i.e., P = F/A.
- However, the cornea is not an ideal sphere; two other forces come into play:
  - Force of capillary attraction between tonometer head and tear film (T)
  - Additional force (C) independent of IOP required to flatten the relatively inflexible cornea opposite to F

- F+T = PA+C
- IOP = (F+T−C)/A

- A is measured along the inner surface of the cornea and is designed such that when A = 7.35 mm, the diameter of corneal flattening is 3.06 mm, and at this value, the opposing forces of capillary action and corneal inflexibility cancel each other out.
- Since displacement of aqueous is 0.5 µl, pressure induced by tonometer tip is negligible; therefore, applanation tonometry is not affected by ocular rigidity.

What is the technique?

- A biprism that contacts the cornea creates two semicircles.
- The edge of corneal contact is made apparent by instillation of fluorescein into tear film while in cobalt blue filter.
- By rotating a dial calibrated in grams, force is adjusted by changing length of spring within the device.
- The prisms are calibrated so that inner margins of semicircles touch when 3.06 mm of the cornea is applanated.

What is the method of applanation tonometry?

- Adjust the patient on slit lamp.
- Put anesthetic drops and fluorescein.
- Adjust angle of 60° between illumination and microscope.
- Open slit lamp light beam to a wide slit.
- Turn to blue filter.
- Set knob at 1 g.
- Set '0' mark of prism with white line on prism; if astigmatism > 3 D, it requires rotation.
- Ideal fluorescein ring: 0.25–0.3 mm.
- Wide rings give underestimation.
- Narrow rings give overestimation.
- Knob is rotated till inner borders of two rings coincide.
- Readings obtained in grams multiplied by 10 = mmHg.

What are the errors in measurement?

- Causes of underestimation:
  - Inadequate fluorescein stain
  - Repeated tonometry
  - Corneal edema

- Causes of overestimation:
  - Elevation of eyes >15°
  - Widening of lid fissure
  - Corneal scar
  - Examiner pressing on globe
  - Squeezing of eyelids
- Thin corneas underestimate IOP, and thick corneas produce overestimation of IOP.
- Quenching of fluorescence: Low fluorescein concentration may cause underestimation of pressures.
- Width of tear meniscus: Wider menisci overestimates IOP, unsatisfactory vertical alignment of semicircles produces erroneous overestimation of IOP.
- Corneal curvature:
  - Rise of 1 mmHg with every 3 D change in corneal astigmatism. More fluid is placed under a steep cornea. Steeper the corneal curvature, more the cornea must be indented to produce standard area of contact.
  - IOP is underestimated by 1 mmHg for every 4 D with the rule astigmatism and overestimated by same amount for against the rule astigmatism—minimized by rotating the prisms so that the flattest meridian is opposite the red-line on the prism holder.
- Corneal epithelial edema: IOP underestimated.

How does one sterilize the applanation tonometer?

- Washing with water
- Wiping with isopropyl alcohol
- Ethylene oxide gas
- Formalin gas chamber
- Disinfection with 2% glutaraldehyde in suspected HIV-positive cases
- Soaking in household bleach 1:10 dilution (sodium hypochlorite) exposure to ultraviolet light
- Using disposable film covers for applanation tips
- 5-to-10-minute soak in fresh 3% hydrogen peroxide or 70% ethanol or isopropanol

How do you calibrate this Haag–Streit Goldmann applanation tonometer?

- One has to use the calibration error check weight bar.

- Bar has five markings:
  - Central marking = Level 0
  - Two on either side = Level 2 (20 mmHg)
  - Two outermost markings = Level 6 (60 mmHg)
- Calibration must be conducted at all these levels.
- Method:
  - At setting 0, if the dial position is moved to –0.05, the feeler arm should fall toward the examiner; if the drum is moved to position +0.05, the arm should fall toward the patient.
  - To check settings 2 and 6, the calibration error check weight bar provided by the manufacturer is used.
  - The calibration error check weight bar has 5 markings on it. The central marking corresponds to level 0. Two on either side of it represent level 2 and the two outermost markings represent level 6. These markings correspond to 0, 20, and 60 mm Hg of IOP, respectively.
  - The calibration error check weight bar and holder are fitted into the slot provided on the side of the applanation tonometer. After setting the mark on the weight bar corresponding to position 2 or 6 on the index mark of the weight holder, the measuring drum is rotated forward. The reading at which the feeler arm with the prism in place moves forward freely is recorded. The difference of this reading from the respective test position is the positive error at that level of testing. Similarly, on rotating the revolving knob in the reverse direction, the reading at which the feeler arm moves backward is noted. The difference between the latter and the testing position is the negative error at that level of testing.
- Acceptable calibration error:
  - Haag–Streit standard: ±0.5 mmHg at all levels of testing (0, 20, 60 mmHg)
  - SEAGIG standard: ±2 mmHg at 0 mmHg, ±3 mmHg at 20 mmHg, ±4 mmHg at 60 mmHg

Identify the tonometer?

Describe it. Mention its uses.

- Goldmann-type applanation tonometer

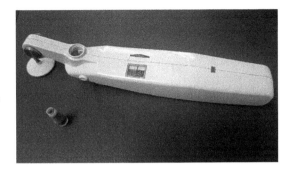

Figure 10.9 Perkins tonometer

- Uses same prisms as Goldmann, but tonometry can be performed in any head position, i.e., sitting or supine
  - It is portable, and its accuracy is comparable to Goldmann.
  - Light source is a battery.
  - Counterbalance ensures accuracy in horizontal and vertical positions.
  - Use: Infants, children, and invalid patients.

Describe Tono-Pen tonometer. Mention its method of use and principle of Mackay–Marg tonometers?

- Handheld and portable and battery-operated
- Uses a principle similar to Mackay–Marg tonometer
- Weight = 16 g
- Method: Brief touch on the cornea obtains 4–10 IOP readings, which are then analyzed by a microprocessor internally and displays a digital reading of the mean of accepted estimations and their coefficient of variance (5%, 10%, 20%, >20%)
- There is good agreement between pressure measurements taken with a Tono-Pen compared with manometric reading in human autopsy eyes
- Principles of Mackay–Marg tonometer:
  - Applanation of cornea via a plunger that moves within a sleeve; the advancing tonometer causes the sleeve to abut the cornea, transferring the force required to flatten the cornea to the sleeve. The pressure tracing then decreases to a level that represents the IOP, which occurs when a corneal diameter of 1.5 mm is applanated. The resulting the excursion of the plunger

is electronically coupled to a transducer and graphically records the movement of plunger on a moving paper records the sum force required to indent the cornea and the IOP.

- Smaller area of 1.5 mm of cornea is applanated and is considered accurate even in scarred and edematous corneas.
- The effects of corneal resistance to deformation and surface tension of tears are less than with a Goldmann tonometry, but it is theorized to be more reliable than Goldmann tonometry.
- The Mackay–Marg, Tono-Pen, and pneumotonometers can measure IOP through soft contact lenses with reasonable accuracy.

What is non-contact tonometer?

- The non-contact tonometer deforms the corneal apex by means of a jet of air.
- The force of air jets increases linearly over time.
- The time elapsed is related to the force of air necessary to flatten the cornea and the IOP.
- The accuracy of NCT is diminished in higher-pressure ranges and in eyes with abnormal fixation and irregular corneas.

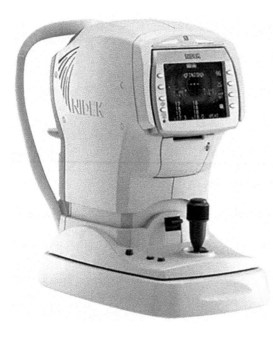

Figure 10.10 Non-contact tonometer (NCT)

- Eliminates corneal abrasions, reaction to topical anesthetics, and transmission of infectious agents.

Classify tonometry.

- Direct
- Indirect:
  - Palpation
  - Contact:
    - Indentation
    - Applanation
- Variable force:
  - Goldmann (prototype)
  - Goldmann type: Perkins, Draeger
  - Mackay–Marg
  - Mackay–Marg type: Tono-Pen
- Variable area:
  - Maklakov
  - Maklakov type: Tonomat, Barraquer
  - Non-contact: Keeler Pulsair tonometer

10.4.2 Gonioscopy

What is gonioscopy?

- It is a method of examination of anterior chamber, specifically catering to the anterior chamber angles using special lenses and viewing systems.
- Principle:
  - Light reflected from the angle reaches the cornea-air interface at an angle exceeding the critical angle and is therefore totally internally reflected
  - Critical angle = 46°
  - By using a contact lens, corneal refractive power is neutralized so that angle can be visualized.
- Gonioscopy lenses are of two types:
  - Direct gonioscopy lenses allow direct visualization of the angle; the lenses have a steeper curvature than the cornea; light rays are refracted at the cornea-air interface such that critical angle is not reached.
  - Indirect gonioscopy mirrors allow visualization through reflection in a mirror-mounted lens, the mirror is mounted on a gonioprism; light rays are reflected from the mirror and leave the lens at nearly right angles.

Figure 10.11 Koeppe lens

What are the indications for gonioscopy?

- Diagnostic:
  - Narrow peripheral anterior chamber angle (VH <2)
  - Neovascular glaucoma
  - Angle recession glaucoma
  - History of inflammation within the eye
  - Developmental anomalies of the angle
- Therapeutic:
  - Argon laser trabeculoplasty
  - Laser goniotomy
  - Reopen a closed trabecular opening

Identify the lens.

What is the Koeppe lens?

- Diameters: 16 mm, 17 mm, 18 mm, 19 mm, 22.5 mm
- 50 D is the power
- Does not have attached rod
- Material: Plastic or glass
- Image: Upright, virtual, and magnified
- Uses principle of simple reflection
- Saline/viscous solution is used as a coupling medium

Mention the advantages and disadvantages of direct gonioscopy?

- Advantages:
  - Panoramic view
  - Patient comfort
  - Simultaneous lens placement on each eye and easy comparison between two eyes
  - Bedside examination
  - Binocularity for lateral angles
  - Transillumination
  - Teaching situation
  - Pediatric examination
  - Goniotomy and goniosynechiolysis
- Disadvantages:
  - Time-consuming
  - Requires large working area and an assistant

- Separate illumination and magnification for best results
- Lacks magnification and illumination compared to slit lamp
- Cannot create optic section to localize Schwalbe's line
- Angle appears more open as patient lies supine

Mention some other lenses for direct gonioscopy?

- Richardson Shaffer: It is used for infants
- Layden
  - Used for premature infants
  - Diameter: 10.5 mm, 11.5 mm
- Hoskins–Barkan
  - No rod attached
  - Used during operative goniotomy
- Thorpe
  - Used in operating room both as surgical and as well as a diagnostic lens
  - Usually has a rod
  - Dome-shaped
- Swan–Jacob
  - It has an attached rod.
  - Viscoelastic is used as a coupling agent.
  - Uses: Goniotomy, ab interno trabeculotomy, while using trabectome, putting I-stent or Cy Pass suprachoroidal device.

Identify the lens. Describe each in detail.

- One-, two-, and three-mirror: Goldmann three-mirror
- Goldmann three-mirror
- Three-mirror lenses: Angles 59°, 67°, 73°
  - 59°—for angle visualization; tongue-shaped
  - 67°—for mid-peripheral fundus and equator; trapezoid
  - 73°—for peripheral fundus and ciliary body and pars plana; rectangular
  - One- and two-mirror lenses: Mirror inclined at 62°, smaller diameter, mirror higher
- Four-mirror lenses: Zeiss, Posner, Thorpe, Sussman
  - Zeiss: Mirror angled at 64° is similar to the Posner lens but is made of glass instead of plastic. It is no longer commercially available.

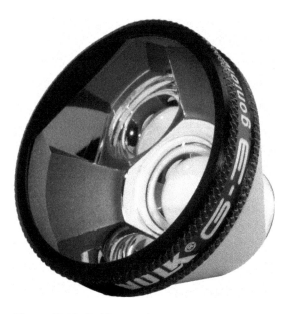

Figure 10.12 Goldmann three-mirror

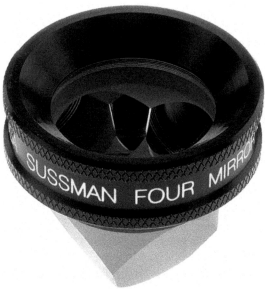

Figure 10.14 Sussman four-mirror

- Incorporates four prisms, not mirrors, to allow the four ocular quadrants to be examined simultaneously
- Usually comes with a frame and a spring which helps to keep the lens stable between the lids
- Needs methylcellulose as coupling agent
- Other benefits of the four-mirror lens:
  - By rotating the lens through only 11°, small areas between the mirrors can be brought into view.
  - Because the lens has a small (9 mm) area of contact with the cornea, the angle can be deepened by pushing on the lens (indentation gonioscopy).
  - Coupling agent: Natural tears or topical anesthetic is usually enough. Hence no viscous fluids are needed, and allows clearer examination as well as photography of the optic nerve head following gonioscopy.

What are the advantages and disadvantages of Goldmann-style one- and two-mirror lenses over three-mirror lenses? (Table 10.6)

What is their use?

- Goldmann style one and two mirror lenses used for Gonioscopy in: Patients with small aperture

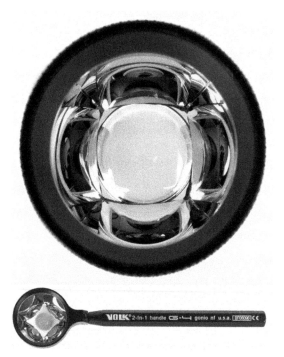

- Sussman four-mirror lens: Similar to Zeiss or Posner lens but without a handle. Preferred by those examiners who hold the lens directly on the cornea.
- Allen–Thorpe gonioprism:
  - Mirror angled at 62°

Table 10.6 Advantages and Disadvantages of Goldmann-Style One- and Two-Mirror Lenses over Three-Mirror Lenses

Advantages	Disadvantages
Higher vantage, good for narrow angles	Foreshortened view
Applicable with handheld slit lamp	Cannot use for peripheral retinal examination
	Can cause partial vacuum causing distortions

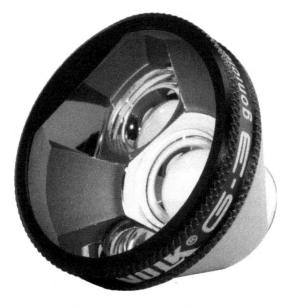

Figure 10.15 Goldmann three-mirror lens

- Patients with deep-set eyes
- Patients who squeeze

Describe the Goldmann three-mirror lenses.

- Contact lens: Multipurpose.
- Anterior surface flat.
- Corneal diameter: 12 mm; radius: 7.4 mm.
- Curve: Steeper than cornea, coupling fluid is required
- Image: Central: Virtual and erect, located near posterior surface of crystalline lens.
- Peripheral: Vertical meridian—upside down.
- Horizontal meridian—laterally reversed.
- Modifications:
  - Goldmann one or two mirror (62°)

- Uses:
  - Diagnostic: For accurate diagnosis of retinal and angle pathology
    - Documentation: Photograph
    - Magnification: Can be increased
  - Therapeutic: Laser delivery
  - Advantages:
    - Parallel view, good for detail
    - Causes less vacuum than smaller lenses
    - Good for neonates
    - Can use for retinal exam
    - Stable view
    - Easier to handle
  - Disadvantages:
    - Contact lens
    - Limited field of view without rotation
    - Indentation gonioscopy not possible

Compare Goldmann single-mirror, Goldmann three-mirror, and Zeiss four-mirror (Table 10.7).

What are the advantages and disadvantages of four-mirror gonioscope (Table 10.8) (flat base curve lenses)?

What are the advantages and disadvantages of indirect gonioscopes? (Table 10.9)

What is indirect gonioscopy?

- Indirect gonioscopy eliminates total internal reflection at the surface of the cornea.
- Light which has been reflected from the angle of the anterior chamber passes through the indirect gonio lens.
- It is reflected by a mirror within the lens.
- Uses illumination and magnification provided by a slit lamp.
- Requires a gonio lens, which contains mirrors.
  - Horizontal mirror
  - Vertical mirror
- Image: Inverted and view is slightly foreshortened of the opposite angle.

What is dynamic gonioscopy?

- Indentation gonioscopy
  - Can be done with four-mirror lenses (as they don't vault the cornea)
  - Compresses the central cornea that causes stretching of limbal ring
  - Straightens the corneo-scleral angle with partial rotation of iris and ciliary body
  - Aqueous forced out of the angle into the AC

Table 10.7 Comparison of Goldmann Single-Mirror and Three-Mirror versus Zeiss Four-Mirror

Type of Lens	Goldmann Single-Mirror	Goldmann Three-Mirror	Zeiss Four-Mirror
Diameter of corneal contact (mm)	12	12	9
Overall diameter (mm)	15	18	9
Size of rim (mm)	1.5	3	None
Mirror angulation (°)	62	59	64
Mirror height (mm)	17	12	12
Distance from central cornea (mm)	3	7	5
Coupling fluid	Required	Required	Not required
Dynamic gonioscopy	Manipulation	Manipulation	Indentation

Table 10.8 Advantages and Disadvantages of Four-Mirror Gonioscope

Advantages	Disadvantages
No gonio solution	Requires excellent manual dexterity
Good for screening	More awareness of lens
Easy to implement	Corneal folds causing clinical practice distortion
Indentation gonioscopy possible	Difficult to see over bowed iris
Unstable view	

Table 10.9 Advantages versus Disadvantages of Indirect Gonioscope

Advantages	Disadvantages
1. Focal lines for localization of Schwalbe's line	Poor lateral view
2. Magnified view	Patient discomfort
3. Excellent for small details	Difficult for repeated examination
4. Use of laser treatment	Small field of view
5. Easy to implement in clinic	Reversed view

- Iris is pushed posteriorly
- Can open up an appositionally closed angle
- Therefore, helps differentiate appositional and synechial angle closure
- Indications:
  - Suspected cases of intermittent angle closure
  - To view the trabeculum in eyes without much pigmentation
  - Idea about the iris insertion
  - Synechial closure
  - Therapeutic modality to relieve an acute attack of acute angle closure glaucoma
- Manipulation gonioscopy:
  - "Over the hill" view or "dive bombers" view

- Patient looks in the direction of mirror
- Mirror is tilted toward angle to be viewed
- Therefore, helps view above a convex iris configuration

What is the normal gonioscopic anatomy?

- Cornea
  - Schwalbe's line: The anterior termination of the trabecular meshwork, junction between anterior chamber angle structures and the cornea. Noted as SL. To visualize, use a thin slit beam at a slightly oblique angle, this line can be identified by the corneal wedge noted using by "light wedge" formed at the junction between the inner

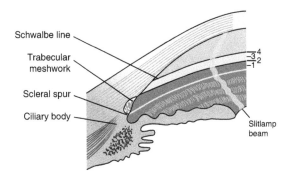

Figure 10.16 Normal gonioscopic anatomy

light beam along the cornea endothelium and the outer light beam along the corneo-scleral junction.

- Prominent Schwalbe's line is called posterior embryotoxon; it can be normal variation but can also be seen as a component of Axenfeld–Rieger anomaly.
- Increased pigmentation is seen in pigmentary glaucoma and PEX along Schwalbe's line, known as Sampaolesi's line.
- Trabecular meshwork (TM): Consists of anterior (between Schwalbe's line and anterior edge of the Schlemm's canal) and posterior part or functional TM (remainder of the meshwork, especially the part adjacent to Schlemm's canal), noted as anterior TM (ATM) and posterior TM (PTM), respectively.
  - Pigmentation: Common in inferior and nasal angle
- Scleral spur: Posterior lip of scleral sulcus. Noted as SS.
  - Seen as prominent white line between ciliary body band and functional TM
  - Most definite landmark of the angle, usually denoted angle being open.
- Ciliary body band: Portion of the ciliary body visible in the anterior chamber as a result of iris insertion into ciliary body. Noted as CBB. Usually noted as a gray or dark brown band.
  - Wide CBB: Myopia, aphakia, angle recession, cyclodialysis
  - Narrow CBB: Hyperopia, anterior iris insertion
- Iris: Noted at the beginning of the gonioscopy process, to check for pupillary edge, contour

of iris, site of insertion and angulation between iris insertion and the slope of the inner cornea.

- Convex: Hyperopia, pupillary block
- Concave: Pigment dispersion syndrome
- Sine wave configuration: Plateau iris syndrome (it is type of primary angle-closure glaucoma caused by a large or anteriorly positioned ciliary body)

What are the abnormal gonioscopic findings in the angle?

- Peripheral anterior synechiae versus iris processes:
  - ACG: Broad synechiae at all levels
  - Uveitis: tented synechiae
  - Neovascular: Broad synechiae, full width, new vessel
  - ICE syndrome: Synechiae onto the peripheral cornea
  - After ALT: Small synechiae, irregular, up to posterior trabeculum
- Increased trabecular meshwork pigment:
  - Uveitis
  - ACG
  - Pigmentary glaucoma
  - Pseudoexfoliation
  - Tumors
- Normal versus new vessels in the angle:
  - New vessels: Finer, lacy, bridge across the trabecular meshwork
  - Normal vasculature: Circular, broader, do not bleed on gonioscopy
- Poor view of scleral spur:
  - Narrow angle
  - Synechiae
  - Inflammatory exudates
- Prominent spur:
  - Cyclodialysis
  - Angle recession
- Blood in Schlemm's canal:
  - External pressure from gonioscopy
  - Increased episcleral venous pressure
  - Thyroid eye disease
  - Carotid cavernous fistula
  - Sturge–Weber syndrome
  - Low IOP
- Widened ciliary body band:
  - Angle recession
  - Cyclodialysis

Mention some common errors during gonioscopy?

- Peripheral anterior synechiae versus iris processes
- New vessels versus true vessels
- Misinterpretation of pseudo angle versus true angle
- Convex iris obscuring the angle:
  - Ask patient to look in direction of mirror.
  - Avoid indenting the peripheral cornea.
  - Do not tilt the gonio mirror.
- Iris surface flat: Poor view of the angle:
  - Ask patient to look away from the mirror.
- Differentiating pseudo from true angle:
  - Cut parallelopiped.
  - Note where parallelopiped loses its three-dimensionality.
  - Indentation of peripheral cornea.

What are the methods of angle assessment?

- Slit lamp
  - Van Herrick (Table 10.10):

Table 10.10 Grading Van Herrick

Grade	Relation between Corneal Slit Image and Anterior Chamber Depth	Interpretation
4	1: 1 or higher	Angle closure very unlikely Chamber angle approx. 35–45°
3	1/2	Angle closure unlikely Chamber angle approx. 20–35°
2	1/4	Angle closure possible Chamber angle approx. 20°
1	1:<1/4	Angle closure likely Chamber angle approx. 10°
0	Closed	Angle closure Chamber angle approx. 0°

- A narrow-slit beam is placed perpendicular to the most peripheral part of the cornea.
- The oculars are adjusted to give a view at an angle of about 60° from the light beam.
- The depth of the anterior chamber is graded in comparison to the thickness of the cornea.
- Smith system (Table 10.11):

Table 10.11 Smith Grading

Grade	Angle Width	Description	Risk of Closure
4	45–35°	Wide open	Impossible
3	35–20°	Wide open	Impossible
2	20°	Narrow	Possible
1	<10°	Extremely narrow	Probable
Slit	Slit	Narrowed to slit	Probable
0	0°	Closed	Closed

- Beam of 1.5 mm is horizontally cast on the cornea
- Procedure involves focusing a slit beam on the corneal surface with the out of focus image of slit beam on iris and lens
- Length of the slit beam when the two are just touching
- Gonioscopy: Grading of the angle is done as follows:

Table 10.12 Scheie Grading

Grade	Structures Seen	Risk of Angle Closure
0	CBB seen	No angle closure
1	CBB narrow	No angle closure
2	CBB not seen, SS seen	Rarely closure possible
3	Post TM not seen	Closure likely
4	Schwalbe's line not seen	Gonioscopically closed

- Scheie system (Table 10.12): On the amount of angle structure visible.
  - Hence, Scheie's grade IV denotes a closed angle; on the Shaffer scale, grade 4 refers to a wide-open angle.
- Shaffer system (Table 10.13):

Table 10.13 Grading Shaffer

Grade	Angle Width	Description	Risk of Closure
4	45–35°	Wide open	Impossible
3	35–20°	Wide open	Impossible
2	20°	Narrow	Possible
1	<10°	Extremely narrow	Probable
Slit	Slit	Narrowed to slit	Probable
0	0°	Closed	Closed

- On the angle created by peripheral iris and corneo-scleral wall.
- This system describes the degree to which the angle is open rather than the degree to which it is closed.
- Whereas Scheie's grade IV denotes a closed angle; on the Shaffer scale, grade 4 refers to a wide-open angle.
- Spaeth system: Grades the three of the angle's anatomy:
  - The level of iris insertion
  - The width of the angle
  - Configuration of the iris
- Grading per Spaeth system
- Iris configuration:
  - q: Queer (concave peripheral iris)
  - r: Regularly straight iris
  - s: Steeply convex iris
- Angular width: 10°, 20°, 30°, 40°
- Level of iris insertion:
  - A: Anterior to Schwalbe's line
  - B: Just behind Schwalbe's line
  - C: At the scleral spur
  - D: Deep angle CBB seen
  - E: Extremely deep angle
- Iris
  - U: Along angle recess
  - V: Up to trabecular meshwork
  - W: Up to Schwalbe's line

- Pigmentation of posterior trabecular meshwork (12 o'clock)
  - 0: No visible pigmentation
  - 1+: Just perceptible pigmentation
  - 2+: Definite but mild
  - 3+: Moderately dense
  - 4+: Dense black pigmentation
- RPC (Rajendra Prasad Centre grading) system
  - Grade 0: Closed
  - Grade 1: Schwalbe's line
  - Grade 2: Anterior (non-pigmented) TM
  - Grade 3: Posterior pigmented TM
  - Grade 4: Scleral spur
  - Grade 5: Ciliary body band
  - Grade 6: Root of iris
- Other investigations for grading angles
  - Ultrasound biomicroscopy (UBM)
  - Anterior segment OCT (AS-OCT)
  - Corneal topography with Scheimpflug photography
  - Scanning peripheral ACD analyzer
  - Optical biometry: ACD measurements

10.4.3 Other lenses in glaucoma

Identify the following lenses used for iridotomy. Mention their characteristics and uses.

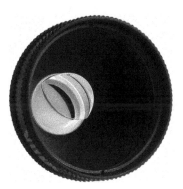

Figure 10.17 Iridotomy lenses

- Abraham lens
  - Contact diameter: 15.5 mm
  - Lens height: 16.5 mm
  - Lens magnification: 1.5 ×
  - Laser spot: 0.67 ×
  - Has a 10 mm diameter 66 D planoconvex magnifying button in the anterior surface

of the lens positioned over the peripheral iris to give a clear view of the iridectomy site.
- The use of the lens increases the laser power at the iris by four times
- Uses:
  - Provides magnification of the target site
  - Increases the power density at the iris and decreases it at the cornea
  - Acts as a heat sink thereby minimizing corneal burns
  - Keeps the lids separate
  - Controls the eye movements
- Other Variants for Iridotomy Lens
- Wise lens: 103 D optical button, at iris reduces size and increases power
- Volk Blumenthal:
  - Newer lens
  - Allows indentation to open up the angle and flatten the peripheral iris
  - Magnification: 1.54×
  - Spot size 0.65×
  - Aspheric lens element provides superior optical quality for sharply focused laser spots

Identify the following lenses used in trabeculo-plasty? Mention their characteristics.

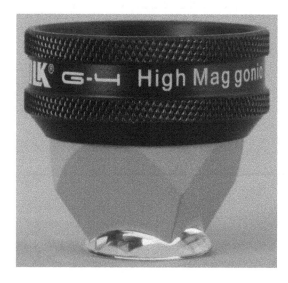

Figure 10.18 Ritch lens

- Four mirrors, two at in 59° and two at 62°
- 17 D planoconvex button in the mirrors
- 1.4× magnification

- Contact diameter: 18 mm
- Lens height: 23 mm
- Latina lens (for SLT): It is made of quartz and has a single mirror at 63° angle with 1× magnification
- Thorpe four-mirror gonioscope: Has four mirrors inclined at 62°

Identify the following lenses used for laser suturelysis.

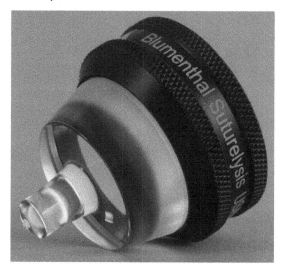

Figure 10.19 Suturelysis lens A

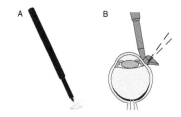

Figure 10.20 Suturelysis lens B

- Hoskins lens: Its 120 D lens causes 1.2× magnification and has flanges
- Other lenses used: Blumenthal lens, Ritch lens, Layden lens, Mandelkorn lens

10.4.4 Optic disc evaluation

What are the factors to be evaluated during optic disc evaluation?

- Disc size
  - It depends on overall size of eyeball and refractive error.

- Normal size 1.5
- Extremely variable. Ranges from 0.96 to 2.91 mm.
- So cup disc ratio varies from 0.1 to 0.5.
- Optic disc size measurement can be done by:
  - Direct ophthalmoscopy
  - Slit lamp with indicator of vertical light beam
- Optic cup:
  - Cup: disc ratio: Variable from 0.1 to 0.9
  - Anything >0.4 is suspicious
  - Shape of the cup: Vertically oval is suspicious
  - Position of the cup: Eccentric is suspicious
  - Lamina cribrosa: Visibility of dots
  - Depth of cup: Deep cup indicates possible glaucoma
  - Asymmetry of cup: Difference of 0.2 is suspicious
- Neuro-retinal rim:
  - ISNT rule (Inferior rim > superior rim > nasal rim > temporal rim)
  - Rim thickness decreased
  - Rim disc ratio is decreased
  - Color changes from pink to pale
- Vascular changes:
  - Nasal shift
  - Bending
  - Baring of vessels
  - Overpass phenomenon
  - Splinter hemorrhages on disc (Drance hemorrhage) characteristic of suspected NTG
- Peripapillary area:
  - Atrophy
  - Alpha zone: Reflects RPE
  - Beta zone: Choroidal atrophy and hence scleral ring is visible, do not confuse with neuro-retinal rim
- Nerve fiber layer
  - Examine in red-free light
  - Seen as slit or wedge-like defect
- To document progression: Handwritten drawing or fundus photograph

What is the differential of a deep cup?

Deep cup differentials to be kept in mind are:
- Physiological
- Myopic fundus

- Compressive lesion on optic nerve or optic chiasma
- Optic pit
- Optic disc coloboma
- Tilted disc
- Morning glory syndrome
- AION
- Methanol alcohol poisoning
- LHON (Leber's hereditary optic neuropathy)
- Radiation neuropathy

10.5 SQUINT AND NEURO-OPHTHALMOLOGY

10.5.1 Definitions

Give the definitions of the following:

- Optic axis (anatomic):
  - Line passing through center of cornea and lens OR
  - Line joining all the Purkinje images
- Pupillary axis: Line perpendicular to cornea center and passing through pupillary center
- Visual axis: Line joining object of fixation to fovea
- Angle kappa: Between visual and pupillary axis, subtended at anterior nodal point
- Angle lambda: Between visual and pupillary axis subtended at pupillary entrance
- Angle alpha: Between optical and pupillary axis
- Horopter: Imaginary surface in space, all points on which stimulate corresponding retinal points
- Pannum's area: Imaginary volume in space surrounding horopter, where objects are seen single though they may stimulate non-corresponding retinal points
- Strabismus or squint: An ocular condition in which the visual axes of the two eyes do not meet at the point of regard (misalignment of the visual axes), or alignment occurs only if the subject is using compensatory mechanism (fusion, etc.) beyond the normal physiological limits

How do you evaluate a patient for strabismus?

- Patient presents because of:
  - Manifest strabismus
  - Deficient ocular movement

- Nystagmus
- Compensatory head posture
- Defective vision
- Subjective symptoms
- History taking:
  - General:
    - H/o trauma
    - H/o previous illnesses
    - H/o treatment taken (glasses, patching, surgery)
    - H/o drugs (alcohol: Wernicke's; smoking: paraneoplastic syndrome)
    - H/o associated features: Variability, neurological features, weight gain, weight loss
  - Squint:
    - What is the problem?
    - Why has the patient come to your chair?
    - Direction of squint/limitation of movement
    - Which eye squints; if it is unilateral (diagnostic amblyopia)
    - Age at which it was noticed (indicates level of development)
    - Onset
    - Duration
    - Constant/intermittent (gives fusional potential)
    - Has it worsened/improved
    - Head posture
    - Whether for near/far
    - Eye closed or not
    - Any nystagmus
    - H/o diplopia
  - Specific history in children:
    - Obstetric history (child's birth weight, gestational age, mother's health during pregnancy and neonatal history of resuscitation)
    - Milestones
    - Recent illness
    - Trauma
  - Examination:
    - General:
      - Children:
      - Hydrocephalus
      - Microcephalus
      - Albinism
      - Down's syndrome
      - Cerebral palsy
      - Craniofacial anomalies
      - Adults:
      - Seventh-nerve palsy
      - Tremor
      - Ataxia
      - Deafness
      - Thyroid Disease
    - Facial appearance:
      - Epicanthus
      - Telecanthus
      - Facial asymmetry
      - Loss of facial expression
      - Vertical gaze palsy
      - Steel Richardson syndrome
      - Enophthalmos
      - Ptosis
    - Head posture:
      - Chin up: Bilateral ptosis, Brown's syndrome
      - Chin down: B/L superior oblique (SO) palsy
      - Head tilt/turn:
      - Paretic squint:
      - If sixth nerve is involved, toward the direction of paralyzed muscle
      - Unilateral SO palsy: Chin down, contralateral head tilt with ipsilateral head turn
      - Restrictive squint:
      - DRS 1: Ipsilateral face turn
      - DRS 2: Contralateral head turn
    - Others:
      - Nystagmus
      - Torticollis
      - Unilateral deafness
      - Habit
- Squint examination (summary):
  - Sensory tests
  - Motor tests
  - Tests related to visual acuity
  - Tests related to extraocular muscle movements (EOMs)
  - Special tests for nystagmus

10.5.2 Squint evaluation sequence

What is the sequence for strabismus examination?

Strabismus or squint evaluation involves detailed tests beyond a routine comprehensive eye examination, which is must in all cases. The following sequence is a systematic approach, though neither exhaustive nor absolute, as there are many ways to approach such patients.

- I] Sensory tests for squint
  - Observe
  - Visual acuity
  - Cover test
  - Synoptophore
  - Stereopsis
  - Fusion
  - Retinal correspondence
  - Suppression
  - Four-prism test
  - Near point of convergence
  - Near point of accommodation
- II] Motor tests for squint
  - Cover
  - Hirschberg test
  - Krimsky's test
  - Prism cover
  - Cover-uncover test
  - Alternate Cover test
  - Synoptophore
  - Maddox wing
  - Maddox rod test
  - Double Maddox rod test
- III] Other related tests to visual acuity:
  - Contrast sensitivity
  - Visually evoked potential (VEP)
  - Electroretinaogram (ERG)
- IV] Movement-related tests for squint
  - Eye movement related
    - Duction
    - Version
    - Vergences
    - Diplopia evaluation
    - Hess chart
    - Lee chart
  - Special tests for eye movements
    - Parks three-step test
    - Forced duction test (FDT)
    - Force generation test (FGT)
    - Electrooculogram (EOG)
    - Electromyography (EMG)
    - Saccades
    - Smooth pursuit movements
    - Vestibulo-ocular movements
    - Optokinetic movements

- I} Sensory examination:
  - I} A] Observe:
    - General:
      - Head posture
      - Squint
      - Nystagmus
      - Epicanthus/telecanthus
      - Palpebral aperture asymmetry (ptosis/retraction)
      - Pen light/corneal reflex related tests
    - Evaluation of angle kappa:
      - Target torch light distance 33 cm and observe corneal reflection: If fovea is temporal to pupillary axis, corneal light reflection will be nasal to center of cornea. This is positive-angle kappa.
      - If fovea is nasal to pupillary axis, corneal light reflection will be temporal to center of cornea. This is negative-angle kappa.
      - Large-angle kappa: Pseudoexotropia, ROP with temporal dragging of macula.
      - Large-angle kappa: Pseudoesotropia.
      - Bruckner's light reflex test: Used in small infants.
        - Eye where brighter the glow from direct ophthalmoscope, it is more deviated/amblyopic eye.
  - I} B] Visual acuity:
    - Distance: 6 m (far), 33 cm (near)
    - Uniocular/binocular
    - With correction
    - a) In small children: (<1 year)
      - Assessment of fixation
        - Aim: Ability to fix target
        - Steadiness and persistence of fixation
        - Target: Toy/light
        - Note:
          - Position of corneal reflection
          - Manifest strabismus: Unilateral/alternating
          - Speed of fixation
          - Reaction of occlusion
          - Ability to pick up small objects
          - Distance: 33 cm
          - Use hundreds and thousands Sweet test

- Result: Location and attempt to pick up when vision ≥6/24
- Forced preferential looking (FPL) test:
  - Teller's acuity cards (TAC)
  - Distance: 38 cm, 55 cm, 84 cm
  - Method: Binocularly first followed by uniocular.
  - Correlation between TAC and Snellen's acuity is at present unreliable

- b) In children >2 years of age
  - Quantitative tests
    - Distance: 6 m
    - Test used:
      - Snellen's
      - Sheriden–Gardiner singles matching card
      - Kay's picture
      - Mentor BVAT (Baylor Video Acuity Tester)
      - Refraction: Manifest cycloplegia, fogging

- I} C] Cover tests
  - Cover test: Should be performed at a distance of 6 m and 33 cm
  - Target: Depends on age and vision
  - For distance: Snellen's, spot light, remote control toy
  - For near: Spot light, small toy, fixational stitch with letters (to stimulate and control accommodation)
  - Occluder: Opaque, frosted, or hand especially in a child
  - Patient should wear full refractive correction
  - Cover-uncover test:
    - Aim: Detection of manifest deviation (heterotropia)
    - Method: Patient fixes on required target
    - One eye is occluded—uncovered eye observed as the cover is placed over fellow eye
    - Results:
      - If no movement of uncovered eye to take up fixation, then patient was fixing with fovea.
      - Any movement of uncovered eye to take up fixation indicates a manifest deviation of that eye.

- Test repeated making same observation while covering the other eye.
- Watch only uncovered eye as the cover is being placed in front of the other eye.
- If neither eye has moved to take up fixation, then the patient is bifoveally fixing. A latent deviation should then be looked for.
- Recording

Cover Test (CT)	For Near (N)	For Distance (D)	Fixation
With glasses	Orthotropia	Constant Right ET	Not holding fixation
		Right/alt ET	Can hold fixation Right

- Alternate cover test (cross cover test)
  - Aim: Diagnose latent deviation
  - Patient fixes on latent target
  - Method:
  - Occluder transferred from one eye to the other without any interval and examiner watches the eye that is behind the cover as the occluder is being transferred to the other eye
  - Longer occluder is left over one eye—more disruptive is the fusion revealing full extent of squint
  - Recording:

Cover uncover test	For near (N)	For distance (D)
Using glasses	Small exophoria	Moderate exophoria with poor recovery

- Information provided by cover test:
- Direction of deviation
- Difference in angle from (N) to (D) fixation
- Effect of accommodation and of patient refractive error
- Concomitance or incomitance in primary position compared to in all positions of gaze and deviation fixing with either eye

- Other characteristics of manifest strabismus
  - Constant or intermittent
  - Unilateral or alternating
  - Estimation of VA in a constantly squinting eye by a study of fixation.
- Speed of recovery in latent strabismus is an indication of fusion amplitude.
- Presence of latent or manifest latent nystagmus
- Recording:
  - Type of deviation
  - Estimation of its size
  - Whether manifest squint is constant or intermittent—which eye deviates
  - Speed of recovery
  - Any special feature, e.g., DVD
- I} D] Synoptophore: (see details in "Instrument" chapter 9)
  - Uses:
    - To check grade of binocular vision:
      - Simultaneous macular perception (SMP)
      - Fusion
      - Stereopsis (There are simultaneous paramacular, macular and foveal perception slides)
    - Measure of angle of deviation in all 9 gazes:
      - a. Objective
      - b. Subjective
      - c. Normal retinal correspondence: If objective = subjective
      - d. Abnormal retinal correspondence: If objective > subjective
        - Difference between objective and subjective = Angle of anomaly
        - If angle of anomaly = Objective; it is a harmonious ARC
        - If angle of anomaly < Objective; it is a non-harmonious ARC
        - Bielschowsky's after-image test slides are used to diagnose ARC
    - Range of suppression scotoma
    - Measurement of angle kappa (angle between optic axis and visual axis, rarely exceeds 5–7 degrees)
      - + = When visual axis cuts nasal to optic axis
      - – = Opposite

- For these slides number, alphabets (43210 ABCDE), animal pictures are put.
- When patient looks at the light, examiner looks at the corneal reflections
- Measurement of IPD
- Range of fusion or version
- To measure convergence, tubes are moved toward each other. Fusion breaks when diplopia is present.
  - Arms are moved back so that fusion is regained.
  - Similarly, range of divergence is estimated.
  - To check the amplitude for near, –3 D lens is placed before each eye.
  - Similarly vertical and torsional range of fusion estimated.
- I} E] Stereoacuity: (see details in "Instruments chapter 9"):
- I} F] Fusion:

Table 10.14 Normal Fusional Amplitudes

Distance	Convergence	Divergence	Vertical
6 m	14 PD	6 PD	2.5 PD
25 cm	38 PD	16 PD	2.6 PD

- Stereopsis can indicate fusion and therefore BSV
- Worth's four-dot test
  - Aim: To diagnose fusion and dominance of eye
  - Distance: 6 m, 33 cm
  - Method: Patient wears red/green glasses and is asked how many lights he sees at 6 m and 33 cm
  - Very dissociative test
  - Responses:
    - i. Four lights: one red, two green, one pink or green depending on dominant eye: Indicates bifoveal or peripheral fusion
    - ii. Five lights: two red, three green: Indicates diplopia: may be crossed (heteronymous) or uncrossed (homonymous)

- iii. Two lights or three lights: Suppression of one eye
- There may be alternation between two or three lights indicating alternating suppression.
- Dissociating tests Suppressing patient may sometimes give diplopia response because of disruption or suppression or dissociation caused by red/green glasses.
- Test recorded as fusion, diplopia or suppression and distance tested.
- At distance: four dots cover 1.25° area
- At near: four dots cover 6° area (which will cover tiny foveal scotoma)
- Fusional amplitudes (Table 10.14):
- Can be assessed using
  - Synoptophore
  - Prisms in free space
  - Prisms in free space:
    - Using prisms bar or rotation prism: Can be used in combination with Worth's four-dot test
    - Endpoint: Diplopia
    - Distance: 6 m, 33 cm
    - Fixation target: Gradually increasing strength of prisms until diplopia is experienced subjectively or watch for break in either eye (objectively)
    - Use: "Base out" followed by "base in," then "base up," and finally "base down"
    - If manifest squint present: Correct deviation
    - Then, assess amplitudes using additional prisms
- I} G] Retinal correspondence (see details in "Chapter 9 – strabismus and orthoptics" chapter):
  - After-image test—synoptophore
  - Bagolini's glasses Least dissociative test
  - Test of foveal to extra-foveal—correspondence in cases of strabismus by providing images that fall on the fovea of the fixing eye and on foveal area of the deviating eye
- I} H] Suppression:
  - Synoptophore

- Worth's four-dot test
- Bagolini's glasses
- Four-prism test
- Red filter ladder test:
  - Detects degree of depth of suppression
  - Filters of increasing density kept over seeing eye till its image is degraded to such an extent that it allows the suppressed image in strabismic eye to be perceptible and the patient c/o diplopia.
- I} I] 4 D prism test:
  - Aim: Confirm presence of mono-fixation syndrome
  - Method: Patient fixes on a penlight or small target for distance. A 4 D base out prism is introduced from temporal side in front of the eye suspected of having foveal suppression.
  - Results:
    - Positive test: Indicative of foveal suppression shows no movement of the fellow eye.
    - If there is bifoveal fusion and no suppression, the fellow eye makes a small corrective movement.
- I} J] Near point of convergence:
  - Method: Objects moved toward the patient in the midline from about 50 cm away.
  - Apparatus: Interesting object, RAF rule.
  - Results: When near point of convergence has been reached and fusion is lost, one eye will diverge. Patient may or may not indicate when object appears double. If they suppress, it may indicate a longstanding convergence problem.
  - Recording:
    - Convergence to nose or left eye breaks at 10 cm c/s diplopia
    - Normal: 8–10 cm or less
- I} K] Near point of accommodation:
  - Apparatus: RAF (Royal Air Force) ruler
  - Method: Tested binocular and uniocular

- Appropriate optical correction for distance
- Reading target that patient can see clearly at the end of the rule is moved toward the fixing eye until the patient first notices that the print is blurred.
- Special tests:
  - Contrast sensitivity
  - VEP
  - ERG
- II] Motor examinations:
  - II] A} Cover tests (covered previously)
  - II] B} Hirschberg's test (corneal reflections test)
    - Distance: Near fixation
    - Method:
      - Spotlight held in front of the patient at 33 cm from his eyes
      - Examiner must be directly behind the light
      - Position of light's reflection on each cornea checked
      - 1 mm displacement = 7° of strabismus
    - Pitfall: Slight displacement from the center nasally (+ angle kappa) or temporally (– angle kappa) may occur giving the impression of a strabismus when in fact the eyes are correctly aligned, as test is for near only
    - Use: Rough estimate of angle of deviation
  - II] C} Krimsky's test (prism reflex test)
    - Carried out in the same way as Hirschberg
    - Prisms are used to move the corneal reflection in the deviating eye to a position similar to that of the fixing eye
    - Apex of prism in direction of squint
    - Right esotropia = Base out prism right eye
    - Modified Krimsky:
      - If squinting eye is densely amblyopic or blind—prism placed in front of fixing eye until corneal deviation in the deviating eye becomes central.
      - Modified Krimsky cannot be done if squinting eye has resistance of movement.

- Disadvantages:
  - Krimsky underestimates in deviation >15 PD (in comparison to PBCT).
  - It measures only near deviation.
  - Uncontrolled accommodation and wrong interpretation in presence of angle kappa.
- II] D} Prism cover test:
  - Method of measuring angle of deviation
  - Measures horizontal, vertical deviation—latent, manifest, and combined manifest and latent deviation at any distance, with either eye fixing, in any gaze position
- II] E} Prism cover-uncover test:
  - Measures manifest squint
  - Prism placed before deviating eye at the same time as the fixating eye is covered
  - End-point: No movement of squinting eye
  - Simultaneous prism introduction and cover test (prism cover-uncover test):
    - Measures the manifest strabismus only
    - Prism should be placed before the deviating eye at the same time as the fixing eye is covered—allows the measurement of the deviation with the minimum of dissociation
  - Essential to do this part of the test before doing the prism and cross-cover test in the monofixation syndrome and accommodative esotropia
- II] F} Prism and cover-cross-cover test (alternating cover test):
  - Measures manifest and latent component of squint as well as total deviation.
  - Distance: Near and distance
  - Target: Toy/Snellen/Torchlight
  - Method: Patient fixes on chosen target
    - Prism placed in front of deviating eye
    - Fixing eye covered and eye behind the prism is watched to see if it makes any movement to take up fixation
    - Strength adjusted until no movement is detected, or just a flick movement in opposite direction
    - Apex of prism in the same direction as the squinting eye is pointing
    - Right esotropia—base out right eye

- Prerequisites and cautions:
  - Central steady fixation
  - Vision—enough to see the target
  - EOM—normal, no restriction or limitation
  - Cooperative patient
  - Target—to control accommodation
  - Position of prism held
  - Do not stack prism
  - Both eyes should not be uncovered at the same time till deviation is neutralized
  - High refractive errors in spectacles can induce prism and measurements in PBCT in positive lenses decreases and negative lenses increases the deviation measured on PBCT, especially if lenses > ±5 D
- Advantages:
  - Measures total angle of deviation
  - Most accurate and widely used
- II] G} Synoptophore (covered previously)
- II] F} Maddox Rod:
  - Principle: Dissociation of vision in two eyes
  - Uses:
    - Measures deviation in combination with prism at any distance or in any direction of gaze
    - Commonly used for diagnosis of phoria for far
  - Method:
    - Patient fixes a small light and rod is placed in front of the deviating eye.
    - Grooves are placed horizontally to measure horizontal deviation. Patient sees vertical line. Two eyes see dissimilar images and are dissociated, allowing muscle imbalance to become manifest.
  - Instrument: Made of multiple cylindrical lenses
    - Red in colour and hence white light appears as red line
    - Vertically placed grooves—horizontal line for vertical deviation
  - Test only measures deviation present—does not differentiates heterotropias and heterophorias

- II] I} Maddox wing:
  - Aim: Diagnose and measure heterophorias at near
  - Measures deviation (tropias) only
  - Cannot differentiate between heterophorias and heterotropias
  - Principle: Dissociation of vision in two eyes: Right eye sees arrows, left eyes sees scales
  - Three scales: Horizontal, vertical, and torsional
  - Method:
    - Patient asked to indicate the position of the vertical arrow on the horizontal scale to record the horizontal deviation.
    - Position of horizontal arrow on the vertical scale to measure vertical deviation.
    - Torsion: Indicated if the horizontal arrow is not parallel to the horizontal measurement scale. The arrow adjusted until patient sees it parallel.
  - On the horizontal scales:
    - Even number—exophoria
    - Odd number—esophoria
  - On the vertical scales:
    - Even number—left hypertropia
    - Odd number—right hypertropia
  - Red arrow:
    - Tilted superiorly—incyclophoria
    - Tilted inferiorly—excyclophoria
    - 1 line = 2° incyclophoria
- II] I} Double Maddox rod:
  - Used to detect and measure torsion
  - Requisites: Two differently coloured Maddox rod (red and white) preferable with good and near equal vision in each eye
  - Method: Maddox rod with grooves placed vertically to form a pair of horizontal lines when patient looks at spotlight
  - Distance—near and far
  - Patient asked if lines are parallel or not
    - If parallel—no torsion
    - If either one or both lines appear tilted—torsion present
    - Patient asked to adjust position of rods until lines appear parallel

- Results: Amount of axis change read off scales
  - If lines are tilted toward nose—excyclotorsion
  - >10° excyclodeviation—bilateral SO paresis
  - <10° excyclodeviation—unilateral SO paresis
- III] Other tests
  - Prisms:
    - Light reflex displacement in degrees
    - Same principles and quantitative measurement of the area over which a patient can maintain binocular fixation with the head held still
  - Perimeter used:
    - Maintains fixation on the target as it moves from the center to the periphery—until diplopia is appreciated
    - If diplopia present straight ahead—target is moved to an area where the patient can fix binocularly
  - Hess or Lee chart:
    - Test for paresis:
    - Comparing the deviation of fixing either eye in primary and secondary deviations. If paretic element suspected—do PCT with fixing right and fixing left.
    - Deviation fixing with eye (secondary deviation) will be greater than that fixing with the unaffected eye (primary deviation).
  - Neutral density filters:
    - Differential between organic and strabismic amblyopia. Visual acuity in cases of organic amblyopia is reduced by diminishing the illumination with a neutral density filter, whereas the visual acuity in an eye with strabismic amblyopia remains relatively unchanged.
    - Not useful in cases of anisometropia amblyopia because there is a depression of sensitivity throughout the visual field and not mainly at the macula, as in cases of strabismic amblyopia.

- IV] Ocular movements:
  - Versions: Done in each diagnostic gaze positions (binocular)
  - Ductions: Checked to determine if there is any weakness of a muscle or restrictive Syndrome (uniocular)

Mention special points in examination for Vertical strabismus and incomitant strabismus.

- History: Including assessment of diplopia: Monocular/binocular
- Assessment of any head posture
- Look for:
  - a) In case of vertical squint: (in addition to usual tests):
    - DVD
    - Nystagmus
    - IOOA
    - SOUA/SOOA
    - A or V patterns
  - b) In case of constant ET/XT:
    - DVD
    - IOOA
    - Nystagmus
    - A/V pattern
    - Cross fixation in ET
  - c) In case of accomodative esotropia:
    - Use accommodative target: Use a reading chart
    - In case of toy: Concentrate on fine details like nose
    - Cycloplegic refraction must
  - d) In case of intermittent exotropia (IXT):
    - Stereoacuity for distance and near
    - Control and recovery of squint
    - A and V phenomenon
    - Lateral gaze incomitance
  - e) In case of paralytic squint:
    - Head posture
    - Deviation more when fixing with paretic eye
    - DVD
    - IOOA
    - Nystagmus
    - A/V pattern
    - Park's three- step test: To detect single cyclovertical muscle paresis
    - It does not hold true in: More than one cyclovertical muscle paresis
      - Restrictive squint
      - DVD

- Myasthenia
- Previous surgery on vertical recti
- Skew Deviation
- Test:
  - 1.) Which eye is hyper in primary?
  - 2.) Which horizontal gaze vertical deviation is more?
  - 3.) Which head tilt vertical deviation is more?
- Torsion:
  - Bagolini glass test
  - Double Maddox rod
  - Rotation of optic disc and fovea
- Forced duction test: (FDT)
  - Aim: To differentiate between paresis and restriction
  - Anesthesia:
    - General: Below age of 7 years (avoid succinyl choline)
    - Topical: Above age of 7 years
  - Technique:
    - Hold the eye to be tested with fixation forceps at the limbus. Do not push or pull the globe.
    - Patch the other eye or use for fixation.
    - Patient is asked to look in direction innervational of gaze limitation to eliminate inn. Flow to antagonist muscle.
    - Rotate the globe with the forceps at limbus further than the patient can using his maximal innervation in that gaze.
  - Interpretation:
    - Absolute restriction: Browns, TRO
    - Progressive restriction: Muscle scarring
    - Leash and reverse leash phenomenon: If the muscle after feel of "tether" on the stabilizing forceps gives a brisk, normal velocity, saccadic movement in either direction
    - If globe is fully rotated: no paresis
    - If globe cannot be rotated further than voluntary gaze: restrictive
    - If in between: Combined
  - Indications:
    - Suspected restrictive squint
    - Blow out fracture orbit

- DRS
- Brown
- Strabismus fixus
- Mobius
- TRO
- Postoperative following scleral buckle, squint, transposition procedure, glaucoma implant.
- Long-standing deviation with secondary muscle contracture
- Intraoperative FDT should be done:
  - Before and after peritomy
  - Before and after muscle disinsertion/reinsertion
  - Before and after recession
  - Before and after resection
- Disadvantages:
  - Patient may squeeze and tighten the muscle
  - Doing the test if globe is pushed back: false negative
  - Doing the test if globe is pulled out: false positive
  - Contracture may release after FDT
  - Posterior restrictions may not be detected
  - Conjunctival hemorrhage/tear may occur
- Exaggerated FDT:
  - In this the globe is retracted to exaggerate the restriction of the obliques
  - a) Inferior oblique traction test:
    - The limbus is held at inferotemporal and superior nasal quadrant positions.
    - The globe is pushed back into orbit in full adduction position maintaining intorsion of the globe.
    - Then globe is brought temporally while continuing to push it backwards
    - If inferior oblique normal or taut: the globe is seen to "pop up" and a click is felt.
    - If inferior oblique lax or weak: above response absent.
    - If test positive after muscle weakening procedure: insufficient weakening.
  - b) Superior oblique traction test:
    - Limbus is held in the superotemporal and inferonasal quadrant position.

- The globe is pushed back into orbit in full adduction, maintaining full extorsion of the globe.
- The globe is then brought temporally while continuing to push it backwards.
- If superior oblique normal or taut: the globe is seen to "pop up" and a click is felt.
- If test positive after muscle weakening procedure: insufficient weakening.
- Active force generation test: (AFGT):
  - Aim: To detect muscle action in presence of restriction, i.e., whether underaction because of restrictive element or combined restriction + paresis
  - Technique:
    - Patient is asked to look into opposite direction to relax the muscle to be assessed.
    - Globe is held with the forceps and examiner assess the tension.
    - Now the patient is asked to look in the direction of the paretic muscle and examiner feels the tug. This tug can be quantified by Scott forceps of muscle transducer.
  - Interpretation of AFGT with Scott forceps:
    - Normal: 60–80 grams
    - Paresis: 30–80 gm
    - Paralytic: < 5 gm
  - Uses of AFGT:
    - Helpful in surgical planning
    - a) In case of complete paralysis/muscle transposition
    - b) Moderate to good force present—resection/recession procedure
  - Disadvantages:
    - Need awake and co-operative patient
    - Muscle to be free from anesthesia effect
    - Can be done under topical only
- AC/A ratio:
  - Relationship of accommodation and convergence
  - AC/A ratio is the ratio between accommodative convergence and accommodation. The normal range is between 3–5 PD convergence per diopter of accommodation

- Measurement of AC/A ratio:
- Heterophoria method:
  - It involves changing distance of fixation from distance to near.
  - The IPD is first measured.
  - The patient is made to wear his refractive correction.
  - Deviation is first measured by PBCT by asking patient to fixate at 6 m distance, and then again deviation is measured by asking patient to fixate at 33 cm.
  - Calculation from above previous measurements as follows:
    - AC/A = IPD + (N − D)/P, where
    - IPD is in cm
    - N = Near deviation in prism diopters
    - D = Distance deviation in prism diopters
    - P = Lens power used for testing
- Gradient method:
  - The fixation distance is kept constant, and the spherical lenses are changed to increase or decrease accommodation effort.
  - Done at fixed distance of 6 m with concave lenses or at 33 cm with convex lenses.
  - Patient made to wear his correction and deviation is measured for distance (= D).
  - Deviation is again measured after giving him −3 D concave lens and asked to fix on same accommodative target at 6 m (= N).
  - Calculation from above previous measurements as follows:
    - AC/A = N − D/3.
    - If other than -3 D lens is used, then change denominator accordingly.
    - Similarly, this method can be done at 33 cm also using convex lenses.
- Graphic method: Graph is plotted for convergence against different spherical glasses
- Fixation disparity method: Used in experimental settings.
  - Uses of AC/A ratio:
    - To study accommodative esotropia to understand the different types

- To study exodeviations with simulated divergence excess exotropia to be differentiated from true divergence excess exotropia
  - Changes in AC/A ratio: Agents like miotics, convex glasses, prisms, and surgery can artificially change the AC/A ratio.

10.5.3 FAQs on strabismus entities

What is infantile esotropia?

- Definition: Constant esotropia with an onset from birth to 6 months
- Rarely present at birth (therefore congenital esotropia—misnomer)
- Characteristics:
  - Large angle (30 PD or more)
  - Stable angle (initial alternation with crossed fixation)
  - Neurologically normal
  - Asymmetric optokinetic nystagmus
  - Naso-temporal asymmetry indicates onset during infancy
- Associations:
  - Amblyopia
  - Abduction defective
  - Adduction excess
  - IOOA/SOOA
  - Dissociated deviations (vertical or horizontal)
  - A/V pattern
  - Torticollis
  - With best correction: Subnormal vision
- Differential diagnosis:
  - Sixth-nerve palsy:
    - Very rare
    - Check for doll's eye movement
    - Check for duction with one eye patch
  - Nystagmus blockage syndrome:
    - Nystagmus intensity is inversely proportional to ET angle
    - Often overdiagnosed
  - ET with CNS abnormalities: Variable angle and surgical results
  - Refractive accommodative esotropia: Usually late onset, rarely early
  - Sensory esotropia: Check for unilateral visual loss

- DRS type I:
  - Incomitance present
  - Palpebral aperture abnormalities
- Etiology:
  - Delayed maturation/defect in vergence mechanism in patients with initial normal sensorial system including normal stereopsis
- Presurgical evaluation:
  - Check for following
  - Equal visual acuity?
  - Is any hypermetropic refractive error above +2.5 D fully corrected?
  - Is the fundus normal?
  - Is the angle stable?
  - Has Duane syndrome type 1 been ruled out?
  - Are there dysfunctions of the oblique muscles?
  - Are there dissociated vertical OR horizontal deviations?
  - A or V pattern?
  - General health of patient?
- Patient should have:
  - Alternating vision
  - Completed motor analysis
  - Timings of surgery:
    - Very early (3 months)
    - Optimal (6–12 months)
- Disadvantages of very early surgery:
  - Risk of overcorrection
  - Growth of globe size possible
- Advantages of very early surgery: Better binocularity
- Non-surgical management:
  - Botulinum toxin under EMG control:
    - Mechanism: Neutralizes the abnormal dynamics and is the least invasive alternative for surgery
    - Does not change the arc of contact and changes the abnormal motor mechanism
    - Bilateral low dose of botulism in MR muscle: Positive results within 2–3 days
    - Disadvantages:
      - Unstable results
      - Temporary results
      - Need for surgery in later life

- Surgical options:
  - B/L medial rectus recession
    - One can combine with obliques/for residual squint correction, LR resection
    - Need for reopening in 20–50%
  - Results:
  - 1) Cure of squint: Unattainable in 100%, as long-term variability is possible even during later years.
  - Ideal is orthotropia with
    - Normal visual acuity
    - Normal stereopsis
    - Normal sensory and motor fusion
    - Normal retinal correspondence
  - 2) Subnormal binocular vision: Reduced or absent stereopsis
  - 3) Microtropia:
    - Insignificant on cover test
    - Mild amblyopia
    - Parafoveal fixation
    - Reduced stereopsis
    - No further treatment except for amblyopia
      - Stability of alignment may be altered after decades, but usually good
  - 4) Monofixation syndrome:
    - ET <10 PD
    - Harmonious ARC
    - Alternation on amblyopia
    - Fusional amplitudes
    - Stable angle
    - Results depend on:
      - Age of onset
      - Time elapsed between onset and completed surgical correction
      - A good result may deteriorate years after surgery
  - 5) Small-angle esotropia or exotropia: <10 PD
    - Acceptable result
    - No additional correction necessary
    - Cosmetically acceptable

What is Ciancia syndrome?

- Ciancia syndrome:
  - Tight medial rectus holding the eye in adduction
  - Limitation of abduction
  - Face turn toward the fixing eye

- Exaggerated end-point nystagmus occurs on attempted abduction
- Treatment:
  - Maximum—7 mm B/L medial rectus recession

Classify acquired esodeviations.

- Classification of acquired esodeviations: based on . . .
- Comitance:
  - Comitant
  - Incomitant:
    - Paralytic-paretic deviations
    - Non-paralytic:
      - Alphabetic patterns
      - Retraction syndrome of DUANE
- Comitant deviations:
  - Accommodative ET:
    - Refractive accommodative ET (normal AC/A ratio)
    - Non-refractive accommodative ET (high AC/A ratio)
      - Hypoaccommodative ET
      - Partially accommodative ET
- Non-accommodative ET:
  - Infantile:
    - Basic
    - Non-accommodative convergence excess
    - Nystagmus compensation (blockage) syndrome
    - Microtropia
    - Esotropia of myopes
    - Acute ET
    - Recurrent ET
    - Divergence insufficiency or paralysis
    - Secondary ET:
      - Consecutive
      - Sensory
- Accommodative ET:
  - Refractive accommodative ET:
    - Onset typically 2–3 years but may be during infancy
    - ET fully corrected with hypermetropic spectacles
    - Surgery is unnecessary and contraindicated
  - Non-refractive accommodative ET:
    - Unrelated to refractive errors
    - Caused by abnormal near reflex:

- Near deviation > distance deviation due to high AC/A ratio
- Indication for bifocals:
- Small ET or orthophoria at distance
- ET at near eliminated by additional plus lenses
  - Hypoaccommodative ET (Costenbader)
    - May have reduced NPA
    - Accommodative effort elicits hyperconvergence
- Non-accommodative ET
  - Non-accommodative convergence excess
    - Unrelated to refractive error
    - Near deviation > distance deviation but normal AC/A ratio
    - Surgery: Recession MR OU or Faden operation
    - Nystagmus compensation "blockage" syndrome
      - Pseudo-abducens paralysis
      - Nystagmus intensity inversely proportional to ET angle
      - ET increases with increased visual acuity
      - Convergence damping of manifest congenital nystagmus
      - Often misdiagnosed: Infantile ET with nystagmus in abduction
      - Surgery: Recession MR OU combined with Faden operation
  - Microtropia (Lang):
    - Synonym: Monofixation syndrome of Parks
    - Primary and secondary forms
    - ET with negative or inconspicuous cover test
    - Border between microtropia and small-angle ET is poorly defined
    - Mild amblyopia with parafoveal fixation
    - ARC occurs frequently
    - Significance: Explains amblyopia in absence of manifest strabismus or anisometropia
  - Esotropia in high myopia:
    - Non-specific: May need "sutureless" muscle surgery
    - Slowly progressive large-angle ET: Consider orbital restriction
  - Recurrent ET: Definition: Return to original angle after multiple surgery

What is dissociated vertical deviation (DVD)?

- Dissociated vertical deviation (dissociated strabismus complex) (DVD)
  - This is a sensory anomaly characterized by elevation, excyclotorsion and lateral movement of the eye under cover.
  - Characteristics:
    - Violates Herring's law
    - Does not cause diplopia (due to poor fusion and suppression)
    - DVD can be either phoria or tropia
    - Usually bilateral, asymmetric, and more profound in non-dominant eye
    - Most commonly associated with ET
    - Usually associated with ET, IXT, and latent nystagmus
    - May be associated with head posture. Head tilt on opposite side indicates poor control or large magnitude DVD
  - Problems with DVD:
    - Longstanding DVD leads to SR contracture and true hypertropia
    - Amblyopia
    - Cosmetic
    - Difficult to measure vertical deviation
  - Classification:
    - A) Types:
    - Comitant: when vertical deviation measures same in abduction, primary gaze, and adduction
    - Incomitant: DVD is incomitant when there is difference in magnitude in these three positions
    - B) Severity:
    - Mild: 0–9 PD
    - Moderate: 10–19 PD
    - Severe: 20 PD (±7 PD)
  - Evaluation:
  - Measurement of deviation:
    - PBUCT: Keep increasing base down prism in front of deviated eye till no movement is seen on alternate cover
    - Hirschberg's: Gives gross estimate
    - Bielschowsky's phenomenon:
    - Present in 50% DVD
    - Decrease in intensity of light in the fixing eye: Dissociated eye gradually comes down
    - Impression: Gives measures of the depth of DVD

- Red glass test: Red glass in front of either of the eye. Red light is always perceived below white light. This is important to differentiate DVD from hypertropia.
- In hypertropia, red light is perceived below or above white light depending on whether kept in front of hypertropic/hypotropic eye.
- DVD can coexist with IOOA (Table 10.15).

Table 10.15 DVD Comparison with Inferior Oblique Overaction

	DVD	IOOA
Elevation present in	Abduction, adduction primary position	Only adduction
SOOA	Maybe (+/−)	Never
V pattern	−	+
Contralateral SR pseudoparalysis	−	+
Bielschowky's phenomenon	+	−
Red Glass test	Always below white	Can be above or below white
Saccadic velocity of refixation	Slow 10–200°/sec	Fast 200–400°/sec

- Rapid refixation movement of hypotropic eye can be measure with PBCT. Then total upward deviation may be measured using PBUCT.
- Management:
  - Conservative:
    - a) Observation
    - b) Correction of refractive error (image blur, so it breaks fusion and worsens DVD)
    - c) Correction of amblyopia
    - d) Correction of squint by: Prism/surgery (improves peripheral fusion)
    - e) Switching fixation to non-dominant eye
  - Surgical management:
    - In 90% of patients, surgical correction of horizontal deviation will correct DVD

- Bilateral surgeries are usually required
- Indications:
  - Increase in frequency of DVD
  - Manifest DVD (especially in children, risk of amblyopia present)
  - Head posture
  - Cosmetic
- Selection of surgery depends on:
  - Severity of DVD
  - Associated IOOA
  - Associated SOOA
- Severity of DVD:
  - Moderate: (<5 PD in abduction)
  - Severe: (>5 PD in abduction)
- Various surgeries are (Table 10.16):

Table 10.16 DVD Surgical Treatment Options

DVD	IOOA	SOOA	Surgery
Moderate (<5 PD in Abduction)	+	−	IO recession with anterior positioning.
Severe (>5PD in Abduction)	+	−	IO recession with anterior position + SR recession
+	−	−	SR recession (5–7 mm) + inferior rectus resection (5 mm)
+	−	+	SR recession 7–10 mm, SO post tenectomy

- IO recession with anterior positioning of IO
- SR recession (7–10 mm) with/without Faden
- IR resection 5 mm

What is Duane's syndrome?

- It is a restrictive squint due to innervational anomaly
- Etiology: Absence of sixth-nerve nucleus and aberrant innervation of LR from branch of third cranial nerve

- Type I (esotropia):
  - Commonest
  - Associated with Goldenhar syndrome, Wilderwanck syndrome
  - Deficit in abduction
  - Ipsilateral face turn
  - Esotropia in primary position
  - Narrowing of palpebral fissure on adduction and widening in abduction
- Type II:
  - Deficit in adduction and exotropia; very rare
- Type III:
  - With exotropia in primary position (can occur with esotropia or no squint)
  - Contralateral face turn
  - Deficit in adduction and abduction
  - Lid fissure narrowing in adduction, widening in abduction
  - Upshoot and downshoot is frequent
- DRS plus: DRS plus vertebral, limb, and ear defects
- Variant of DRS:
  - 1) Vertical retraction syndrome:
    - Limitation of elevation or depression with palpebral aperture anomaly
    - Congenital Adduction deficit with divergence
- Associations of DRS:
  - Ocular:
    - Nystagmus
    - Goldenhar syndrome—epibulbar dermoid
    - Anisocoria
    - Ptosis
  - Non-ocular:
    - Goldenhar:
      - Epibulbar dermoid, facial hypoplasia
      - Pre-auricular skin tag
      - Vertebral anomaly
      - First and second branchial arch defect
    - Klippel–Feil anomaly:
      - Cervical vertebrae anomaly
      - Web neck
      - Facial asymmetry
    - Wilderwanck syndrome: Klippelfiel + sensorineural deafness
- Indications of surgery in Type I:
  - Significant face turn
  - Esotropia in primary position

- Choice:
  - Recess ipsilateral MR
  - Degree of recession depends on magnitude of face turn
  - Moderate face turn (15–20°): 5.5–6 mm
  - Large face turn (25–40°): 6.5–7 mm
  - Other option is adjustable suture taken
  - In case of residual face turn after maximum MR recession, consider a Hummelsheim transposition
- Disadvantage of transposition in 10–15% patients can lead to induced hypertropia and fear of anterior segment ischemia.
- DRS Type III:
  - Management options:
  - Surgery:
    - Contralateral face turn: Ipsilateral LR recession
    - Severe co-contraction and lid fissure narrowing on adduction and face turn: Ipsilateral MR recession and LR recession
    - If upshoot and downshoot: Y split of LR
    - Faden: On lateral rectus, to treat upshoot and downshoots with LR recession
- DD of DRS:
  - LR palsy
  - Mobius syndrome
  - Oculomotor apraxia
  - Congenital esotropia

10.5.4 Classify exodeviations

- XT classification by:
  - According to fusional control:
    - Exophoria
    - Intermittent or constant XT
  - According to near/distance variation of the angle:
    - Divergence excess type (D>N)
    - Pseudo-divergence excess type (D=N after patching)
    - Basic XT (D=N)
    - Convergence insufficiency type (N>D)
  - Dissociated exodeviation
  - Consecutive exodeviation
  - Primary (very rare)
  - After surgery for ET

- Etiology:
  - Unknown
  - Possibly a combination of innervational and orbital factors
  - Burian: basis misalignment of the eyes (basic deviation) upon which innervational factors (dynamic deviation) are superimposed
- Symptomatology:
  - Asthenopia (with exophoria or intermittent XT)
  - Improvement of asthenopia may be a sign of progression
  - Crossed diplopia
  - Photophobia
  - Occasionally: micropsia
- Clinical characteristics:
  - Prevalence
  - Age of onset
  - Progression in 75%
  - Female sex preponderance (2/3 are female)
  - Anomalies of ductions:
    - Defective adduction
    - Excessive Abduction
  - Sensorial adaptations:
    - Suppression (frequent)
    - Abnormal retinal correspondence (frequent)
    - Amblyopia (rare)
    - Panoramic vision
- Examination and special tests:
  - Choice of the fixation target:
    - Stimulate accommodation at near fixation
    - Relax accommodation at distance fixation
  - Variability of fusional control
  - Examine children before and after school
  - Anxiety effect influences preoperative measurement
  - Examine while fixating on objects in the far distance
  - Occlusion test:
    - Assesses the role of fusional convergence in controlling XT at near
    - Determines the surgical management
    - Avoid binocular input during the cover test
  - +3.00 DS test
    - Determines role of accommodative convergence in reducing near deviation

- - Predicts effect of postoperative bifocals in case of overcorrection
- Lateral incomitance:
  - Reduce amount of recession LR OU when XT decreases in lateral gaze
- Conservative therapy:
  - Full correction of myopia
  - Overcorrection with minus lenses?
  - Alternating occlusion?
  - Convergence training?
  - Other orthoptic training?
- Indications for surgery:
  - Constant large-angle exotropia: We can operate between 1 and 2 years of age
  - Intermittent XT
  - When manifest least 50% of the time
    - When symptomatic
    - We operate rarely prior to age 4
    - End target of surgery: small-angle consecutive ET
- Goals of surgery:
  - Stable fusion at near and distance
  - Asymptomatic patient
  - Aim for 12–15 PD overcorrection
- Types of surgery
  - Basic XT (N=D): Recess LR, Resect MR
  - Pseudo-divergence excess type: Recess LR, Resect MR
  - Divergence excess type: Recess LR OU (Table 10.17)
  - Convergence insufficiency type: Resect MR OU
- Amount of surgery:
  - Depends on type of deviation
  - Examination of ductions and versions
  - Lateral incomitance
  - Sensory state (amblyopia, sensory XT)
- Results of surgery:
  - Criteria for success: Stable and comfortable binocular vision
  - Literature lists 60–90% success rate

Table 10.17 Dosage for Recession LR OU

ANGLE (PD at distance)	LR Recession (mm)
15	4
20	5
35	7
40	8
50	7 + resection LR

- Prevention of large overcorrections:
  - Full correction of high hypermetropia
  - Avoid excessive resection of MR
  - Do forced duction in the operating room
  - Do spring-back balance test
- Management of consecutive esotropia:
  - Duction exercises
  - Alternating patching
  - Correct hypermetropic refractive error
  - Prisms
  - Benefit of sensory "jolt"?

What is convergence insufficiency type of XT?

- Convergence insufficiency:
  - Asthenopia
  - Occurs most often in students
  - Reduced convergence amplitude
  - Remote NPC, normal NPA
  - Therapy: Orthoptics
  - Rarely ever needs surgery: Resection MR OU
- Accommodation—convergence insufficiency:
  - Young adults
  - Remote NPC and NPA
  - Orthoptics is not of much benefit
  - Treat with base out prisms and bifocals
  - Surgery: Resection MR OU

What is intermittent exotropia (IXT)?

- Normal newborn 60–70% small-angle exotropia present
- Resolves in 4–6 months
- 50–90% of all exotropia
- Important characteristics:
  - Variable angle of deviation
  - Good binocular vision
  - Amblyopia and ARC rare
  - Progression unpredictable
- Clinical presentation:
  - Usually present by 6–12 months
  - Onset rare after 4 years
  - Manifests with fatigue/evening/daydreaming
  - Diplo-photophobia—one eye closed in bright light to avoid diplopia because of loss of fusion control due to light
- Classification types (Table 10.18):
  - a) Burian's classification:
    - According to distance and near measurements:
      - Basic: N = D (with 10 PD)
      - Divergence excess: D > N by 10 PD
      - Convergence insufficiency: N > D by 10 PD

- Pseudo-divergence excess: D = N after patch
- b) Kushner's classification:
  - High proximal convergence
  - Pseudo-high AC/A ratio: Tenacious proximal fusion
  - High AC/A ratio
  - Low AC/A ratio—fusional convergence insufficiency
  - Pseudo-convergence insufficiency
- A) Measurement of angle of deviation:
  - 1) Prolonged alternate patch test:
    - To overcome tonic fusional convergence during ACT
    - The ocluder placed for sufficient duration
  - 2) Patch:
    - Either eye for 30–60 min
    - To differentiate true/pseudo-divergence excess type
  - 3) High AC/A ratio: (+3 D test/lens gradient test)
    - Put + 3 D: Near increases by 20 PD or more than distance deviation
    - Diagnosis: Divergence excess of high AC/A ratio
  - 4) Distance measurement: (in feet)
    - Very far = 100–200
    - D = 20
    - N = 2
  - Important to gauge variability and to show patient and relative with photographic documentation about the possible decompensation later; prefer to document with each eye fixating, if alternating.

Table 10.18 Phases: Calhounz's Classification of XT

	Deviation	Sensory
I	Exophoria—Distance, Ortho—Near	No symptoms
II	Intermittent Exotropia—Distance, Ortho/exophoria—Near	Symptomatic for Distance
III	Exotropia—Distance, Exophoria/Intermittent Exotropia—Near	BV—Near, Suppression Scotoma—Distance
IV	Exotropia—Distance, Exotropia—Near	No binocularity

- B) Fusional control (Table 10.19):
  - Clinical control (ease of drifting into exotropia) and recovery (ability to regain fusion):
  - Graded for both distance and near
  - Home control XT manifesting >50% of waking hours—poor control
- C) Stereoacuity (for distance and near):
  - Is objective indicator of:
    - Fusional control and control of deviation
    - Measurement of distance stereoacuity: Random dot E test
- Treatment (Table 10.20):
  - Conservative
    - 1. Correct refractive error
    - 2. Occlusion:
      - Part-time
      - Dominant or alternate
      - 4–6 hours
      - Prevents suppression
    - 3. Overcorrection with minus:
      - Stimulates accommodative convergence, decreases exotropia (–1D to –4D over patient's cycloplegic refraction)
    - 4. Prisms (relieving prisms—base in):
      - Decreases deviation
      - Increases fusional vergence and bifoveal fixation
    - 5. Orthoptic treatment and anti-suppression exercises:

Table 10.19 Grading of Fusional Control in XT

Grade	Control	Recovery
Excellent	Is not tropic	Within seconds after cover, before blink
Good	Is not tropic spontaneously, briefly tropic after cover	Quick recovery <5 s after cover/exo
Fair	Occasional spontaneous tropia	With blink or change in fixation distance
Poor	Tropic frequently, nearly all the time	May stay tropic even after blink or change in fixation distance

Table 10.20 Newcastle Scoring—NCS

1. Home Control	
0	Squint/monocular eye closure never noticed
1	Squint/monocular eye closure seen occasionally (50% of time child observed) for distance
2	Squint/monocular eye closure seen frequently (50% of time child observed) for distance
3	Squint/monocular eye closure seen for distance & near fixation
ADD	
2. Clinical Control Near	
0	Manifest only after cover test and resumes fusion without need for blink or refixation
1	Blink or refixate to control after CT
2	Manifest spontaneously or with any form of fusion disruption without recovery
ADD	
2. Clinical Control Distance	
0	Manifest only after cover test and resumes fusion without need for blink or refixation
1	Blink or refixate to control after CT
2	Manifest spontaneously or with any form of fusion disruption without recovery

NCS total = Home + Clinic near + Clinic distance

- Convergence exercises (for convergence insufficiency)
- Pencil push-ups:
  - Focus on pencil tip holding at arm's length, keeping an index card (placed on wall 6–8 feet away).
  - While bringing pencil close to bridge of nose, attempt to keep tip single, if one of the cards at wall behind disappears, stop moving

pencil, blink once or twice till card image at back becomes two.
- Continue moving the pencil slowly toward nose until it could no longer be kept single and then to try to regain single vision.
- If able to regain single vision, continue bringing pencil close to bridge of nose till becomes double.
- If cannot regain single vision, start the procedure again.
- Schedule: 20 push-ups per day at home, 5 days per week for 12 weeks, and this treatment required approximately 15 minutes per day.
- Prism convergence exercises (exercising prism for IXT—base out).
- Synoptophore exercises
- Computer-based vision therapy: Exercises are done on a computer using software designed to improve convergence, with or without special glasses.
- Indications of conservative treatment:
  - Young patients (4–5 years)
  - Control of deviation better
  - Angle of deviation: 20–25 PD
- Observe for progression: Signs of progression:
  - Increased frequency of tropia
  - Increases size of deviation
  - Decreases stereoacuity
  - Increasing suppression, i.e., absence of diplopia in manifestation phase
- Surgery:
  - Improve binocularity
  - Cosmetics
  - Indications for surgery:
    - Large-angle deviations >20 PD
    - Deviation present >50% of waking hours
    - Signs of progression
    - Failure of conservative treatment
  - Timing of surgery:
  - Early:
    - Advantage: Prevents sensory changes

- Disadvantage: Risk of consecutive esotropia: Leading to monofixation
- Delayed (Jampolsky):
  - Advantage: Accurate diagnosis and measurement of amount of deviation
  - Risk of consecutive ET decreases
- Defer surgery: If angle of deviation ≤ 20 PD, if age ≤ 4 years
- Choice of procedure:
  - Symmetric bilateral LR recession preferred in all except:
  - Convergence insufficiency—where bilateral MR resection done
- Goal:
  - <10 years: Avoid consecutive ET (fear of amblyopia and loss of binocularity)
  - >10 years: Orthotropia
  - Adult: Undercorrect. If overcorrection: Symptomatic diplopia
  - Undercorrection common in myopia/large-angle deviation
  - Overcorrection: 10–15 PD in visually mature patient
  - Undiagnosed lateral incomitance: Risk factor for large-angle ET
  - High AC/A ratio: Risk factor for large-angle ET
- Factors affecting surgical outcome:
  - Age
  - Degree of control
  - Lateral gaze incomitance (decrease the amount of LR recession)
  - Proximal fusion

What is Brown's syndrome? (Table 10.21)

- Brown's syndrome is a restrictive squint characterized by restriction of active and passive elevation in adduction. Frequently unilateral, rarely bilateral.
- Clinical features:
  - Elevation in adduction deficient
  - Elevation in midline less deficient
  - In abduction, there is no deficit of elevation
  - No superior oblique overaction
  - V or Y pattern
  - FDT positive in elevation in adduction

- Downshoot in adduction
- Intorsion on attempted upgaze
- Widened palpebral aperture in adduction
- Primary position: hypotropia
- Anomalous head posture (chin up due to primary position hypotropia)
- Face turned away from affected eye
- Variable head tilt
- Can be associated with horizontal squint
- First 6 points: Must for definitive diagnosis
- Types:
  - Congenital
    - Constant
    - Stable
    - Can resolve spontaneously
    - Because of stiff superior oblique tendon complex
    - Surgery may be required
    - Could be seen with anomalous superior oblique tendon/trochlea
  - Acquired:
    - Because of restriction within/around trochlea
    - Trauma (Brown's with ipsilateral superior oblique paresis = canine tooth syndrome)
    - JRA (tenosynovitis)
    - Myositis
    - Ethmoid sinus surgery
    - Sinusitis
    - Frontal sinus surgery with abscess formation and metastasis in region of trochlea
    - After superior oblique surgery (after SO tucking)
    - After orbital/retinal surgery
    - Usually resolves spontaneously—anti-inflammatory agents
- Differential diagnosis:
  - Double elevator palsy (elevation deficit more in abduction than adduction)
  - Congenital fibrosis syndrome
  - SO overaction with/without IO palsy
  - Blowout fracture
  - Adherent syndrome in SO surgery (elevation deficit more in abduction)
- Conservative treatment:
  - Most common management of Brown's: Observation and counselling

Table 10.21 Brown's Syndrome Features

	Restriction of Elevation in Adduction	Down Shoot in Adduction	Hypotropia in Primary Position
Mild	+	–	–
Moderate	+	+	–
Severe	+	+	+

- Corticosteroid injection into the region of trochlea may be attempted in inflammatory causes of Brown's syndrome
- Surgery indications:
  - Severe degree of elevation deficit in adduction (primary position hypotropia) >20 PD
  - Abnormal head posture
  - Patient demanding despite being counselled
- Principles of surgery:
  - SO tendon is divided into:
  - Anterior third: Responsible for intorsion
  - Posterior third: For depression and abduction
  - Both components of the SO tendon are theorized to be tight in Brown's syndrome; hence, it must be either tenotomized or lengthened (silicone expander, split lengthening, chicken stitch).
- Management:
  - A segment of 240 silicon band is placed between 2 cut ends of SO tendon
  - SO tenotomy with silicone expander (6–12 mm)
  - SO tenotomy with ipsilateral IO recession (undercorrection is common)
  - Ipsilateral SO tenotomy (increases incidence of SO palsy)

What is double elevator palsy?

- Double elevator palsy or monocular elevation deficit syndrome is a term used to describe diminished ocular elevation present in all fields of gaze, usually said to be having weakness of the two elevators of one eye—superior rectus and inferior oblique.
- Clinical features:
  - Elevation deficit in abduction and adduction

- Hypotropia
- Chin elevation
- Implies paresis of SR and IO
- Actually, there is tight inferior rectus in 70%
- Associated features:
  - True ptosis in 50%
  - Pseudoptosis in almost all patients
  - Jaw winking
  - Duane's syndrome
  - Other misdirection syndrome
- Indications of surgery: Hypotropia in primary gaze causing chin elevation
- Goal of surgery:
  - To increase the field of binocular vision
  - Surgical management depends on FDT to determine SR function
  - Good SR function with tight inferior rectus muscle: ipsilateral IR recession
  - Poor SR function (SR palsy): Ipsilateral IR recession and split tendon transfer 1/2 MR and 1/2 LR to SR muscle (vertical Hummelsheim)
  - Treatment of ptosis after 6 months
- Differential diagnosis: IR cysticercosis

10.5.5 Pupil testing

Mention the pathways of the following light reflexes.

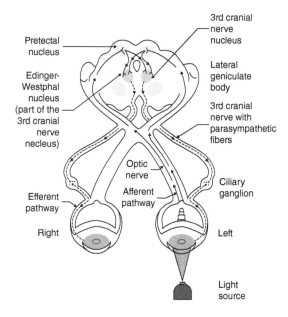

Figure 10.21 Pupillary light reflex

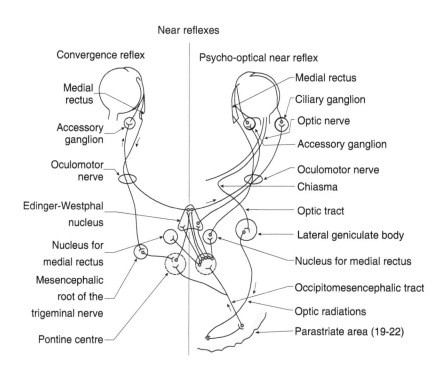

Figure 10.22 Convergence reflex and Psycho-optical near reflex

How does one go about pupillary evaluation? (Table 10.22)

Evaluation of pupil can be as follows:
PERRCA: Pupils equal, round, reacting to light, central accommodating

- Size: If equal or anisocoria is present, if aniso-coria mention whether it is in light or dark?
- Response to light—direct/consensual
- RAPD
  - Whether constricts with same velocity: Pharmacological or Adie's tonic pupil
  - Whether it re-dilates with same velocity
- Light near pupillary assessment
- Reporting of pupillary examination should be as follows

Table 10.22 Pupillary Examination Documentation

	OD	OS
Dark	5 mm	5 mm
Light	3 mm	3 mm
Reaction to light	Brisk	Brisk
RAPD	No	No
Dilatation in dark	Normal	Normal
Reaction to Near	2 mm	2 mm

- Physiological anisocoria of <0.4 mm is present in 20% of population.
- Always ask the patient to look at far and throw the light from below.

Pupillary reactions are controlled by which muscles?

- Sphincter pupillae:
  - For constriction
  - Parasympathetic nerve supply
- Dilator pupillae:
  - Causes dilatation
  - Sympathetic nerve supply

How is pupillary size checked?

- Handheld pupil gauge
- Handheld pupil camera
- Infrared pupillometry (most sensitive)
- With torch
  - Measure in dark and light (labeled aniso-coria if difference is >0.4 mm)
  - Assess with near stimulation

How do you test pupillary reaction to light?

- Patient must fix on distant target (eliminates accommodation).
- Room must be dimly lit.
- Primary light source should be bright enough to produce constriction of the pupil.
- Secondary light source may be used to assist in viewing the pupillary reflex in darkly colored irides (obliquely illuminated).
- Position yourself within 25 cm of the patient, but not in his line of sight (i.e., off to one side, sitting or standing).
- Instruct the patient to remove his spectacles.
- Direct light reflex: Record the response to light on the pupil, which is directly illuminated, by light in terms of briskness of response. Can use grading from 0 to 4, where 0 is no response and 4 is brisk constriction.
- Consensual light reflex: Similar record as mentioned, but the response to light is checked in the non-illuminated pupil. If possible, use barrier to prevent light from the other eye illuminated the study pupil. The rapidity of response and change in amount of pupil size should normally correspond to that of the direct response. Can be graded in similar manner.

How does one check for the pupillary response to near?

- Must have room light that is adequate to fix-ate on an accommodative target (avoid a very brightly lit room).
- Do not use a non-accommodative target (such as pen).
- When a person looks at a near, accommodative target, three responses are noted during the near synkinesis.
  - Accommodation (contraction of ciliary muscle leading to increase lens thickness and curvature but decrease length)
  - Convergence (contraction of medial rectus muscle)
  - Miosis (contraction of pupillary sphincter)
- The near reflex is nearly always normal if the light reflex is normal, but not otherwise.
- Hence, near reflex testing is usually avoided when light reflex is normal.

How does one test for light near dissociation?

- Light near dissociation is said to occur when the near reflex is significantly better than the light reflex.
- Always check near response if abnormal light reflex or asymmetric light reflex.
- Document with grading if possible.

What is RAPD? (Table 10.23)

Relative afferent pupillary defect (RAPD)
- Measurement of RAPD can be done by neutral density filter over the normal eye.
- We can neutralize the RAPD and quantify it in log units.
- Availability of filters range is 0.3, 0.6, 0.9, and 1.8 log units (0.3—mild, 0.6–0.9—moderate, 1.8—severe).

Table 10.23 Quantification of RAPD

Disease	Quantification of RAPD (log units)
Optic neuritis	0.3–3
Optic tract disease	0.4–0.6 contralateral eye (temporal field loss)
Pre-tectal lesion	Contralateral RAPD (no field loss)
Anisocoria	0.1 log unit for every mm
CRVO	Ischemic: 0.9–1.2 Non-ischemic: <0.6
RD	• 1 quadrant: 0.3 • 2 quadrant: 0.6 • 3 quadrant: 0.9 • Total RD: Up to 2
RP	<0.3
Amblyopia	<0.5
Patching	Up to 1.5 log unit in non-occluded eye

- RAPD does not cause anisocoria.
- Causes:
  - With visual loss:
    - Unilateral or asymmetric optic neuritis/optic neuropathy/AION
    - Severe unilateral retinopathy
    - Maculopathy with VA <6/60 (small RAPD because of involvement of papillomacular bundle)
  - Without visual loss: Lesion of pretectal nucleus (causes contralateral RAPD)

What are the causes of contralateral RAPD?

Contralateral RAPD
- Without visual loss: Lesion of pretectal nucleus or brachium of the superior colliculus (because the afferent pupillary fibers leave optic tract before reaching LGB)
- With visual loss (the reason is the retina is dark adapted and therefore causes excess retinal stimuli on the side of dense cataract/prolonged patching):
  - Dense unilateral cataract
  - Prolonged patching of one eye/complete ptosis
  - Optic tract lesion
- If a patient has no RAPD but is suspected to have optic neuropathy, then the differentials are:
  - Bilateral optic neuropathy
  - No optic neuropathy
  - Infiltrative optic neuropathy
  - Prior sphincter damage or another pathology

How does one test for RAPD?

- Under dim room illumination with the patient fixating a distance target, illuminate the patient's right eye directly with a bright hand-held light, in a manner identical to that used when testing the light reflex. Note the pupillary constriction in both eyes.
- Move the light beam immediately and swiftly over the patient's nose to the left eye, simultaneously noting the pupillary response in that eye. Ensure you illuminate each pupil from the same angle.
  - Normally, the pupil will either constrict slightly or remain at its previous size.
  - If the pupil dilates when it is illuminated, a relative afferent pupillary defect is present, which usually indicates a disorder of the optic nerve or severe retinal pathology. This means the direct light reflex is weaker than the consensual light reflex.
- Quickly the light is swung back to the right eye. One should normally see a mild constriction or no change in size at all. Net pupillary constriction or dilation is an abnormal response.
- Steps 1–3 must be repeated rhythmically, spending equal time illuminating each pupil,

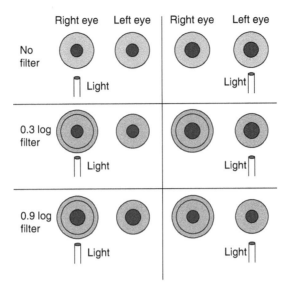

Figure 10.23 Assessment of a Left Relative Afferent Pupillary Defect

until it is clear whether pupillary responses are normal or abnormal relative afferent pupillary defect (RAPD) is recorded as 1+ to 4+, with 1+ indicating a mild afferent defect and 4+ indicating an amaurotic pupil, a severe defect in which the affected eye shows no direct light response.

- (A) The light before the healthy right eye causes a direct constriction and a consensual constriction in the left. Swinging the light from the healthy to the affected eye, a dilation is seen in the affected eye as the direct reflex is weakened allowing the consensual from the good eye to override.
- (B) Placing filters before the healthy eye allows the depth of defect to be assessed. A 0.3 filter does not change to pupil activity.
- (C) A 0.9 filter before the healthy eye reduces the consensual signal from the healthy eye to a level that allows the weaker direct reflex in the affected eye to dominate. This is the filter that first shows this reversal so may be recorded for this RAPD.

What are the grades of RAPD? (Table 10.24)

Table 10.24 Grade of RAPD Using Neutral Density Filter

Grade	Neutral Density Filter (log units)	Pupillary Response
1	0.4	A weak initial pupillary constriction followed by greater redilation
2	0.7	An initial pupillary stall followed by greater redilation
3	1.1	An immediate pupillary dilation
4	2	An immediate pupillary dilation, following 6 seconds of illumination
5	Infinity	Immediate pupillary dilatation with no constriction at all

How does one evaluate a case of anisocoria?

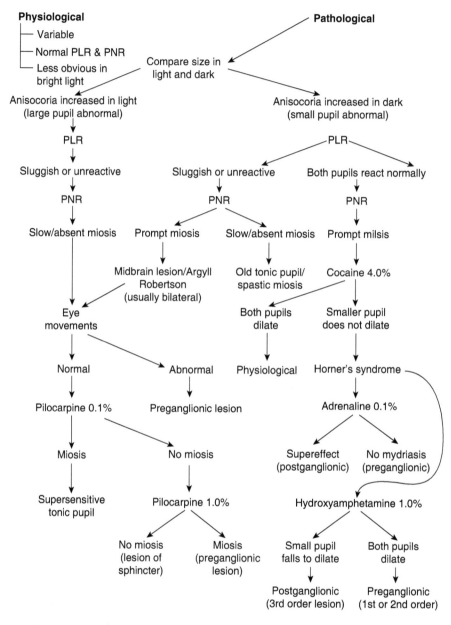

Figure 10.24 Flowchart for evaluation of anisocoria
PLR = Pupillary Light Response
PNR = Pupillary Near Response

What are the causes of anisocoria greater in dark?

- Simple anisocoria
- Horner's syndrome
- Pharmacological (thymoxamine, cocaine, adrenergic drugs)
- Pharmacological stimulation of parasympathetic pathway (organophosphate esters, pilocarpine, methacholine, arecoline)

What are the causes of anisocoria greater in light?

- Third-nerve paresis
- Tonic pupil (Adie's pupil)
- Trauma to the iris sphincter
- Glaucoma
- Siderosis
- Pharmacological inhibition of parasympathetic pathway (atropine, scopolamine)

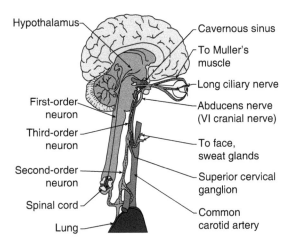

Figure 10.25 Sympathetic pathway

What is Horner's syndrome?

- It is an oculo-sympathetic paresis.
- A combination of ptosis, miosis, and anhydrosis is called Horner's syndrome.
- It occurs due when sympathetic innervation to the eye is interrupted so that the dilator muscle of the eye is weakened causing the pupil to decrease in size.
- Horner's syndrome is localized based on the order of sympathetic neurons affected.
- First order: Central
- Second order: Preganglionic
- Third order: Postganglionic

Describe the sympathetic pathway?

- Origin is in the hypothalamus.
- First-order neuron: Hypothalamus to ciliospinal center of Budge at the level of C8–T2
- Second-order neuron: Through dorsal root along the brachial plexus over the apex of lung, ascends to superior cervical ganglion, which is placed near the angle of mandible at the bifurcation of common carotid artery
- Third-order neuron: From superior cervical ganglion along the adventitia of internal carotid artery through the cavernous sinus along the first division of the fifth cranial nerve, supplies—dilator, Muller's muscle in upper and lower lids
- Fibers for facial sweating branch at superior cervical ganglion from the remaining sympathetic fibers

What are the signs of Horner's syndrome?

- Mild ptosis (upper lid and lower lid)
- Miosis due to palsy of the dilator muscle (pupil dilated widely after adrenergic stimulation due to denervation hypersensitivity); in light, both pupils constrict due to normal sphincter pupillae, but in the dark, the weakness of the dilator muscle is more apparent.
- Pseudoenophthalmos (decreased palpebral aperture)
- Dilatation lag in dark: Horner's pupil dilates more slowly
- Ipsilateral anhydrosis (in first- and second-order neuron lesions)
- Loss of ciliospinal reflex
- Heterochromia (congenital Horner's affected iris is lighter)
- Small or sunken eye (apparent enophthalmos)
- Slightly elevated lower eyelid (upside-down ptosis)
- Vasomotor and sudomotor changes of the skin on the affected side seen in central and preganglionic Horner's syndrome

When does a painful Horner's syndrome occur?

- Always rule out carotid dissection of ipsilateral internal carotid artery unless proved otherwise
- Recurrent cluster headache
- Redness, paratrigeminal syndrome (diagnosis of exclusion)
- Facial pain

Table 10.25 Pharmacological Tests for Horner's Syndrome

Drug	Normal Pupil	Horner's Pupil	Anisocoria
Cocaine 4–10%	Dilates	Doesn't dilate well	Increases
Apraclonidine 0.5–1%	Does not dilate	Dilates	Decreases
Palpebral fissure will improve with apraclonidine only, not with cocaine			
Phenylephrine 1%	Does not dilate	Established (10 days) post-ganglionic lesion, Horner's pupil will dilate and ptosis may be temporarily relieved	Decreases
		Central or preganglionic Horner pupil does not dilate	Remains same

What are the tests for diagnosis of Horner's syndrome? (Table 10.25)

- Cocaine blocks reuptake of norepinephrine; therefore, with intact sympathetic innervation, it will cause pupillary dilatation and have no effect with impaired sympathetic innervation regardless of location because there is no release of norepinephrine into the synaptic cleft.
- Apraclonidine is an α-2 agonist that has no effect on intact sympathetic innervation and causes mild pupillary dilatation with impaired sympathetic innervation regardless of level of lesion. Because of denervation hypersensitivity, α-1 stimulation dilates Horner's syndrome and elevates ptotic lid.
- Phenylephrine 1%
  - Easily available than hydroxyamphetamine and adrenaline, with comparable effect.
  - Typically prepared by dilution of commercially available 2.5% or 10% solution.
  - Effect: Established post-ganglionic lesion Horner's pupil will dilate.
  - Reason: In post-ganglionic Horner's, the dilator pupillae muscle develops denervation hypersensitivity to adrenergic neurotransmitters.
- Adrenaline 0.1%: Similar mechanism to phenylephrine
- Hydroxyamphetamine 1%
  - Slightly more sensitive than phenylephrine
  - Effect: Normal or preganglionic lesion dilates, post-ganglionic does not
  - Reason: It potentiates the release of noradrenaline from functioning postganglionic nerve ending. In a lesion of third order, no release hence no effect.

How does one localize the lesion?

- Pharmacological:
  - Hydroxy amphetamine test (1%)
  - Normal pupil dilates
  - Horner's pupil dilates: First- or second-order neuron lesion
  - Horner's pupil does not dilate: Third-order neuron lesion
- Assessment of sweating with iodine and starch:
  - Ipsilateral loss on the whole body: First order
  - Ipsilateral loss on face: Second order
  - No Loss: Third order
- Clinical:
  - Adult:
    - First order:
      - Hypothalamus lesion/tumor: Will have associated contralateral hemiplegia
      - Brain stem: Wallenburg's syndrome, MS, tumor: Patients will have altered pain and temperature sensation over face, limb ataxia and bulbar disturbance causing dysarthria, dysphagia, and Horner's syndrome
      - Spinal cord: Trauma, tumor, MS, myelitis, AV malformations, syringomyelia
      - Association of contralateral fourth CN with Horner's: Lesion is midbrain, lesion maybe at fourth-nerve nucleus or ipsilateral fascicle before decussation
    - Second order:
      - Pancoast syndrome
      - Malignancy from lung or breast cancer can sometimes spread

behind the carotid sheath at level of C6 associated with phrenic, vagus, and recurrent laryngeal nerve palsy called Rowland Payne syndrome
- Brachial plexus injury
- Cervical spine disease
- Thyroid lesion
- Sympathetic chain schwannoma
- Subclavian artery aneurysm
- Iatrogenic trauma/surgery (C8–T1)
- Pneumothorax
- CABG, pacemaker insertion
  - Third order:
    - Internal carotid artery dissection/aneurysm (traumatic/spontaneous)—associated with sudden severe ipsilateral facial and neck pain
    - Neck dissection
    - Skull base/nasopharyngeal lymphoma
    - Cavernous sinus lesions such as tumors, aneurysms or infection associated with ipsilateral ophthalmoplegia, pain or dysesthesia of the face
    - Carotid aneurysm/pituitary
    - Cluster headache
    - Basal skull fracture
    - Giant cell arteritis
    - Tumors of nasopharynx or jugular foramen
- Children:
  - Congenital (presents within 4 weeks of birth):
    - Trauma
    - Cervical rib
    - Neuroblastoma
    - Agenesis of internal carotid artery
  - Idiopathic
  - Acquired:
    - Neuroblastoma
    - Rhabdomyosarcoma
    - AVM
    - Glioma
    - MS
    - Trauma
    - Surgery
    - Carotid artery dissection (isolated Horner in child: Rule out neuroblastoma)

Treatment of Horner's syndrome?

- Treat the cause
  - Spontaneous resolution
  - Apraclonidine: Gives temporary relief
  - Ptosis surgery: Fasanella–Servat procedure

What are the causes of a miotic pupil?

- Pupil size ≤2 mm
- Ocular:
  - Hypermetropic: Physiological
  - Chronic pilocarpine treatment
  - Acute iridocyclitis
  - Congenital
  - Pseudoexfoliation syndrome
  - Congenital rubella syndrome
  - Lowe's syndrome
- Systemic:
  - Opium poisoning
  - Pontine hemorrhage

What are the causes of a mydriatic pupil?

- Ocular:
  - Physiological: Myopia
  - Angle-closure glaucoma
  - Mydriatic drops
  - Sphincter tear (post-traumatic)
  - Congenital familial iridoplegia
  - Postsurgical
- Systemic:
  - Third-nerve palsy
  - Head injury
  - Coma
  - Barbiturate poisoning

What are the causes of dyscoria (abnormal shape)?

- Congenital malformation
- Post-inflammatory—posterior synechiae
- Coloboma: Traumatic/congenital
- Hypoplastic iris: Axenfeld–Rieger
- Lens subluxation

What are the causes of corectopia?

- Abnormal displacement of pupil is called corectopia
- Normal pupil 0.5 mm infero-nasal to center
- Causes:
  - Sector iris hypoplasia
  - Coloboma

Table 10.26 Heterochromia Causes

Congenital		Acquired
Hypochromia	**Hyperchromia**	• Trauma
Congenital Horner's	Oculodermal melanosis (associated with glaucoma with increased incidence of ocular/orbital melanoma)	• Rubeosis • Iridocyclitis (HZO) • ACIOL • Post intraocular operation
Fuchs heterochromic iridocyclitis	Pigmented tumor	• Anterior segment ischemia post muscle handling
Incontinentia pigmentii	Melanosis oculi	• Siderosis
Waardenburg–Klein syndrome	Nevus of Ota	• Rubeosis
Hypomelanosis of Ito		• Iris ectropion syndrome
GCC (glaucomatocyclitic crisis)		• Leukemic infiltration • ICE syndrome

- Lens subluxation
- ICE syndrome
- Axenfeld–Rieger syndrome

What are the causes of heterochromia? (Table 10.26)

- Important to rule out Horner's syndrome:
  - Benign shoulder dystocia
  - Life-threatening neuroblastoma of sympathetic chain
  - Heterochromia iridium: Unilateral
  - Heterochromia iridis: Sectorial
  - Bilateral heterochromia
  - Hirschsprung's disease (aganglionic megacolon)
  - Waardenburg's syndrome

What are the causes of ectropion of iris?

- Congenital:
  - Rubeosis
  - Congenital iris ectropion syndrome: Ectropion, glassy smooth iris, high insertion of root, angle dysgenesis, glaucoma
  - Neurofibromatosis
  - Facial hemi atrophy
  - Prader–Willi syndrome

What are the causes of iris transillumination?

- Trauma, post intraocular operation, uveitis
- Albinism
- Hypoplasia

- ICE syndrome
- Marfan's syndrome
- Subluxation of lens
- Microcoria
- Axenfeld anomaly
- PDS—pigment dispersion syndrome (mid-peripheral iris)
- Pseudoexfoliation—peripupillary
- Fuchs heterochromic iridocyclitis

What are the causes of iris nodules?

- Lisch: Tan color: Neurofibromatosis, increases with age
- Xanthogranulomatous: Yellowish/red, vascular
- Brushfeld s: Down's syndrome, hypopigmented (25% normal)
- Koeppe's nodules
- Busacca nodules
- Iris pearls: Leprosy
- Sarcoid
- HIV
- Lymphoma

10.5.6 Confrontation test

How is confrontation testing performed for gross visual field examination?

- Recording confrontation visual field results.
  - Normal result: the patient counts fingers in all quadrants of both eyes.

- Bitemporal hemianopia: The patient fails to count fingers in the temporal quadrants of each eye.
- Homonymous hemianopia: The patient fails to count fingers in the temporal quadrants of one eye and the nasal quadrants of the other eye.
- CF = Counts fingers
- Steps:
  - Introduce yourself to the patient.
  - Patient sits directly across one arm's length away.
  - Make sure you are sitting such that your eyes are at the same level as the patient; this ensures your visual field is similar to the patients.
  - Prior to testing peripheral fields, ensure central vision is intact with prior visual acuity testing.
  - After closing your right eye and the patient's left eye with their palm (not fingers), ask the following questions:
    - Ask the patient to look at your nose.

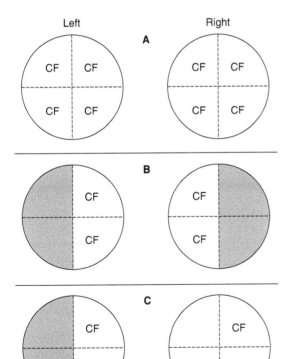

Figure 10.26 Confrontation visual field recording

- Central vision: Ask whether the examiner's entire face is clear or if there is any part that is blurry or missing, and if so, which part. This gives an idea about gross visual field defects. Alternatively, an Amsler's test can be performed to check central vision.
- Static testing: Show fingers in each quadrant, in a plane equidistant from patient and examiner, and ask the patient to mention the number of fingers he sees.
- Kinetic testing: Can also perform this examination by asking the patient to inform you when they see your finger wiggling or a white pin, which is brought in from outward, inward from non-seeing into seeing field and the results are compared with when the target is seen by the examiner
- Always test all four visual field quadrants.
- More sensitive and central defects can be tested with a red pin.
- Red desaturation test: This is done to detect hemianopic defect.
  - Occlude the eye and ask patient to look at examiners nose.
- A bright red object is presented to the patient in two different quadrants in front of the eye to be tested and asked if there is any difference in the brightness of the color in any quadrant.
- Can alternately push the red object across the vertical meridian and ask the patient when it becomes less red.
  - Same procedure is repeated in the other eye.

10.5.7 Optic disc-related

Q. How do you evaluate the optic disc clinically?

- Disc size:
  - It depends on overall size of eyeball and refractive error
  - Normal size around 1.5 mm
  - Extremely variable; ranges from 0.96 to 2.91 mm
  - So, cup disc ratio varies from 0.1 to 0.5

- Optic disc size measurement can be done by:
  - Direct ophthalmoscopy: The spot size of the particular DO is usually mentioned by the company of having a standard size.
  - Slit lamp with vertical light beam, measuring graticule used and correcting factor of the lens used.
- Optic cup:
  - Cup: Disc ratio: Variable from 0.1 to 0.9
  - Anything >0.5 is suspicious
  - Shape of the cup: Vertically oval is suspicious
  - Position of the cup: Eccentric is suspicious
  - Lamina cribrosa: Visibility of dots
  - Depth of cup: Deep cup indicates glaucoma
  - Asymmetry of cup: Difference of 0.2 is suspicious
- Neuro-retinal rim:
  - Area between cup and the edge of optic disc
  - ISNT rule (thickness maximum of inferior quadrant)
  - Rim thickness decreased
  - Rim: disc ratio is decreased
  - Color changes from pink to pale
- Vascular changes:
  - Nasal shift
  - Bending
  - Baring of vessels
  - Overpass phenomenon
  - Splinter hemorrhages on disc (Drance hemorrhage) characteristic of suspected normal tension glaucoma (NTG)
- Peripapillary area:
  - Atrophy
  - Alpha zone: Reflects RPE
  - Beta zone: Choroidal atrophy and hence scleral ring is visible. Do not confuse with neuro-retinal rim.
- Nerve fiber layer:
  - Examine in red-free light
  - If the nerve fibre layer is affected then seen as a slit or wedge like defect
- To document progression: Handwritten drawing or fundus photograph. Gold standard—stereo photography pair

Q. What are the differential diagnosis of deep cup?

- Physiological
- Myopic
- Compressive lesion on optic nerve or optic chiasma
- Optic pit
- Optic disc coloboma
- Tilted disc
- Morning glory syndrome
- AION
- Methanol alcohol poisoning
- LHON (Leber's hereditary optic neuropathy)
- Radiation neuropathy

Q. What is the definition and clinical features of papilledema?

- Definition: It is a non-inflammatory disc edema due to increased intracranial pressure.
- Pathogenesis is usually theorized to be due to partial arrest of fast axoplasmic flow (fast 500 mm/24 hr, slow 2 mm/24 hr).
- Symptoms:
  - Transient blurring of vision (early no changes except if hemorrhage at macula, later due to ON compression)
  - Headache, worst in recumbent position
  - Vomiting
  - Diplopia
  - Gradual diminishing of vision
- Signs:
- Fundus in general:
  - Bilateral
  - Opacification of NFL
  - Disc:
    - Hyperemic and elevated; 3 mm elevation corresponds to 1 D on direct ophthalmoscopy
    - Margins blurred; starts nasally; if temporal margins blurred first, then think of tumor or juxta-papillary choroiditis
    - Venous dilation (other causes: DM, dysproteinemia, glaucoma, CRVO, CCF, angiomatosis)
    - Venous pulsation absent (if present CSF pressure >200 mm of H_2O) 20% of normal patients it's absent
    - Splinter hemorrhage

- Exudates
- Cotton wool spots
- Haziness of retinal blood vessels at disc margin due to swelling of NFL
- Paton's lines (circumferential retinal folds) in peripapillary region, surest sign of true disc edema, present in early stages, disappear in late stages and are present because of temporal retinal displacement
- Obliterated cup
- Vascular signs:
  - Venous congestion of arcuate and peripapillary blood vessels
  - Peripapillary and papillary hemorrhage (if extensive think of CRVO/HTN)
  - Cotton wool spots (NFL infarcts)
  - Hyperemia of optic nerve head
  - Hard exudates
- Non-fundus signs:
  - Enlarged blind spot
  - No pupil abnormality except in supratentorial masses
  - Kernohan's syndrome: Pupil involvement with LMN signs same side
  - Terson's syndrome: Papilledema with preretinal hemorrhage is almost always due to subarachnoid bleed (i.e., r/o CRVO, PDR)
  - Foster–Kennedy syndrome: Disc edema in one eye and optic atrophy in the other eye
    - Causes: frontal lobe glioma, olfactory lobe meningioma, active AION in one eye and old AION in the other eye

What are the causes of unilateral papilledema?

- Unilateral papilledema: True raised ICT having disc edema only in one eye

- Optic atrophy in one eye
- Foster–Kennedy
- One-eyed

How to assess optic disc clinically in a case of papilledema?

- A 2–6 D difference needed to focus vessels at the surface of optic disc when compared to those on retina, using a direct ophthalmoscopy
- In phakic eyes: 2 D ≈ 1 mm, in aphakic eyes 3 D ≈ 1 mm elevation
- Hence papilledema ≈ 0.75 to 2 mm elevation

What is the classification of papilledema? (Table 10.27)

What are the stages of papilledema?

- Early:
  - Hyperemia of disc
  - Indistinct disc margins
  - NF swelling of disc
  - Paton's lines
  - Peripapillary hemorrhage and flame-shaped hemorrhage
- Acute decompensated—advanced:
  - Grossly swollen hyperemic disc
  - Masking of blood vessels
  - Grossly dilated blood vessels
  - Hemorrhage
  - Cotton wool spots
  - Hard exudates
  - Retinal striae
- Chronic (late):
  - Champagne cork appearance (long-standing cases)
  - Fewer hemorrhages
  - Cup obliterated
  - Macular star
  - Hyperemia decreased

Table 10.27 Classification of Papilledema

Author				Staging		
Hoyt	Early	Fully developed	Chronic			
Sanders	Early	Fully developed	Chronic	Vintage		
Frison	0	1	2	3	4	5
	Normal	C-shaped halo	Complete halo	Vessels off disc obscured	Vessels on the disc obscured	Mushroom disc

- Arcuate field loss
- Hard exudates within nerve head
- Terminal:
  - Pale atrophied flat disc
  - Secondary optic atrophy
  - Arteriolar attenuation and sheathing
  - Poor vision
  - Gliosis
  - Disc dirty gray
- Frisen scale for grading papilledema
  - Stage 1: Nasal halo of disc blurring
  - Stage 2: Circumferential halo of swelling; cup maintained
  - Stage 3: Elevation of disc with obscuration of one or more segments of blood vessel at disc margin
  - Stage 4: Almost complete obscuration of major blood vessels on disc
  - Stage 5: Partial or total obscuration of all disc vessels

What is the management of papilledema?

- Counsel patient about the grave nature of the sign and possible neurological complications associated with the same
- Investigations:
  - Visual fields; enlarged blind spot early, later peripheral field constriction
  - MRI/CT to rule out intracranial masses/ bleeds
  - Bedside USG is useful in detecting optic disc edema if optic nerve sheath diameter is greater than 5 mm
  - Lumbar puncture with manometry (fear of coning) with CSF studies
  - To regularly check progression on visual fields and vision is important
- Treatment:
  - Neurology reference with vital monitoring.
  - Treat the underlying cause
  - Diuretics, carbonic anhydrase inhibitors
  - Repeated lumbar puncture (LP)
  - Optic nerve sheath decompressions
  - Lumbo peritoneal shunts

Discuss in brief about optic nerve sheath decompression.

- Optic nerve sheath decompression involves slitting of ON sheath and scleral ring.

- Indications:
  - ON sheath hematoma
  - Pseudotumor cerebri (benign intracranial hypertension)
  - Compression of ON ex: Diffuse meningioma which is not resectable
  - Papilledema (especially in acute)
  - Low-grade brain infection, e.g., treated cryptococcal infection
- Contraindications: Patient not fit for GA
- Preoperatively: Neurosurgical and ophthalmic evaluation
- Anesthesia:
  - GA is better.
  - Manipulation is easy.
  - Pupils can be checked.
- Approaches:
  - Medial orbitotomy (Smith)—not popular
  - Lateral orbitotomy (Davidsons)
  - Transconjunctival (Galbraith and Sulliva)—popular
  - Combined
  - Lateral canthotomy (Korsten and Kolvin)—recent
- Technique of OTN decompression:
  - Under microscope
  - Linear slit incision
  - 3 longitudinal slits in dura with lysis of subarachnoid adhesions
  - Excision of rectangular window in dura
- Optimum site:
  - Just behind the globe where the optic nerve is bulbous (subarachnoid space is wider); hence, damage to pial blood vessels is less, so safer
  - Arachnoid in the dural window is also excised and gives good outflow of CSF
- Precautions: Avoid injury to nutrient blood vessels to optic nerve
- Technique:
  - Reverse Trendelenburg position
  - Speculum
  - Keep checking pupil (if it dilates, decrease the pressure on the globe)
  - Transconjunctival approach:
    - Peritomy—medially with radial cuts
    - MR—hooked and disinserted
    - Expose optic nerve by globe rotation laterally with traction suture and using malleable retractors medially

- Displace posterior ciliary blood vessels
- Decompression:
  - 4 mm behind the globe—4 mm long incision is made
  - Parallel smaller incision can be made
  - Two rectangular windows of dura made
- Reattach medial rectus
- Close conjunctiva
- Advantages over the lateral orbitotomy approach:
  - Quick access
  - Retrobulbar anesthesia enough
  - Skin incision not required
  - Less complications
  - Avoid temporal posterior ciliary artery (hence, blood supply to choroid in macular region less affected)
- Disadvantages:
  - MR disinsertion
  - Excess traction on globe required
  - Additional lateral orbitotomy may be needed
- Complications:
  - Visual loss (permanent) if:
  - CRAO
  - BRAO
  - AION
  - Direct trauma
  - Choroid infarction
  - Optic nerve sheath hematoma
  - Motility defect
  - Pupillary abnormalities
  - Dellen
- Trials:
  - IONOT: Ischemic optic neuropathy decompression trial in NAION
  - Result: ON sheath decompression in NAION not effective
  - In papilledema, 70% patients relieved from headache and papilledema
  - Hence recommended in pseudotumor cerebri patients with progressive vision loss and headache in spite of medical treatment

What are the causes of pseudo-papilledema?

- Disc edema without raised ICT
- Causes:
  - Inflammatory: Optic neuritis, neuro-retinitis, papillo-phlebitis, uveitis, focal choroiditis
  - Peri-optic meningitis, glioma, mass lesion (orbit)
  - Infiltrative: Lymphoma, leukemia, reticulo-endothelial cell carcinoma
  - Vascular: AION, CRVO, systemic malignant HTN
  - Metabolic: Dysthyroid eye disease, DM
  - Neoplastic:
    - Hemangioma, glioma, metastasis (disc)
    - Intracranial masses, sphenoidal ridge meningiomas
  - Systemic: Anemia, hypoxemia
  - Ocular hypotony
  - Miscellaneous causes:
    - Hypermetropia
    - Narrow optic canal
    - Optic disc drusen
    - Myelinated nerve fibers
    - Glial veil

What is optic neuritis? Classify.

- Inflammation of optic nerve
- Classification:
  - Anatomical
    - Papillitis with ON edema
    - Retrobulbar neuritis without ON edema
    - Neuro-retinitis with macular star (can never be due to MS)
  - Etiological:
    - Demyelinating
    - Infections:
      - Bacterial: TB, syphilis, Lyme
      - Viral: Measles, mumps, chickenpox, HZO
      - Fungal: Cryptococcal
      - Contagious from sinus/orbit/cranium
    - Intraocular inflammation
    - Autoimmune: SLE, Wegner's syndrome, sarcoidosis

What are the clinical features of optic neuritis?

- Typical:
  - Females > males
  - Age 20–40 years
  - White race

- Onset: Sudden painless decreased vision with retrobulbar pain increasing on eye movements
- O/E:
  - Signs and symptoms of optic nerve dysfunction: Vision from no PL to 6/6
  - Peak loss: 2 weeks
  - Starts improving after 2 weeks
  - Decreased contrast: Out of proportion to vision loss
  - Decreased color vision
  - RAPD
  - Disc normal/swelling
  - Vitreous mild inflammation
  - Retinal venous sheathing present, indicates increased risk of MS
  - Vision starts improving after 2 weeks
  - Almost complete recovery by fifth week
  - Uthoff's phenomenon: Worsening of symptoms with rise in body temperature
  - Residual effects:
    - Decreased color
    - Decreased contrast
    - Mild RAPD

What is the differential diagnosis of optic neuritis? (Tables 10.28 and 10.29)

- AION: Papilledema, altitudinal field defects, FFA—no leak
- LHON: Telangiectatic blood vessels around disc, no leak on FFA
- Devic's disease: MRI cavitation + (in MS—gliosis) + Myelitis
- Schilder: Generalized weakness, progressive, <10 years death follows

Table 10.28 Typical versus Atypical Optic Neuritis

Typical	Atypical
Unilateral	Bilateral
Age 20–40	Older patients
Females > males	No predilection
Vision loss within 2 weeks	Beyond 2 weeks
Vision improvement after 2 months	Fails to improve
Painful	Painless

Table 10.29 Difference between Optic Neuritis and Papilledema

	Papilledema	Optic Neuritis
Vision	Normal till secondary optic atrophy sets in	Usually decreased
RAPD	Nil till secondary optic atrophy sets in	Always present
Color	Normal	Decreased
Contrast	Normal	Decreased
Disc edema	Present	Present in 30%
MRI	Cause	Periventricular demyelination

- CRION (chronic inflammatory optic neuropathy):
  - Bilateral, painful, optic neuropathy with blood investigations, CSF, MRI normal
  - Long-term immunosuppression required
- If no improvement on steroids, r/o compressive/infiltrative lesion

What is multiple sclerosis?

- Idiopathic demyelination of CNS
- Does not involve PNS
- Lesions are separated in time and space
- Diagnosis: Two or more neurological events separated in time and space
- Ocular features
  - Sensory:
    - Optic neuritis is the presenting feature in up to 20% of MS patients.
    - Two-thirds will develop it during course of disease.
    - Visual field defects.
    - Will never present as neuro-retinitis (rule out intermediate uveitis/retinal vasculitis).
  - Motor:
    - Inter nuclear ophthalmoplegia (INO)
    - Horizontal gaze palsy

- One and a half syndrome
- Duchenne Muscular Dystrophy (DMB)
- Ocular dysmetria
- Skew
- Nystagmus
- Isolated cranial nerve involvement
- Other CNS lesions:
  - Hemisphere: Dementia, dysphagia, hemiparesis
  - Brain stem: Dysarthria, dysphagia, ataxia, nystagmus
  - Spinal cord: Motor/sensory/bladder + Bowel + Sexual dysfunction
- Transient disturbances:
  - Lhermitte's sign: Pain on neck flexion
  - Uthoff's sign: Symptoms increase on exercise due to raised temperature
  - Trigeminal neuralgia

Explain risk factors and prognosis for multiple sclerosis.

- Positive risk factors are:
  - Patient:
    - Age: 20–40
    - Sex: Female
    - Race: White
    - Family history: Present
  - Ocular:
    - Uthoff's phenomenon present
    - FFA shows a leak present at disc margins
    - Optic neuritis in fellow eye
    - Recurrences positive
  - Systemic:
    - Other CNS symptoms/signs present
    - HLA DR 2 positive
    - CSF: Oligoclonal bands
    - MRI: Peri-ventricular lesions (≥3, each ≥3 mm in size)
- Prognosis: 3R's
  - Recovery from MS
    - 100% show some recovery
    - 75% show full recovery
  - Recurrence of MS—75% have no recurrence
  - Risk of MS
    - 75% females develop MS
    - 35% males develop MS

What is the management of MS? Explain prognosis along with risk factors as well as possibility of future development of lesions?

- Investigations required in a case of MS depends on type of MS:
  - Typical:
    - Routine investigations not required
    - MRI indicated
  - Atypical, recurring, and in children:
    - Routine investigations required
    - Mantoux and X-ray chest (TB)
    - VDRL, FTA-ABS (syphilis)
    - Immunofluorescence and ELIZA (Lyme disease)
    - ANA (sarcoidosis)
    - TORCH titers (toxoplasma)
    - Viral markers (HIV)
    - CSF
    - MRI
- Role of MRI (preferred over CT):
  - Rules out other causes, such as compressive lesion
  - Diagnosis of PNS involvement
  - MRI has excellent ability to show demyelinating plaque
  - Size >2 mm, site and number of plaques identified
  - Guides re-treatment with interferon to delay MS
- MRI criteria for diagnosis of MS:
  - At least three lesions, out of which two will abutt lateral ventricles
  - Will have diameter ≥5 mm
  - Will be infratentorial
- On MRI:
  - Ovoid periventricular and corpus callosum plaque with long axis perpendicular to ventricular margin
- On CSF:
  - Oligoclonal bands
  - Not necessary in routine evaluation of typical optic neuritis
  - Indicated in atypical cases
- Natural course:
  - Vision worsens for two weeks, then improves
  - Almost complete recovery by five weeks

Summarize various studies as well as newer treatments for MS?

- Studies:
  - ONTT (optic neuro-retinitis treatment trial)
  - CHAMPS (the controlled high-risk Avonex MS trial)
  - ETOMS (early treatment of MS study)
  - Champions (controlled high-risk Avonex MS prevention surveille)

1) ONTT:
- Aim:
  - Efficacy of steroid treatment
  - Relationship between MS and optic neuritis
- 457 patients enrolled, randomized to three treatment regimes
- Treatment given:
  - IV steroids—IV methyl prednisolone × 3 days + Oral steroids × 11 days
  - Oral steroids—14 days
  - Placebo—14 days
- Results: For recovery from MS
  - IV steroids vs. placebo
    - Faster recovery
    - Final vision outcome same
    - Though visual fields, color, contrast better
  - Oral steroids vs. placebo: No difference
- Results for recurrence of MS:
  - IV steroids vs. placebo: No difference
  - Oral steroids vs. placebo: Higher recurrence
- Results for risk of MS:
  - IV steroids vs. placebo: Lower risk at 1 year but same after that
  - Oral steroids vs. placebo: No difference
- MRI: Important predictor of MS (≥3 mm, each ≥3 mm in size, increases risk by 12 times)

2) CHAMPS:
- Aim: Effectiveness of (Avonex) interferon beta 1a in patients with one demyelinating episode in decreasing likelihood of CDMS or worsening of MRI
- All patients received IV prednisolone (3 days) + 14-day oral steroids
- Then randomized to 2 groups:
  - Interferon intramuscular injection once/week
  - Placebo injection
- Results:
  - Risk of developing fresh newer episode decreased (at the end of 2 years)
  - Worsening of MRI decreased

3) ETOMS:
- Aim: Early treatment of MS with interferon beta-1b is effective in delaying CDMS (after 1st attack)
- MRI diagnosis required
- IFN beta-1a: 22 g subcutaneously weekly for 2 years vs. placebo given
  - Conclusion: Risk of CDMS is much less in interferon treated group

4) CHAMPION:
- Controlled high-risk Avonex (IFN beta-1a) multiple sclerosis prevention surveillance
- Aim: Results of Avonex given as "immediate" or "delayed" (after 30 months) was compared
- IT (immediate treatment): As in Champ study
- DT (delayed treatment): After 3 months
- Results:
  - IT (compared to DT):
    - Recurrence less
    - CDMS developed less
    - MRI changes were less
- Newer treatments:
  - Immunosuppressive: Azathioprine + Cyclophosphamide/methotrexate/cladribine
  - Immunomodulators: Anti-CD4 monoclonal antibodies, IV immunoglobin, Copolymer 1
  - Stem cell transplant (not proven)

What are the other causes of antigen-specific central nervous system (CNS) inflammatory demyelinating autoimmunity manifesting optic neuritis? (Table 10.30)

Table 10.30 Optic Neuritis Manifestation of Autoimmune Diseases with Inflammatory and Demyelinating Antigen-Specific CNS

Disease	Clinical Features	Biomarker	MRI and Imaging	Treatment
NNeuromyelitis optica (NMO) or Devic's disease	Rare but major cause of acute or subacute unilateral or bilateral vision loss. Transverse myelopathy often precedes or follows vision loss, other neurological signs maybe present.	AQP4IgG positive, negative for anti-MOG Ab. II 6 and IL 6 receptor markers are increased in NMO. GFAP + in highly active inflammatory NMO.	Spinal cord: Involvement of long segment of cord (>4 vertebral bodies) and extending more than 2/3 of cross-section. Brain: peri-ependymal lesions surrounding third ventricle and cerebral aqueduct, thalamus, hypothalamus, and midbrain.	High-dose intravenous steroids (1gram IV methylprednisolone daily for five days) followed by a slow taper of oral prednisone and long-term immunosuppressive therapy. Plasmapheresis for acute symptoms.
MOG Ab associated Optic neuritis	Rare, but important cause of significant vision loss, though usually recovers. Diverse and recurrent course. Optic disk edema, may be severe, bilateral, and recurrent optic neuritis. Variable neurological signs.	MOG Ab positive, negative for AQP4IgG	Long segments of optic nerve enhancement, enhancement with extension to the peribulbar fat may be seen. MRI also shows periorbital involvement commonly in acute attack.	Corticosteroids (prolonged treatment), plasmapheresis if severe acute presentation.

AQP4 IgG = Aquaporin 4 immunoglobulin G
MOG Ab = Myelin oligodendrocyte glycoprotein antibody

What is optic atrophy? And how do you diagnose the same?

- Definition: Abnormal pallor of the disc as a result of damage to the ganglion cells and axon of the reticulo-geniculate pathway leading to loss of conducting function of the optic nerve.
- Pathogenesis: Involves two processes, degeneration of optic nerve fibers and proliferation of astrocytes and glial tissue
- Pathology:
  - Proliferation of glial tissue
  - Decreased number of capillaries
  - Destruction of nerve fibers

- Volume of nerve fibers decreased
- Diagnosis:
  - Fundus appearance of a pale disc
  - Optic nerve dysfunction: Decreased vision, color desaturation, RAPD, visual fields, and VEP changes
  - Increased excavation
  - Abnormal disc pallor

What is the mechanism of pallor noted in optic atrophy?

- Normal optic disc is pink
- Pallor occurs when:

- When light falls on a normal disc the transparent axons, conduct the light while the capillaries reflect it back making it appear pink.
- Atrophic disc is mainly glial tissue, which is not transparent, and hence, no light is reflected back.
- Thus, appears pale.

What is the classification of optic atrophy? (Tables 10.31 and 10.32)

- Classification:
  - Pathological:
    - Ascending: Wallerian degeneration—primary lesion is in the choroid, retina, optic nerve
      - Causes are RD, CRAO, glaucoma, choroiditis, trauma, toxins, PRP, papilledema.
    - Descending: Primary lesion is in the brain, chiasma, optic tract, LGB lesions

Table 10.31 Types of Optic Atrophy

Type	Primary	Secondary	Cavernous (Schnabel's)	Segmental	Consecutive
Definition	Orderly degeneration of ON fibers replaced by alteration in the architecture of ON head	Marked degeneration of the optic nerve fibers with proliferation of glial tissue ONH architecture is lost	Axonal degeneration without any glial tissue proliferation Caverns filled with hyaluronic acid	Temporal Degeneration of the axial fibers or papillomacular bundle which enters temporally (Nissl's degeneration)	Following diseases of retinal nerve fibers Choroid, ganglion cells
Disc appearance	Chalky white color Sharp margins Normal retinal blood vessels Normal surrounding and peripheral retina	Dirty gray with poorly defined margins Cup obliterated by glial tissue Peripapillary sheathing, arterial narrowing, drusen around the disc	Cup vertical increased in size NR rim notch Pallor of the rim Laminar dot sign Backward bowing of lamina cribrosa bayoneting sign baring of circumlinear vessels Peripapillary atrophy and halo Disc saucerization	Temp pallor Margins clear Blood vessels normal No other fundus pathology	Waxy color Normal margins Arterial attenuation Normal cup with some retinal pathology

Table 10.31 (Continued) Types of Optic Atrophy

Type	Primary	Secondary	Cavernous (Schnabel's)	Segmental	Consecutive
Causes	ON injuries ON tumors Pituitary tumors Optic neuritis Tabes dorsalis Band/bowtie: Chiasmal syndrome with bi-temporal defect	Papilledema papillitis	Glaucoma, methyl alcohol poisoning, demyelination, tabes dorsalis, chronic ischemia	Temporal pallor: Toxic optic neuropathy Altitudinal: AION, Wedge: BRAO	RP, Choroditis, PRP, myopia, CRAO, quinine, cerebro-macular degeneration, myopia, long-standing retinal detachment

Table 10.32 Other Types of Optic Atrophy

Pressure/traction	Toxic	Nutritional	Traumatic
Glaucoma	Tobacco, pipe smoking and alcohol	B12, B6, B1, B2 deficiency	Tear in nerve fiber
Post-papilledema	Drugs:	Bilateral decrease vision	Due to fracture fragment compressing the nerve fiber
Sclerotic calcified arteries causing pressure on the optic nerve	Ethambutol, quinine, INH, sulfa	Post-column sensory loss	Hematoma
ICA-optic chiasma	Chloramphenicol	Ataxia motor neuron disease decreased tendon reflexes	Concussion ON avulsion
Ophthalmic artery optic foramen Aneurysmal ICA Basal arachnoiditis	Central or centro-cecal scotoma		

- Clinical:
  - Primary
  - Secondary
  - Consecutive
  - Cavernous (glaucomatous)
  - Segmental: Temporal, altitudinal, wedge-shaped
- Etiological
- Consecutive: Due to lesions of ocular tissues: Retina, choroid, optic disc
  - Circulatory: CRAO, arteriosclerosis, AION, NAION
  - Post-inflammatory
    - Local: Intraocular, optic neuritis
    - Septicemia, TB, syphilis
    - CNS: Multiple sclerosis, encephalitis
- Metastasis
  - Metabolic: DM, thyroid, nutritional
  - Traumatic
  - Hereditary:
    - Autosomal Dominant optic atrophy
    - Leber's hereditary optic neuropathy (LHON)

What are the causes of opto-ciliary shunt vessels?

- Meningioma
- Glioma
- Old CRVO
- Chronic papilledema
- Idiopathic

10.6 RETINA-RELATED

10.6.1 Lenses used for fundus biomicroscopy

Which are the lenses used in indirect fundus biomicroscopy?

- Non-contact
  - Concave lenses: Hruby lens
  - Convex lenses: +60 D, +78 D, +90 D
  - Indirect lenses: +30 D, +40 D, +14/+15 D
- Contact
  - Modified Koeppe's lens
  - Goldmann three-mirror lens

Identify and state the characteristics of the following lens.

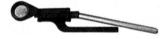

Figure 10.27 Hruby lens

- Power: −58.6 D (concave lens)
- Non-contact
- Slit-lamp mounted for stability
- Image: Inverted, real, minified
- Advantage: Good resolution
- Disadvantages:
  - Small field, cannot visualize beyond equator
  - Small magnification (5–8°), i.e., about 1 DD
  - Therefore, used as only diagnostic lens
  - Precise patient fixation is required

Identify and state the characteristics of the following lens.

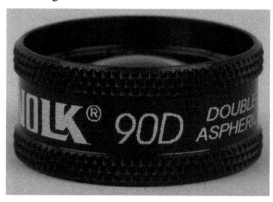

Figure 10.28 +90 D lens

- Non-contact
- Handheld
- Image: Real, inverted, laterally reversed, field wide, magnified
- Working distance from the cornea: 6.5 mm
- Features a small 26 mm diameter ring for dynamic fundoscopy

What is the magnification of the image? (Table 10.33)

- Magnification = Power of the eye × magnification of the slit lamp/power of the lens
- Therefore, magnification of a +90 D lens = 60/90 × 10 = 7.6
- Thus, field of view is directly proportional, and magnification is inversely proportional to the power of the lens
- Stereopsis = Magnification/4
- Field of view = Dioptric power (DP) of the lens × 2
- Lens image magnification working distance (mm)

Identify and state the characteristics of the following lens.

- Working distance from the cornea: 11 mm
- High magnification views of the posterior pole
- Useful in detailed optic disc and macula imaging

Identify and state the characteristics of the following lens.

- Excellent in general diagnosis
- Ideal balance of magnification and field of view
- Working distance from the cornea: 7 mm

Table 10.33 Lens Magnification

Lens	Image Magnification	Working distance (mm)
60 D	1.15	13
Super 66	1	11
78 D	0.93	8
90 D	0.76	7

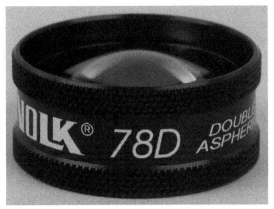

Figure 10.31 +78 D lens

- Powerful convex lens
- Biconvex aspheric with one surface more curved than the other
- Less curved surface toward the patient's eye (silver lined)
- Acts as:
  - Condensing lens for the illuminating system
  - It forms inverted image of the retina in space, which is then focused through the eyepiece
  - Technique is "indirect" because image of the fundus is seen through a condensing lens forming an image in space, which is visualized, rather than the actual fundus
  - Image: Formed close to the principle focus of the lens between lens and observer
  - Retinal magnification: 60/20 = 3×
  - Field of view = 40° (20 × 2)

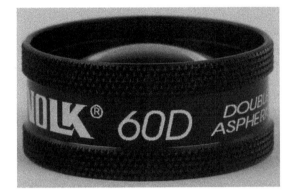

Figure 10.29 +60 D lens

What are the advantages of these lenses?

- Stereoscopic three-dimensional view of the retina
- Binocular viewing through slit lamp
- Can view image through media opacities such as cataract
- Allows for manipulation of images
- Using slit-lamp magnification and filters
- Image size is less affected by patients' refractive error

Identify and state the characteristics of the following lens.

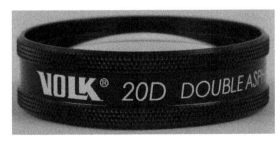

Figure 10.30 +20 D lens

Identify and state the characteristics of the following lens.

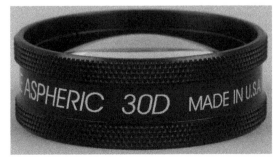

Figure 10.32 +30 D lens

- High dioptric power
- Therefore, least magnification (60/30 = 2×)
- Stereopsis is half that of normal (2/4 = 1/2)
- Field of view is the largest (30 × 2 = 60°)
- Uses:
  - Panoramic view of the fundus
  - Small pupil fundoscopy possible
  - Disadvantage: Fundus details are not seen well as image is minified

Identify and state the characteristics of the following lens.

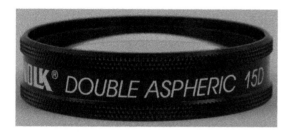

Figure 10.33 +15 D lens

- Low dioptric power lens
- Retinal magnification = 4 × (60/15)
- Stereopsis maximum (4/4)
- Field of view = 30° (15/2)
- Use: Detailed view of macula/optic disc for determining evaluation of retina in shallow retinal detachments

What are the magnifications and stereopsis of these various lenses? (Table 10.34)

What are the various lenses used for contact bio microscopy of the fundus?

- Modified Koeppe's lens
- Goldmann three-mirror contact lens
- Wide-field pan-fundoscopic indirect contact lens

10.6.2 Lenses for lasers

Common characteristics of all lenses

Lenses for retinal laser treatment (PRP/focal laser)
- Surface: Posterior concave to confirm corneal curvature
- Anterior: Flat/convex
- Mirrors: Allow examination of peripheral retina/angle
- Prisms: Allow examination of mid- peripheral retina
- Flange: Stabilization and prevention of blink
- Knurled edge for ease of manipulation
- Shell is conical made of PMMA and Aluminum
- Anti-reflection coating (ARC)
  - Decreases reflected white light from slit lamp
  - Decreases laser light from treatment beam that could pose a potential hazard to an observer standing behind the laser operator
  - ARC decreases reflected light between 400 and 700 nm from approximately 4% to <1%
- Sterilization: ETO

Identify the following lenses used in PRP and focal laser and state their main differences? (Table 10.35)

Table 10.35 Image Characteristics of Laser Lenses

Plano Concave	High plus Power
E.g., Three-mirror	Indirect
Image: Upright	Image: Inverted
Resolution: Good	Resolution: Good
Field: Limited	Field: Wide

Table 10.34 Lens Magnification and Stereopsis

Lens Power (D)	Magnification	Field of View	Stereopsis	Working Distance from Cornea (mm)
+30 D	2×	60°	1/2	26
+20 D	3.25×	40°	3/4	47
+14/+15 D	4.17×	30°	1	72

Identify and state the characteristics of the following lens (Table 10.36).

Figure 10.34 Mainster lens

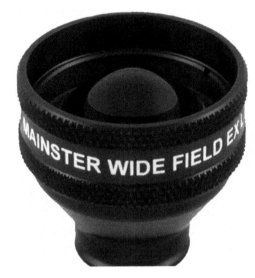

Figure 10.35 Mainster wide-field lens

- Biconvex aspheric anterior lens element and a concave lens to corneal curvature
- Image: Real inverted situation in front of lens

- Advantages:
  - Field: 58% greater than Goldmann
  - But lateral and axial magnification better, therefore good for diagnosis of macular pathology
  - Good resolution

Identify the following lenses and state their differences (Table 10.37).

Identify and state the characteristics of the following lens.

Figure 10.36 Rodenstock pan fundus

- Power: 85 D
- Parts: Biconvex spherical anterior lens element
- Image: Real, inverted inside biconvex lens
- Anterior surface: Convex spherical
- Advantages:
  - Good panoramic view
  - Field 84% greater than Goldmann
  - Magnification 24% less than Goldmann
  - Spot size >40% with conventional CL
  - Precautions: Slit lamp should be pulled away from patient's eye
  - Disadvantage: Peripheral distortion of reflexes, view of periphery difficult

Table 10.36 Differences in Laser Lenses

Type of Lens	Goldmann	Panfundoscopic	Mainster
Anterior surface	Flat	Convex spherical	Convex aspherical
Image type	Virtually erect	Real inverted	Real inverted
Power	−67	85	61
Lateral magnification	0.93	0.71	0.96
Relative magnification	1	0.76	1.03
Axial magnification	0.86	0.51	0.92
Spot size settings (actual in microns) → effective with lens			
100	108	141	105
200	216	282	210
500	541	704	524
1000	1081	1409	1048

Table 10.37 Differences between Mainster Standard, Wide-Field, and Ultra-Wide-Field Lens

	Mainster Standard	Mainster Wide-Field	Mainster Ultra-Wide Field
Field	Post-pole to mid-peripheral (90–121°)	118–127°	165–180°
Image magnification	0.96 times	0.68 times	0.51 times
Laser spot magnification	1.05 times	1.5 times	1.96 times
Anterior surface	Convex aspheric	Convex aspheric	Convex aspheric
Uses	Due to good magnification—good to diagnose Macular edema Macular thickness CNV—focal and grid laser	PRP	PRP

Identify and state the characteristics of the following lenses.

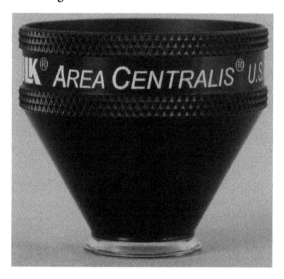

Figure 10.37 Volk area centralis lens

- Indirect contact lens
- Good field of view = 70/84°
- Image magnification is good = 1.06×
- Laser spot magnification = 0.94×

Identify and state the characteristics of the following lenses.

- Field of view = 115/137°
- Image magnification is good = 0.67×
- Laser spot magnification = 1.5×
- Allows CNVM treatment up to maximum spot size of 6400 μm providing excellent visualization

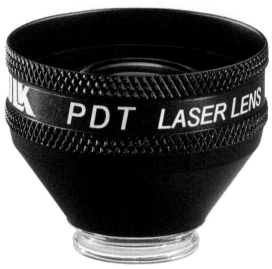

Figure 10.38 Volk PDT lens

- Comes with SupraCoat which covers the 689 nm laser wavelength indicated in this type of procedure

Identify and state the characteristics of the following lenses.

Volk transequator lens
- Designed for focal therapy and mid to far peripheral fundus diagnosis
- It has a wide field of view, which presents a realistic contour of the retina due to the unique optical design of the lens.
- Superior optics allows dynamic globe movements
- Field of view = 110/132°
- Image magnification = 0.70×

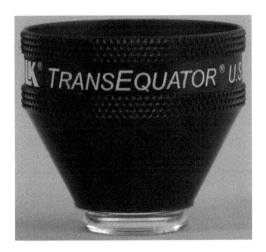

Figure 10.39 Volk trans-equator lens

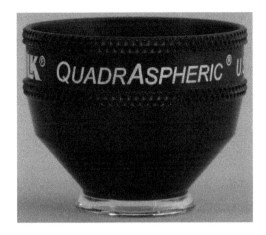

Figure 10.40 Volk quadraspheric lens

- Laser spot magnification = 1.44×
- Image: Real, inverted, and laterally reversed
- Advantages:
  - Small pupil viewing possible
  - Diameter 28.6 mm, therefore good for peripheral viewing
  - Anti-reflective coating
  - Four aspheric surfaces, which decreases astigmatic across entire field
- Uses: PRP, peripheral tears/holes laser

Identify and state the characteristics of the following lenses (Table 10.38).

- Extreme wide-field examination
- Double aspheric
- Have high-grade low-dispersion glass, which gives superior image quality PRP treatments
- Replaced older Superquad 160
- Magnification = 0.5×
- Laser spot = 2.0×
- Field of view = 160°
- Uses
  - HR wide field: Used in PRP
  - Smaller and easier to manipulate in patient's orbit
  - Short length of lens helps to manipulate in front of laser
  - Widest field of view to ora serrata
  - Double aspheric
  - Have high-grade, low-dispersion glass, which gives superior image quality
  - Replaced older Volk optical area centralis
  - Magnification = 1.08×

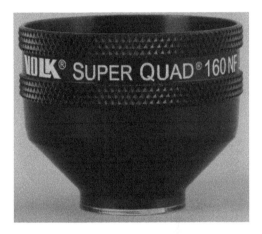

Figure 10.41 Volk super quadraspheric 160 lens

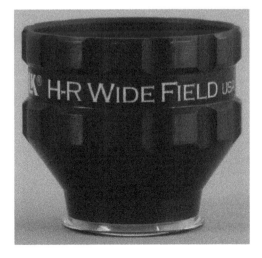

Figure 10.42 High-resolution (HR) wide-field lens

Table 10.38 Volk Quadaspheric versus Super Quad Lens

	Volk Quadraspheric Lens	Volk Super Quadraspheric 160 Lens
Field	130°	160°
Image	Inverted and reversed	Inverted and reversed
Uses	• Four aspheric surfaces and has ARC coatings thereby reducing astigmatism across entire field of view • Enhances visualization through small pupils • Preferred wide-field fundus laser lens for diagnosis and treatment of retina	• Widest field of view • Simultaneous visualization of posterior pole to the peripheral retina • Therefore greater safety margin during extreme wide-angle PRP • Ideal lens for visualization and treatment of PDR, ischemic RVO, peripheral retinal holes and tears
Image magnification	0.51×	0.5×
Laser spot magnification	1.97×	2×

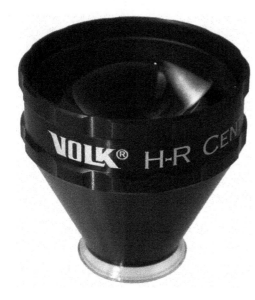

Figure 10.43 High-resolution (HR) centralis lens

- Laser spot size = 0.92×
- Field of view = 74°
- Uses:
  - Used for focal and grid laser
  - Detailed posterior pole examination
  - Better in smaller pupil sizes
  - Reduced size housing helps manipulate within the orbit

How does one clean these lenses?

- Clean with the contact lens cleaner solution or warm water, not hot water

- Dry with soft lint-free cloth
- Never autoclave or boil lenses
- Alternately place the lenses in
- 3% hydrogen peroxide solution
- 2% glutaraldehyde aqueous solution for 20 minutes
- Sodium hypochlorite 1:10 parts for 10 minutes
- Pure 70% isopropyl alcohol for 10 minutes

10.6.3 Retina-viewing systems for surgery

What are the challenges for VR operating viewing systems?

- Many tissues involved are transparent
- Special optical systems needed to re-invert images for practical manipulation during surgery
- Easily obscured view due to blood, air bubbles, altered fluidics during vitreous manipulation
- Peripheral retina and vitreous base at times are difficult to access

What are the various approaches for VR operating viewing systems?

- Initially used plano-concave or biconcave lenses which provided, direct image (no invertor needed) 20–30° field of view (FOV)

- Difficult to manipulate and needed changes for vitreous states
- Various modifications of the classical lenses have been tried to overcome these challenges
  - Small diameter lenses
  - Sewed on contact lenses
  - Handheld irrigating lenses
  - Self-stabilizing systems for lenses (e.g., SSV system by Volk)
  - Two newer approaches
    - Wide-angle viewing systems
    - Endoscopic systems
    - Use of end-aspirating endo illuminator reduces bleeding and other obscurations to viewing vitreous

What are the classical or conventional lenses?

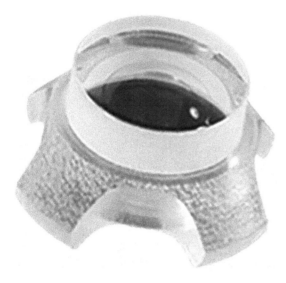

Figure 10.44 Sewed-on contact lenses

Classified based on:
- Optical design
- Anchoring mechanism
- Irrigating method
- Material of manufacture
- Corneal contact lenses usually made of plastic, glass, or quartz
- If >10 mm in diameter, do not move freely; if <9 mm, more prone to displacement
- Posterior concave curvature necessary to neutralize corneal power
- Longer radius of curvature than that of cornea to prevent air bubbles and blood accumulation in between lens and cornea

- Anterior surface usually plano, needs indentation to view beyond equator
- Anterior surface can be inclined to give lens a prism configuration and offer a more peripheral fundus view
- Non-magnified view but microscope compensates
- Types:
  - Small-diameter contact lenses:
    - Diameter: 9.8 mm
    - Stays due to capillary action
    - Lightweight, easy to sterilize
    - No assistant needed
    - Not stable during tilting of eyeball for manipulation
  - Sewed-on contact lenses:
    - Contact lens placed over a metallic ring, sewn at limbus to sclera
    - Lenses directly put into the ring
    - Entire set of lenses can be placed in the same ring, depending on eye state
    - No assistant needed
    - Sutures needed over sclera
    - Can block view to collection of blood and debris between lens and cornea
  - Handheld irrigating lenses:
    - Continuous supply of fluid
    - Assistant must hold the lens and manipulate according to the operating surgeon's direction
    - Does not get blocked by blood or debris
    - Fluid film prevents contact loss
    - Needs good viewing system for assistant as well as experience
    - Can cause epithelial damage to cornea, or excessive pressure

Give examples of direct viewing, conventional lenses.

- Landers system plano concave lens: Core vitrectomy
  - Landers biconcave lens: Visualization in air-filled eye (90 D lens—25° angle field)
  - Machemer's magnifying lens: Surface details on posterior pole (28–30° angle field)
  - Peyman wide-field lens: Equatorial portion
  - Tolentino 20° prism: Periphery
  - Tolentino 30° prism: Extreme periphery

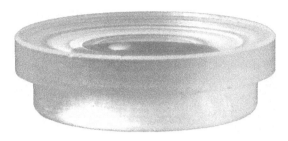

Figure 10.45 Landers system of conventional direct viewing lenses

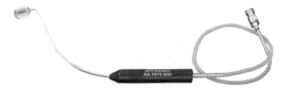

Figure 10.46 Machemer's plano-concave

- Machemer's plano-concave irrigating lens (plano/–45 D) for phakic and pseudophakic lens
  - Field of view = 36°
  - Both for macular and detachments surgeries
- Biconcave irrigating lens (90 D)
  - For air filled phakic and pseudophakic eyes
  - Field of view = 24°

What is the principle of wide-angle viewing system?

- Uses principle of indirect ophthalmoscope (astronomical telescope)
- Objective = Cornea and natural lens
- Eyepiece = High plus condensing lens
- Produces real, inverted, aerial image of retina
- Re-inversion using stereoscopic image inversion systems
- The use of two adjoining but orthogonally oriented prisms
- Can be moved into or out of the viewing path of the microscope in either a manual or mechanized manner.
- Common properties of all contact and non-contact wide-angle systems are an inverted fundus view and a device to convert the image to a normally oriented view of the field

- In an emmetropic eye, parallel rays from the eye, pass through strong convex ophthalmoscopy lens with zero vergence, and focus in the focal plane of the ophthalmoscopic lens that is located 5.8 mm from its principal plane
- Beyond that point, the rays within the rays are divergent
- Aerial image of the patient's fundus is formed in the focal plane of the ophthalmoscopy lens
- This fundus image viewed by surgeon is real and inverted through the operating microscope
- The basic principle is similar to that of indirect ophthalmoscopy

Examples of indirect wide-angle viewing systems.

- Contact type:
  - VPFS (vitreous panfundoscope)
  - CWF (contact wide-field system)
  - AVIS (advanced visual instrument system)
  - ROLS (reinverting operating lens system)
  - Clarivit
  - HRX (Volk Optical)
- Non-contact type:
  - BIOM (binocular IDO): (Oculus)
  - MERLIN (Volk Optical)
  - EIBOS (Erect Indirect Binocular IDO)
  - OFFISS (Topcon)
  - RESIGHT (Carl Zeiss): Peyman–Wessels–Landers

Describe a wide-angle contact viewing system?

- Rodenstock panfundoscope system (PFS)
  - Original Rodenstock panfundoscope lens was designed without invertor, which was later incorporated to serve the need for free-hand vitreous surgery manipulation
  - Inverted image, thus needs SDI (stereoscopic diagonal inverter)
  - Field of view = 120–130°
  - Held by handle or standard lens ring
  - Contact-based wide-angle visualization provides 10° greater field of view than non-contact systems (BIOM and EIBOS)
  - Eliminates corneal asphericity
  - Decreases the need for ocular rotation (tool flex) to view the periphery

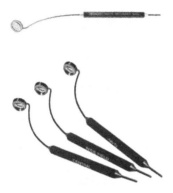

Figure 10.47 Biconcave irrigating lens—90 D

- Although PFS provides a wide field, it is relatively heavy and distorts retinal images especially in air-filled eyes
  - PFS (vitreous panfundoscope)
  - Meniscus lens is coupled with a spherical lens and it gives real, inverted image. The field of view is wide, and the image is small.
- ROLS (Re-inverting Operating Lens System)
  - Single-element re-inverter prism design to correct the inverted image, ensures left/right fusion, high-efficiency light transmission
  - Perfect optical transparency for better view of inferior fundus
  - Provides excellent transparency and stereopsis
  - Fits many microscopes: Zeiss style
  - Wild style fits only Leica/Wild microscope
  - ROLS does not touch the eye; thus, no sterilization is required.
    - Super Macula lens: 60°
    - Mini Quad lenses: 127°
    - Mini Quad XL lenses: 134°
    - Dyna: 156°
- Parts:
  - Lens positioning unit (LPU): Includes the fine focus wheel for precise focusing.
  - ROLS Infinity—powered version of ROLS which auto aligns when the LPU is rotated into place. It has the condensing lens assembly (CLA) system, which, along with the invertor system, aligns into place, with LED indicators for the same.

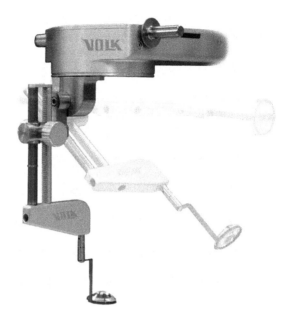

Figure 10.48 Volk's Merlin viewing system

- Three lenses used with the Merlin system (ACS indicated steam autoclavable):
- WIDE ANGLE ACS® LENS: FOV = 102/120°: Widest field of view, allowing visualization of the retina approaching the ora serrata
- MID FIELD ACS® LENS: FOV = 80/95°: Higher magnification lens for clearest views of the macula
- SMALL WIDE-ANGLE ACS® LENS: FOV = 95/112°: Smallest diameter lens, ideal for patients with small pupils or deep-seated eyes, and pediatric cases. Lens fogging is reduced compared to classical wide angle

What are the advantages and disadvantages of wide-angle contact viewing systems?

- Advantages:
  - Easy introduction of instruments without disturbing lens
  - Greater field of view
  - Better clarity
- Disadvantages:
  - Bulky and not very stable on the cornea
  - Hard to maintain a steady view of the fundus because an assistant must hold the lens precisely on the cornea well centered and coaxial with the microscope

- This makes the surgery cumbersome both for the surgeon and for the assistant besides warranting the need for a skilled assistant to hold the lens

Describe the wide-angle non-contact viewing systems for VR surgery?

- Independent Viewing Systems (IVS)
  - Type of system for viewing the intraoperative vitrectomy surgery such that when the IVS lens goes down, the focus is anterior, and while the lens goes up, focus is posterior.
  - Manipulation is easier when IVS lens is away from cornea, but field of view is increased when the lens is closer to the cornea.
  - Or place HPMC onto the cornea.

Table 10.39 Differences between Non-Contact and Contact VR Operative Viewing Systems

Non-Contact System	Contact System
No assistant required	Skilled assistant required
No corneal trauma	Corneal trauma +/− → lens and corneal opacity
Good with FAE	Not easy with fluid air exchange
Good for pediatric cases or in steep cornea	Not easy in pediatric cases and poor in steep corneal curvature
Great depth of focus	Depth not so marked
Can move eye and maintain a good image	Image lost if eye rotated
Has steep learning curve	No learning curve
Less optical resolution than contact systems	Better resolution; gives up to 150° of view
Expensive and may require modification of microscope	Not so expensive

- IVS provides reduced depth perception compared with contact viewing system.
- OCULUS Binocular Indirect Ophthalmomicroscope (BIOM)
  - Invented by Dr Spinatz
  - IO principal with operating microscope
  - SDI is used to invert the image
  - Fast mount and easy shift during surgery
  - A wide angle of view: 90–110°
- Stereoscopic Diagonal Inverter (SDI)
  - It is an inverter system incorporated in the operating microscope to re-invert the inverted image.
  - It was invented by Spitznas and Reiner.
  - It provides a stereoscopic image with good depth of field.

What are the differences between the non-contact and contact VR operative viewing systems? (Table 10.39)

What is the self-stabilizing systems for contact lenses used for viewing during Vitrectomy? (E.g., SSV system by Volk)

- These are modifications for the various types of contact lenses used during visualization for vitrectomy
- Most of the standard lenses are available with special flanges to allow for stabilization over the cornea without the use of assistant using handles
- Uses coupling agent: HPMC
- Creates vacuum like hold, but not very stable for globe manipulation
- Can loose "contact" during indentation for peripheral visualization
- Corneal distortion, similar to other contact lens use

What is the chandelier viewing system?

A self-retaining 27G chandelier endo illuminator was developed by Oshima in 2007.

Figure 10.49 SSV contact-type lenses

- The chandelier illumination system is fixed in the sclera using a separate port and provides wide-angle diffuse lighting.
- Eckardt introduced a 27G dual-light chandelier illumination system, which utilizes two sclerotomies to provide homogenous lighting and minimize shadows seen with single-fiber chandelier systems.
- Advantage of chandelier system: Superior video image quality
- Disadvantage of chandelier system:
  - The distant diffuse fixed illumination may make identifying dissection planes at the surgical point of interest more difficult and cause glare after fluid–air exchange.
  - Diffuse illumination also reduces the ability to see transparent structures, such as ILM, ERM, and the vitreous layers, compared to focal illumination from light pipes.
  - Greater shadows cast by instruments in the path of the light.
  - Thermal buildup.

What are the other advances in VR viewing systems?

- The use of 3D visualization systems using acquisition of two horizontally disparate images using high-dynamic 3D digital cameras and then passively separating them into polaroid 3D glasses displayed on 4K organic light emitting diode (OLED) screens using ultra-HD technology
- This has enabled the development of heads-up display systems like:
  - NGENUITY 3D system (Alcon)
  - Panoramic RUV system (Leica)

10.7 LASERS IN OPHTHALMOLOGY

What is the full form of the word "laser"?

- Light amplification of simulated emission of radiation

What is the principle of laser?

- Energy source: Stimulates active medium, which may be gas/liquid/solid, to emit specific wavelength of light. This light is amplified in an optical feedback system through the active medium and there the emitted light is known as laser beam.

- Projection of laser compared to white light.
- It is monochromatic.
- It is coherent; i.e., there isn't any divergence of beam, so the spot size is predictable.

What are the parts of a laser?

- Lasing medium: The nature of lasing medium decides the wavelength of laser. Lasing medium decides the name of laser.
- Excitation source: Within the lasing medium, i.e., light, electricity, heat, ionizing radiation.
- Amplification: Paired mirrors for optical feedback. One mirror is fully reflective (back mirror), and front mirror is partially reflective.

What are the modes of laser operations?

- Continuous wavelength:
  - A continuous stream of photons is delivered
  - E.g., thermal laser (argon, krypton, infrared diode, and frequency doubled YAG)
- Pulsed laser:
  - Long pulsed laser
    - Energy pulses of tens of microseconds/milliseconds effect:
    - Thermal
    - E.g., argon and pulsed dye laser
  - Short pulsed laser
    - Q-switched:
      - Energy pulses are delivered in nanoseconds. They are photo-disruptive.
      - Very little thermal effect, so called as cold laser
      - E.g., Q-switched ruby and Q-switched Nd:YAG
    - Mode-locked:
      - Energy pulses are delivered as a train of short duration (picoseconds).
      - Cumulative effect of pulses causes photo disruption.

What are the types of fundus pigments?

- Melanin:
  - Absorbs all wavelengths especially green and red
  - Peak: 460–620 nm

- Hemoglobin:
  - Absorbs yellow and green
  - Red not absorbed
  - Peak: 400–580 nm
- Xanthophyll:
  - Absorbs blue
  - Peak: 480 nm

What are the methods of laser delivery? (Table 10.40)

- Transpupillary
- Slit lamp: With and without contact lens
- Laser indirect ophthalmoscope (LIO)
  - Indirect ophthalmoscope used for delivery of either argon green or diode laser
  - Retinal spot size = (Spot size at image plane × Power of indirect lens)/(Refractive power of average eye)
  - Effect of refraction on spot size (Table 10.41):
    - Minus refraction decreases and plus refraction increases spot size as compared to emmetropia
  - Advantages of LIO over slit lamp:
    - Treatment through media opacities/small pupil possible
    - Peripheral treatment especially with scleral depression possible
    - Patients who cannot sit on slit lamp: e.g.: Treatment of ROP or retinoblastoma in pediatric patients
    - Patients in whom contact lenses cannot be put, like recently operated wounds in cataract, sclerocorneal tear or large glaucoma bleb
    - Intraoperative laser following VR surgery
    - In gas-filled eyes easier to treat retinal lesions
  - Disadvantages of LIO:
    - Cannot be used for macular treatment
    - Aiming beam unstable due to movement of head
- Transscleral
- Endolaser:
  - Indications
  - For PRP
  - Around the break
  - Around retinotomy
  - To arrest bleeding
  - Cyclophotocoagulation
  - To destroy epithelial ingrowth

Table 10.40 Laser Delivery Systems Contact versus Non Contact

Contact	Non-Contact
• Goldmann Panfundoscope • Advantages: — Globe Stabilization better — Lid Separation possible — Accurate localization of Laser beam — Anterior to equator treatment possible — Possibility of corneal and lens damage less	• 78 D • 90 D • Advantages: — Useful in corneal pathology like recurrent corneal erosions, postoperative weak wound and with tarsorrhaphy • Disadvantages: — Globe stabilization not possible — Lid separation not possible — Inaccurate localization of laser beam

Table 10.41 Effect of Vitreous Substitutes

Substitute	Spot Size
Air	Decreases
Gas	Decreases
Silicone oil	Increases
PFCL	Increases

- Advantages over endo cryotherapy:
  - Immediate effect
  - Decreased RPE disturbance, therefore reduced incidence of re-PVR
  - Decreased choroidal bleed:
- Advantages over external cryotherapy:
  - Posterior breaks can be treated.
  - Precise treatment of break is possible.
  - Treatment is possible only when retina is flat.
  - Treatment is also possible in air-/gas-filled eye.

Which lasers are used in posterior segment disorders?

- Green laser as frequency doubled Nd:YAG laser (532 nm) or argon green (514 nm)

- Diode laser (810 nm):
  - Start with low power, longer duration. Retinal spot size decreases and intensity increases as the probe nears the retina.
  - Therefore, rupture of Bruch's membrane, choroidal hemorrhage, and retinal break can occur.

Mention the various lasers, their wavelengths and uses?

- Excimer laser (excited dimer)
  - Active medium: Argon fluoride
  - Wavelength: 193 nm
  - Mechanism of action: Photoablation
  - Uses:
    - PRK
    - PTK
    - LASIK
    - Effective in cutting vitreous membrane; cannot be delivered through fiber optic delivery system
- Dye laser
  - Active medium: Gold-copper
  - Mechanism of action: Photodynamic
  - Use: To destroy intraocular tumor (melanoma, retinoblastoma)
- Argon laser
  - Active medium: Argon fluoride
  - Wavelength: 488–514 nm (blue-green)
    - Mechanism of action: Photocoagulative (thermal)
    - Characteristic: Absorbed by hemoglobin and melanin causing thermal destruction
  - Uses:
    - Posterior segment: PRP (scatter); retinal/choroidal tumors
    - Anterior segment: Iridotomy, trabeculectomy (ALT)
    - Advantages:
      - Absorption by hemoglobin and melanin
      - Continuous wave function
    - Disadvantages:
    - Contraindicaticated in macular pathology (xanthophyll absorbs blue and gets heated)
    - Media opacities like cataract, vitreous hemorrhage due to poor penetration

- Krypton laser:
  - Active medium: Krypton red (continuous wave)
  - Wavelength:
    - Krypton (red): 647 nm
    - Red with green: 521, 531 nm
    - Red with yellow: 568 nm
  - Indications:
    - Choroidal neovascular membrane
    - Red with yellow especially useful in macular treatment because of least absorption by xanthophyll
    - Red absorbed in melanin
    - Yellow absorbed in hemoglobin of vessels
    - Advantages:
      - Can be used through cataract and vitreous hemorrhage
      - Does not cause vitreous heating and hence decrease incidence of macular pucker
    - Disadvantages:
      - Pale fundus without melanin: Laser will be ineffective
      - Ineffective in treating vascular abnormalities
      - Increased incidence of pain
- Nd:YAG
  - Solid-state laser in infrared medium
  - Active medium: Yttrium Aluminum Garnett (YAG)
  - Long wavelength: 1064 nm (pulsed Nd:YAG)
    - Mechanism of action: Photo disruption
    - Uses:
      - Capsulotomy
      - Iridotomy
      - Vitreolysis
      - Available as Q-switched and mode locked
  - Short wavelength: 532 nm (frequency doubled Nd:YAG)
    - Mechanism of action: Photocoagulation
    - Uses:
      - PRP
      - Scatter laser
      - Iridotomy
      - Trabeculoplasty
    - Advantage of YAG over argon green laser: Less absorption by xanthophyll in macula

- Semiconductor diode laser:
  - Active medium: Semiconductor crystal (gallium aluminum arsenide)
  - Wavelength: 810 nm (continuous in infrared spectrum)
  - Mechanism of action: Photocoagulation
  - Indications:
    - Retinal tears
    - CSME
    - PRP in PDR
    - PDT
    - Cyclo-destructive procedures
    - Modes of delivery
      - Transscleral
      - Endprobe
    - Advantages:
      - Excellent penetration through media opacities like VH, cataract in comparison to argon green
      - Less electric consumption
      - Portable, lightweight, longer life
    - Disadvantages:
      - Painful
      - Less precise
      - Increased incidence of deeper burns, leading to enhanced Bruch's membrane rupture and choroidal bleed
      - Not absorbed by hemoglobin so ineffective in direct treatment of hemangioma, telangiectasias
- Dye laser:
  - Medium: Liquid
  - Wavelength: Continuous wave
  - Different wavelength output possible
- CO_2 laser:
  - Active medium: CO_2
  - Wavelength: 10,600 nm
  - Mechanism of action: Photo vaporization causing thermal damage leading to denaturation and coagulation of proteins causing an incision
  - Absorbed by both pigmented and non-pigmented layers
  - Uses:
    - For intraocular hemostasis in the management of malignant intraocular tumors
    - Ocular/orbital surgery in infected tissues
    - In NVG

- To segment vitreoretinal membranes
- Especially useful in PDR
  - Disadvantages:
    - During VR surgery, bubble formation can decrease visibility
    - It needs direct contact with membrane for destruction
- Holmium YAG laser:
  - Solid state
  - Wavelength: 2100 nm
  - Active medium: Chromium-sensitized thalium-holmium-doped YAG
  - Mechanism of action: Photocoagulation
  - Indications:
    - Thermal sclerotomy
    - To cut vitreoretinal membrane
    - Scleral buckling: Causes scleral shrinkage to increase buckling effect, especially useful in thin sclera where sutures cannot be taken
  - Advantages:
    - Big peritomy avoided

Mention the uses of neodymium YAG laser?

- Treatment of posterior capsular opacification
  - Postoperative irido-capsular adhesion
  - Iridotomy
  - Iridoplasty
  - Vitreolysis

Identify the lens.

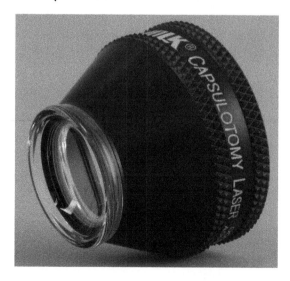

Figure 10.50 Abraham capsulotomy lens

- 10 mm diameter
- 66 D magnifying button in the center of the lens enhances visualization and allows precise laser focus on the posterior capsule
- Use: Stabilizes the patient's eye and minimizes the possibility of pitting the IOL during Nd:YAG laser capsulotomy

Mention the indications and contraindications of this procedure.

- Indications:
  - Decrease in visual acuity or visual function
  - Confirm that PCO is the cause of reduced vision
- Absolute contraindications:
  - Corneal scars/edema that interfere with target visualization
  - Inadequate stability of the IOL
- Relative contraindications:
  - Known or suspected cystoid macular edema
  - Active intraocular inflammation
  - High-risk for retinal detachment

How does on perform YAG capsulotomy?

- Energy settings should be minimum.
- Use contact lens to stabilize the eye, improve laser beam optics, and facilitate accurate focusing.
- Cut across the tension line.
- Cruciate opening to be made: Begin at 12 o'clock position in periphery, progress toward 6 o'clock, and cut across at 3 and 9 o'clock.
- A circular opening can also be made.

- The capsulotomy should be as large as the pupil in mesopic conditions, such as driving at night, when glare from the exposed capsulotomy edge is most likely.

Mention the complications of YAG capsulotomy?

- Elevated IOP
- Cystoid macular edema (CME)
- Retinal detachment
- IOL pitting
- Macular hole and foveal burn (rare)
- Malignant glaucoma (rare)
- Endophthalmitis (propionibacterium acnes) causes an indolent endophthalmitis, which can remain in lens and present as PCO

What are the risk factors for PCO?

- Younger age
- Diabetes
- Uveitis
- Myotonic dystrophy
- Retinitis pigmentosa
- Traumatic cataract

What are the types of PCO?

- Elschnig's pearls: Pearl-type PCO where clusters of residual lens epithelial cells form as round, clear "pearls"
- Soemmerring rings: Rings of residual lens epithelial cells and cortical fibers form between the posterior capsule and the edges of the anterior capsule
- Capsular wrinkling: Broad undulations or fine wrinkles

Index

Note: Page numbers in *italics* indicate a figure and page numbers in **bold** indicate a table on the corresponding page.

For Product Safety Concerns and Information please contact our EU
representative GPSR@taylorandfrancis.com
Taylor & Francis Verlag GmbH, Kaufingerstraße 24, 80331 München, Germany